Lippincott's Primary Care

Psychiatry

Lippincott's Primary Care

Psychiatry

For: Primary Care Clinicians and Trainees, Medical Specialists, Neurologists, Emergency Medical Professionals, Mental Health Providers and Trainees

The Medicine and Psychiatry Advisory Group
University of California, Davis School of Medicine

EDITORS

Robert M. McCarron, DO
Health Sciences Assistant Clinical Professor
Internal Medicine/Psychiatry Residency Training Director
Department of Psychiatry and Behavioral Sciences
Department of Internal Medicine
University of California, Davis School of Medicine
Sacramento, CA

Glen L. Xiong, MD
Health Sciences Assistant Clinical Professor
Department of Psychiatry and Behavioral Sciences
Department of Internal Medicine
University of California, Davis School of Medicine
Sacramento, CA

James A. Bourgeois, OD, MD
Alan Stoudemire Professor of Psychosomatic Medicine
Department of Psychiatry and Behavioral Sciences
University of California, Davis School of Medicine
Sacramento, CA

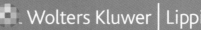
Wolters Kluwer | Lippincott Williams & Wilkins
Health

Philadelphia • Baltimore • New York • London
Buenos Aires • Hong Kong • Sydney • Tokyo

Acquisitions Editor: Sonya Seigafuse
Managing Editor: Kerry Barrett
Marketing Manager: Kimberly Schonberger
Project Manager: Paula C. Williams
Designer: Terry Mallon
Production Services: Cadmus Communication, a Cenveo company

9 8 7 6 5 4 3 2 1

Library of Congress Cataloging-in-Publication Data

Lippincott's primary care psychiatry : for primary care practitioners and trainees, medical specialists, neurologists, emergency medical professionals, mental health providers, and trainees / The University of California, Davis School of Medicine and Psychiatry Advisory Group ; editors, Robert M. McCarron, Glen L. Xiong, James A. Bourgeois.
   p. ; cm.
Includes bibliographical references and index.
ISBN 978-0-7817-9821-1
1. Psychiatry. 2. Primary care (Medicine) I. McCarron, Robert M. II. Xiong, Glen L. III. Bourgeois, James. IV. University of California, Davis. School of Medicine and Psychiatry Advisory Group. V. Title: Primary care psychiatry.
   [DNLM: 1. Mental Disorders—diagnosis. 2. Mental Disorders—therapy. 3. Primary Health Care—methods. WM 140 L765 2009]
   RC454.4.L57 2009
   616.89—dc22   2008047357

To purchase additional copies of this book, call our customer service department at **(800) 638-3030** or fax orders to **(301) 223-2320**. International customers should call **(301) 223-2300**.

Visit Lippincott Williams & Wilkins on the Internet: http://www.lww.com. Lippincott Williams & Wilkins customer service representatives are available from 8:30 am to 6:00 pm, EST.

Foreword

The presentation of patients with psychiatric disorders in nonpsychiatric settings is a phenomenon of growing concern for both primary care and medical subspecialty providers. Indeed, individuals with serious medical conditions are at increased risk for having concomitant psychiatric illnesses. Meeting the complex challenges of those having both general medical and psychiatric illnesses, the University of California, Davis is one of only two universities in the nation to support two thriving combined residency training programs: Family Medicine/Psychiatry and Internal Medicine/Psychiatry.

Lippincott's Primary Care Psychiatry is a timely contribution from our University of California, Davis faculty members, several of whom are dually trained as primary care providers and psychiatrists. These individuals not only have a solid knowledge of psychiatry, but also speak the language of primary care providers and appreciate the unique challenges that nonpsychiatrists face when managing psychiatric disorders. Drs. McCarron, Xiong, and Bourgeois have taken care to distill the most critical information relevant to nonpsychiatric providers. Each chapter contains easy-to-follow diagnostic and treatment algorithms, clinical highlights, case examples, and indications for psychiatric referral. We think that you will find this book an invaluable educational tool and resource—for students, residents, and experienced clinicians.

Frederick J. Meyers MD, MACP
Professor and Chair
Department of Internal Medicine
University of California, Davis School of Medicine

Klea D. Bertakis, MD, MPH
Professor and Chair
Department of Family and Community Medicine
Director, Center for Healthcare Policy and Research
Vice Chair, UCDHS Practice Management Board
University of California, Davis School of Medicine

Preface

Dear Colleague,

Psychiatric disorders such as mood, anxiety, and substance use disorders are among the leading causes of morbidity worldwide. Although primary care practitioners provide over 75% of all mental health services in the United States, most only get a brief exposure to the basics of psychiatry through lectures and clinical rotations. As awareness, recognition, and acceptance of psychiatric disorders increase, the gap between the number of patients who need psychiatric care and the supply of mental health practitioners will continue to grow exponentially. The resultant strain on the public and private mental health systems can, in part, be addressed with a practical, easy-to-use educational tool that will help primary care and mental health trainees and providers feel more comfortable and confident when assessing and treating the most commonly encountered conditions in primary care psychiatry.

Lippincott's Primary Care Psychiatry aims to educate nonpsychiatric health care professionals in the diagnosis, treatment, and general conceptualization of adult psychiatric disorders. All of the editors and primary authors are members of the Medicine and Psychiatry Advisory Group at the University of California, Davis School of Medicine, and many of the authors are dually board certified in psychiatry *and* either family medicine, internal medicine, or psychosomatic medicine. This book illustrates a practical approach to primary care psychiatry because it is principally written by practicing primary care physicians who are also psychiatrists. Because we know first-hand what it is like to work in the primary care setting, we have distilled a large volume of information into a practical and focused overview of primary care psychiatry.

Although psychiatrists write most psychiatric textbooks for psychiatrists, this book is specifically written for health care professionals who have not had extensive training in psychiatry beyond classroom lectures and brief clinical experiences. *Lippincott's Primary Care Psychiatry* is designed to be a user-friendly resource for primary care clinicians, medical specialists (e.g., rheumatologists, endocrinologists, neurologists, emergency medicine providers), mental health providers (e.g., psychologists, social workers, marriage and family therapists), and trainees in these fields (e.g., medical students, internal medicine and family medicine residents, nurse practitioner students, physician assistant students and behavioral health trainees).

Lippincott's Primary Care Psychiatry covers the essential psychiatric conditions found in the primary care setting and can therefore be easily used as part of a psychiatric and behavioral health curriculum for trainees of various clinical disciplines. In the first chapter, we include a practical overview on how to do an efficient and thorough primary care psychiatric interview. We also introduce the *AMPS* screening tool that can easily be used to diagnose the most commonly encountered psychiatric conditions: Anxiety, Mood, Psychotic, and Substance-related disorders. Chapters 2 through 10 cover specific psychiatric illnesses that are highly prevalent in the primary care setting such as mood, anxiety, psychotic, somatoform, substance use, eating, and personality disorders. The second section (Chapters 11 through 14) provides an overview of special topics including suicide and violence risk assessment in the primary care setting, dementias, sleep disorders, and cultural psychiatry. Each chapter includes commonly encountered clinical cases with practical tips, helpful resources for both patients and clinicians, and relevant diagnostic and treatment algorithms. Lastly, the book also has a companion Web site (www.psychforpcp.com) that includes the contents of the book as well as patient education handouts focusing on common psychiatric disorders.

We strongly believe in a biopsychosocial treatment approach that enables patients to learn and utilize lifelong skills that will result in decreased morbidity and often recovery from mental illness. It is our sincere hope that this book gives you the tools you need to provide optimal psychiatric patient care. If you have any suggestions on how we can improve future editions, please let us know.

Robert M. McCarron, DO
Glen L. Xiong, MD
James A. Bourgeois, OD, MD

Dedication

To my beautiful, unbelievably talented, loving wife, and co-editor in life, Marina McCarron
>   RMM

To Donna, my family, my patients, and my teachers
>   GLX

To my wife, Kathleen M. Ayers, PsyD, for her inspiration and partnership, and to the memory of Alan Stoudemire, MD, psychosomatic medicine specialist, Emory University, who, despite his untimely early passing, serves as a continued inspiration to all of us who serve to integrate psychiatry into the practice of medicine by all specialists
>   JAB

Acknowledgments

We would like to thank the following people for their invaluable assistance during the production of Lippincott's Primary Care Psychiatry. We are grateful to the many authors who took the time to share their knowledge. This book would not be in print without their passion to provide empathic, high quality patient care and teaching. We are extremely appreciative of the talented and highly professional LWW editorial staff, particularly Sonya Seigafuse and Kerry Barrett.

We would like to acknowledge the Chairs of Psychiatry and Behavioral Sciences, Internal Medicine, and Family and Community Medicine at UCDMC: Robert Hales, MD, MBA; Frederick Meyers, MD, MACP; and Klea Bertakis, MD, MPH, respectively, whose leadership of these departments fosters a spirit of collegiality and integration in the dual goals of academic progress and patient service.

Robert M. McCarron, DO
Glen L. Xiong, MD
James A. Bourgeois, OD, MD

Contributing Authors

Sergio Aguilar-Gaxiola, MD, PhD
Professor of Clinical Internal
Medicine and
Director, Center for Reducing Health
Disparities (CRHD)
University of California, Davis School
of Medicine

James A. Bourgeois, OD, MD
Alan Stoudemire Professor
of Psychosomatic Medicine
Department of Psychiatry and
Behavioral Sciences
University of California, Davis School
of Medicine

Donald R. Ebersole, MD
Diplomate, American Board of Family
Medicine

Tonya Fancher, MD, MPH
Assistant Professor
Department of Internal Medicine
University of California, Davis School
of Medicine

David Gellerman, MD, PhD
Assistant Clinical Professor
VA Sacramento Medical Center
Northern California Health Care System

Elizabeth N. Gutierrez, MD
Department of Psychiatry and
Behavioral Sciences
University of California, Davis School
of Medicine

Robert E. Hales, MD, MBA
Joe P. Tupin Professor and Chair
Department of Psychiatry and
Behavioral Sciences

University of California, Davis School
of Medicine

Jaesu Han, MD
Training Director
Family Medicine and Psychiatry
Residency
Assistant Clinical Professor
Departments of Family Medicine and
Psychiatry
University of California, Davis School
of Medicine

Kimberly A. Hardin, MD, MS, FAASM
Associate Professor
Department of Internal Medicine
Division of Pulmonary and Critical Care
Medicine
Director, Sleep Medicine Fellowship
Training Program
University of California, Davis School of
Medicine
Medical Director, Sleep Program and
Sleep Laboratory
Veterans Affairs of Northern
California

Tracie Harris, MD
Assistant Clinical Professor
Department of Internal Medicine
University of California, Davis School of
Medicine

Mark C. Henderson, MD, FACP
Vice Chair and Program Director,
Department of Internal Medicine
Associate Dean of Admissions, School
of Medicine
University of California, Davis School of
Medicine

Shelly L. Henderson, PhD
Clinical Psychologist
Department of Family and Community
Medicine
University of California, Davis School
of Medicine

Donald M. Hilty, MD
Associate Professor of Clinical Psychiatry
and Behavioral Sciences
University of California, Davis School of Medicine

Ladson Hinton, MD
Associate Professor
Department of Psychiatry and Behavioral
Sciences
University of California, Davis School of
Medicine

Maga Jackson-Triche, MD, MSHS
Health Sciences Clinical Professor of Psychiatry
Department of Psychiatry and Behavioral
Sciences
University of California, Davis School
of Medicine
Associate Chief of Staff for Mental Health
VA Northern California Health Care System

Pria Joglekar, MD
Assistant Clinical Professor
Department of Psychiatry and Behavioral
Sciences
University of California, Davis School of
Medicine

Joel Johnson, MD
Postdoctoral Scholar
Department of Psychiatry and Behavioral Sciences
University of California, Davis School
of Medicine

Craig R. Keenan, MD
Associate Clinical Professor
Department of Internal Medicine
Director, Primary Care Internal Medicine
Residency Program
Medical Director, General Medicine Clinic
University of California, Davis School
of Medicine

Alan Koike, MD, MSHS
Health Sciences Associate Clinical Professor
Department of Psychiatry and Behavioral
Sciences
University of California, Davis School
of Medicine

Oladio Kukoyi, MD
Assistant Clinical Professor
Department of Psychiatry and Behavioral
Sciences
Department of Family Medicine
University of California, Davis School
of Medicine

Martin H. Leamon, MD
Associate Professor of Clinical Psychiatry
Department of Psychiatry and Behavioral
Sciences
University of California, Davis School
of Medicine

Margaret W. Leung, MD, MPH
Department of Internal Medicine
and Psychiatry
University of California, Davis School
of Medicine

Russell F. Lim, MD
Health Sciences Associate Clinical Professor
Director of Diversity Education and Training
University of California, Davis School
of Medicine
Department of Psychiatry and Behavioral
Sciences

Robert M. McCarron, DO
Health Sciences Assistant Clinical Professor
Training Director, Internal Medicine/Psychiatry
Residency
Department of Psychiatry and Behavioral
Sciences
Department of Internal Medicine
University of California, Davis School
of Medicine

Michael K. McCloud, MD, FACP
Associate Clinical Professor
Department of Internal Medicine
Division of General Medicine
University of California, Davis School of Medicine

L. Joby Morrow, MD
Department of Psychiatry and Behavioral Sciences
Department of Family and Community Medicine
University of California, Davis School of Medicine

John Onate, MD
Assistant Clinical Professor
Department of Psychiatry and Behavioral Sciences
University of California, Davis School of Medicine

Adrian Palomino, MD
Department of Psychiatry and Behavioral Sciences
Department of Internal Medicine
University of California, Davis School of Medicine

Michelle Jo Park
Department of Psychiatry and Behavioral Sciences
Department of Family and Community Medicine
University of California, Davis School of Medicine

Claire Pomeroy, MD, MBA
Vice Chancellor, Human Health Sciences
Dean, University of California, Davis School of Medicine

Cameron Quanbeck, MD
Health Sciences Assistant Clinical Professor
Department of Psychiatry and Behavioral Sciences
Division of Psychiatry and the Law
University of California, Davis School of Medicine

Andreea L. Seritan, MD
Health Sciences Assistant Clinical Professor
Department of Psychiatry and Behavioral Sciences
University of California, Davis School of Medicine

Mark Servis, MD
Professor of Clinical Psychiatry
Roy Brophy Endowed Chair
Department of Psychiatry and Behavioral Sciences
University of California, Davis School of Medicine

Malathi Srinivasan, MD
Associate Professor
Department of Internal Medicine
University of California, Davis School of Medicine

Shannon Suo, MD
Assistant Professor Volunteer Clinical Faculty
Department of Psychiatry and Behavioral Sciences
Department of Family Medicine
University of California, Davis School of Medicine
Medical Director, Northgate Point, RST

Hendry Ton, MD, MS
Director of Education, Center for Reducing Health Disparities
Medical Director, Transcultural Wellness Center
Health Sciences Assistant Clinical Professor
Department of Psychiatry and Behavioral Sciences
University of California, Davis School of Medicine

Glen L. Xiong, MD
Health Sciences Assistant Clinical Professor
Department of Psychiatry
Department of Internal Medicine
University of California, Davis School of Medicine

Julie S. Young, MD, MS
Department of Psychiatry and Behavioral Sciences
University of California, Davis School of Medicine

Abbreviations

AA	Alcoholics Anonymous
ACBT	abbreviated cognitive behavioral therapy
ACT	Assertive Community Treatment
AD	Alzheimer disease
ADHD	attention deficit hyperactivity disorder
ADLs	activities of daily living
AFP	alpha-fetal protein
AMPS	Anxiety, Mood, Psychosis, and Substance Use Disorders
APA	American Psychiatric Association
AUDs	alcohol use disorders
AUDIT	The Alcohol Use Disorders Identification Test
ASD	acute stress disorder
BDI	Beck Depression Inventory
BPD	borderline personality disorder
BZPs	benzodiazepines
CAD	coronary artery disease
CBC	complete blood count
CBT	cognitive behavioral therapy
CDT	carbohydrate-deficient transferrin
ChEIs	cholinesterase inhibitors
CIWA-A	Clinical Institute Withdrawal Assessment for Alcohol
COPD	chronic obstructive pulmonary disease
CT	computerized tomography
CVAs	cerebrovascular accidents
DBSA	Depressive and Bipolar Support Alliance
DBT	dialectical behavior therapy
DCSAD	Diagnostic Classification of Sleep and Arousal Disorders
DLB	dementia with Lewy bodies
DRIs	dopamine reuptake inhibitors
DSD	dementia syndrome of depression
DSM-IV-TR	*Diagnostic and Statistical Manual of Mental Disorders*, 4th edition, text revision
DTs	delirium tremens
DTR	dysfunctional thought record
ECT	electroconvulsive therapy
ED	emergency department
EPS	extrapyramidal symptoms
ERP	exposure response prevention
FGA	first-generation antipsychotics
FTD	frontotemporal dementia
FTLD	frontotemporal lobar degeneration
GABA$_A$	gamma-aminobutyric acid type A
GAD	generalized anxiety disorder
GERD	gastroesophageal reflux disease
GGT	gamma-glutamyltransferase
GI	gastrointestinal
HAM-D	Hamilton Rating Scale for Depression

HD	Huntington disease
HPI	history of present illness
ICD	International Classification of Diseases
ICSD	International Classification of Sleep Disorders
IM	intramuscular
IOM	Institute of Medicine
IPT	interpersonal psychotherapy
LEP	limited English proficiency
LSD	lysergic acid
MAOIs	monoamine oxidase inhibitors
MCI	mild cognitive impairment
MDMA	methylenedioxymethamphetamine
MDQ	Mood Disorder Questionnaire
MET	motivational enhancement therapy
MI	motivational interviewing
MMSE	Mini Mental State Examination
MRI	magnetic resonance imaging
MSE	Mental Status Exam
NAMI	National Alliance for Mental Illness
NIAAA	National Institute on Alcohol Abuse and Alcoholism
NMDA	N-methyl-D-aspartate
NMS	neuroleptic malignant syndrome
NOS	not otherwise specified
NPI	Neuropsychiatric Inventory
NPSs	neuropsychiatric symptoms
OCD	obsessive compulsive disorder
OCF	Outline for Cultural Formulation
OSAH	obstructive sleep apnea-hypoapnea
PCP	phencyclidine
PD	panic disorder
PET	positron emission tomography
PHQ	Patient Health Questionnaire
PLMD	periodic limb movement disorder
PSP	progressive supranuclear palsy
PTSD	posttraumatic stress disorder
RLS	restless leg syndrome
SGA	second-generation antipsychotic
SIDs	substance-induced disorders
SNRIs	serotonin norepinephrine reuptake inhibitors
SP	social phobia
SPECT	single photon emission computed tomography
SRDs	substance-related disorders
SSRIs	selective serotonin reuptake inhibitors
STAR*D	Sequenced Treatment Alternatives to Relieve Depression
SUDs	substance use disorders
TCAs	tricyclic antidepressants
TD	tardive dyskinesia
TSF	Twelve-Step Facilitation
UPS	unexplained physical symptoms
VaD	vascular dementia
WHO	World Health Organization
ZBI	Zarit Burden Interview

Table of Contents

CHAPTER ① The Primary Care Psychiatric Interview

John Onate, MD • Glen L. Xiong, MD • Robert McCarron, DO

A 55-year-old homeless man with type 2 diabetes and hypertension presents for an initial evaluation with a chief complaint of "pain in my feet." A quick review of the chart shows poor adherence to follow-up appointments. The man is disheveled and poorly groomed. He avoids eye contact and looks downward during the interview. The patient says he is not sure when he first noticed the foot pain and states, "I don't know why I came in this time. I'm so far gone it does not matter anyway."

Clinical Significance

Up to 75% of all mental health care is delivered in the primary care setting (1). Unfortunately, reimbursement constraints and limited psychiatric training in most primary care curricula often discourage full exploration and thorough work-up of mental illness (2). Due to the stigma of psychiatric conditions, patients are often reluctant to present to mental health settings and may not seek treatment (3). However, most nonemergent psychiatric conditions can be treated successfully in primary care settings. The ability of the primary care clinician to carefully screen for and evaluate psychiatric symptoms is critical in order to accurately diagnose and effectively treat the underlying psychiatric disorder (4).

Clinical assessment relies heavily on both obtaining the medical history and completing a physical examination for general medical conditions. A similar approach is taken for psychiatric disorders with two main differences. First, the psychiatric interview places additional emphasis on psychosocial stressors and functioning. Second, the mental status examination is analogous to the physical examination for a general medical work-up and is the cornerstone for the psychiatric evaluation. Both of these tasks may be accomplished effectively with improved organization and practice. This chapter divides the psychiatric assessment into three sections: (1) the psychiatric interview, (2) the mental status examination, and (3) time-saving strategies.

The Psychiatric Interview

The initial interview is important as it sets the tone for future visits and will influence the initial treatment (5, 6). While the information obtained

CLINICAL HIGHLIGHTS

- The mental status examination for a psychiatric evaluation is analogous to the physical examination for a general medical assessment.

- The AMPS screening tool (Figure 1.1) includes four primary clinical dimensions of the psychiatric review of systems: Anxiety, Mood, Psychosis, and Substance use. This approach can be easily used in the primary care setting as a starting point

(Continued)

CLINICAL HIGHLIGHTS
(*Continued*)

to develop a reasonable differential diagnosis for common psychiatric disorders.

- The psychiatric interview places an emphasis on psychosocial function and should give a personalized description of the patient from a biopsychosocial perspective.

- One helpful time-saving strategy is the use of the Supplemental Psychiatric History Form to help gather a preliminary psychiatric history. A patient should complete this form either before the first clinic visit or during later visits, if a psychiatric illness is suspected.

from the interview is critical to establish a diagnosis, a collaborative, therapeutic relationship is a key component to a successful treatment plan. Therefore, the clinician should try to balance the urgency to obtain information with the need to establish a positive, trusting therapeutic alliance with the patient. Similar in style and complementary to the general medical history, the psychiatric interview is outlined below (Table 1.1).

CHIEF COMPLAINT AND HISTORY OF PRESENT ILLNESS

The interview starts with a subjective recounting of the presenting problems from the patient's perspective using open-ended questions. Reflective statements may be used to clarify and summarize particular problems (e.g., "You are telling me that you have been depressed for 3 months and because of that you feel like things will never get better."). Clarification and confirmative restatements may also be used (e.g., "You are depressed because you feel that you cannot support your family and not because you lost your house and have to move into a smaller apartment. Did I get this right?").

It is important to organize the sequence of events with each problem individually, giving the most time to the problem with the highest priority. For patients with multiple chronic problems, setting an agenda at the beginning of the encounter will also help them to understand and

Table 1.1 Outline of the Primary Care Psychiatric Interview

Chief complaint and history of present illness (HPI)	• For the first few minutes, just listen to better understand the chief complaint(s) • Make note of changes in social or occupational function • Use the AMPS screening tool for psychiatric symptoms
Past psychiatric history	• Ask about past mental health providers and hospitalizations • Inquire about whether the patient has ever thought of or attempted suicide
Medication history	• Ask about medication dosages, duration of treatment, effectiveness, and side effects
Family history	• The clinician might ask, "Did your grandparents, parents, or siblings ever have severe problems with depression, bipolar disorder, anxiety, schizophrenia, or any other emotional problems?"
Social history	***Socioeconomic status*** "How are you doing financially and are you currently employed?" "What is your current living situation and how are things at home?" ***Interpersonal relationships*** "Who are the most important people in your life and do you rely on them for support?" "How are these relationships going?" ***Legal history*** "Have you ever had problems with the law?" "Have you even been arrested or imprisoned?" ***Developmental history*** "How would you describe your childhood in one sentence?" "What was the highest grade you completed in school?" "Have you ever been physically, verbally, or sexually abused?"

conceptualize their medical problems. The history of present illness (HPI) should include the duration, severity, and extent of each symptom along with exacerbating and ameliorating factors. Patients vary greatly in their recall of subjective historical material, and often vague or contradictory material surfaces. Once consent is obtained from the patient, it is important to follow up on any inconsistencies with the patient and gather collateral information by speaking with family members and other treatment providers.

PSYCHIATRIC REVIEW OF SYSTEMS: AMPS SCREENING TOOL

A thorough review of the major psychiatric dimensions (or "review of systems") should be completed for patients who present with even a single psychiatric symptom. In the time-limited primary care setting, this can be a difficult task. The most commonly encountered primary care psychiatric disorders involve four major clinical dimensions and can be remembered by the **AMPS** mnemonic: **A**nxiety, **M**ood, **P**sychosis, and **S**ubstance use disorders (Figure 1.1). Patients who present with isolated psychiatric complaints such as depression, irritability, anxiety, insomnia, and unexplained physical complaints and those with established psychiatric disorders such as personality or eating disorders should be assessed for the presence of anxiety, mood, psychotic, and

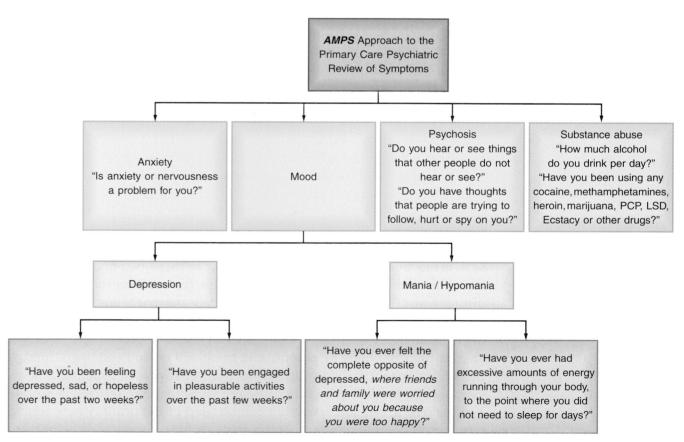

Figure 1.1 Psychiatric review of systems: AMPS screening tool.

CHAPTER 1 Psychiatric Interview

substance use disorders. We recommend incorporating the AMPS screening tool as part of the HPI. The conversation flows more naturally when the practitioner queries the patient comprehensively about both past and current symptoms. When a particular dimension is present and causing distress, further exploration is indicated (Table 1.2).

Anxiety

Anxiety is common in the primary care setting and often comorbid with mood, psychotic, and substance abuse disorders. It is sometimes the primary etiology for a depressive or substance use disorder and the secondary condition(s) will not remit unless the primary anxiety disorder is treated. Anxiety is also a significant acute risk factor for suicide that is commonly underappreciated (see Chapter 14). The quickest and most effective way to screen for an anxiety disorder during the interview is to simply ask, "Is anxiety or nervousness a problem for you?" If the patient reports feeling anxious, it is advisable to say, "Please describe how your anxiety affects you on an everyday basis." Depending on the answer, follow-up questions will help develop a reasonable differential diagnosis.

Mood

The best way to understand a patient's mood is to ask, "How would you describe your mood or emotions over the past few weeks?" The self-reported mood is also an important part of the mental status exam and should be rated as either congruent or incongruent with the corresponding affect. The two main components of mood (depression and mania) should be fully assessed during each primary care psychiatric interview.

Depression is often secondary to and comorbid with primary anxiety, sleep, substance use, and other psychiatric disorders. Depressive symptoms should always be asked about when treating another psychiatric condition—even if the chief complaint is not depression. The two screening questions for a current major depressive episode are: (1) "Have you been feeling depressed, sad, or hopeless over the past two weeks?" and (2) "Have you had a decreased energy level in pleasurable activities over the past few weeks?" The sensitivity and specificity for the detection of a major depressive episode using these screening questions are 96% and 57%, respectively (6). If the answer to either of these two questions is positive, the clinician should have a high index of suspicion for a depressive disorder and probe further. An open-ended approach would be to ask, "What is your depression like on an everyday basis?" or "How does your depression affect your daily life?" In most cases, depressed patients will discuss their troubling symptoms and there will be no need to go through the entire "checklist" for depression (e.g., changes in appetite, energy, sleep, concentration). The Patient Health Questionnaire (PHQ-9) is a nine-item patient self-report form that can be used in the primary care setting to screen for depression or quantify changes in the severity of depression over the course of treatment. All depressed patients should be asked

Table 1.2 The AMPS Screening Tool for Common Psychiatric Conditions

	SCREENING QUESTIONS	FOLLOW-UP QUESTIONS	DIAGNOSTIC AND TREATMENT INSTRUMENTS[a]
Anxiety	"Is anxiety or nervousness a problem for you?"	• "Please describe how your anxiety affects you on an everyday basis." • "What triggers your anxiety?" • "What makes your anxiety get better?"	Generalized Anxiety Disorders Scale (GAD - 7)
Mood	**Depression**[b] 1. "Have you been feeling depressed, sad, or hopeless over the past 2 weeks?" 2. "Have you had a decreased energy level in pleasurable activities over the past few weeks?"	• "What is your depression like on an everyday basis?" • "How does your depression affect your daily life?" • "Do you have any thoughts of wanting to hurt or kill yourself or somebody else?"	Patient Health Questionnaire (PHQ-9) Mood Disorder Questionnaire (MDQ)
	Mania/hypomania 1. "Have you ever felt the complete opposite of depressed, *when friends and family were worried about you because you were too happy?"* 2. "Have you ever had excessive amounts of energy running through your body, to the point where you did not need to sleep for days?"	• "When did this last happen, and please tell me what was going on at that time." • "How long did this last?" • "Were you using any drugs or alcohol at the time?" • "Did you require treatment or hospitalization?"	
Psychosis	1. "Do you hear or see things that other people do not hear or see?" 2. "Do you have thoughts that people are trying to follow, hurt, or spy on you?" 3. "Do you ever get messages from the television or radio?"	• "When did these symptoms start?" • "What triggers your symptoms?" • "What makes your symptoms get better?"	None recommended for the primary care setting
Substance use	1. "How much alcohol do you drink per day?" 2. "Have you been using any cocaine, methamphetamines, heroin, marijuana, PCP, LSD, ecstasy, or other drugs?"	If yes: • "How often do you use?" • "As a result of the use, did you experience any problems with relationships, work, finances, or the law?" • "Have you ever used any drugs by injection?" If no: • "Have you ever used any of these drugs in the past?"	• CAGE[c] • CAGE-AID (adapted to include drugs) • Alcohol Use Disorders Identification Test (AUDIT-C)

[a] These are suggested instruments that could be considered. More details about relevant instruments are available in the corresponding chapters.
[b] If either of these two questions is answered affirmatively, follow-up questions should be asked and a PHQ-9 should be administered.
[c] See Chapters 6 and 7 for details.

CHAPTER 1 Psychiatric Interview

about suicidal thoughts, plans, and intent, with documentation of answers in the medical record.

After screening for depression, one should automatically search for evidence suggestive of a past or current manic or hypomanic episode. Bipolar disorder is important to screen for, as the comorbidity with some psychiatric disorders is more than 50% to 80% (e.g., attention deficit hyperactivity disorder and substance use disorders). Also, it is important to screen for bipolar disorder when starting an antidepressant, because antidepressants may increase the risk of inducing a manic episode in patients with undetected bipolar disorder. Hypomanic and manic episodes should be screened for in patients who present with depression, anxiety, irritability, and insomnia, and whenever antidepressants are considered. Once a patient has had one clearly defined hypomanic or manic episode, the lifelong diagnosis of his or her mood disorder becomes bipolar disorder with the appropriate specifier for each mood episode (e.g., "bipolar disorder, most recent episode depressed," rather than "major depressive disorder").

Upon examination, it may be obvious when a manic episode is present. However, it can be quite a challenge to elicit manic symptoms from the past. Asking questions such as, "Have there been times when you have had a lot of sex or shopped excessively?", "When is the last time you felt very happy, like you were on top of the world?", or "Did you ever stay awake for 2 or more consecutive days?" may confuse the patient and can lead to diagnostic uncertainty. It is preferable to include the opinions of the patients' family and friends, as they may have different perspectives. If collateral history from friends and family is not available, the practitioner can ask, "Have you ever felt the complete opposite of depressed, when friends and family were worried about you because you were too happy?" or "Have you ever had excessive amounts of energy running through your body, to the point where you did not need to sleep for days?" With the last question, it is important to differentiate primary insomnia from a lack of need for sleep due to a manic episode. If the patient answers yes to either question, the follow-up questions should be, "When did this last happen?" and "What was going on at that time?" This type of questioning should cover both past and present manic or hypomanic episodes.

Psychosis

Psychotic symptoms such as disorganized speech and behavior, paranoid delusions, and hallucinations do not commonly present in the primary care setting. These symptoms are, however, important to assess, as they are often associated with mood disorders and substance misuse disorders or are secondary to a general systemic medical condition. The following questions can be used to evaluate psychosis: (1) "Do you hear or see things that other people do not hear or see?" and (2) Do you have thoughts that people are trying to follow, hurt, or spy on you?" These questions will identify a history of hallucinations or delusions (also known as positive symptoms), while disorganized speech or behavior will usually be evident during the mental status examination and during collection of the collateral history. In general, persistent psychotic symptoms of unclear etiology warrant further psychiatric consultation and evaluation for schizophrenia.

Substance Use

Comorbid substance use, abuse, and dependence are common in primary care patients presenting with psychiatric symptoms. Substance use disorders mimic nearly all psychiatric symptoms, especially anxiety, depression, insomnia, hyperactivity, irritability, and hallucinations. Clues to substance use may include social factors such as inability to maintain employment, interpersonal and financial problems, repeated legal offenses, and poor adherence to treatment. Key aspects of a substance abuse history include specific substance(s) used; quantity; frequency; total duration; means of getting the drug; impact of drug use on personal, family, and work functioning; and previous sobriety and treatment history. Priority should be placed on active drug use, especially that which negatively impacts medical treatment and adherence.

PAST PSYCHIATRIC AND MEDICATION HISTORY

The structure and content of the psychiatric history is essentially the same as the medical history. Past diagnoses, treatments, hospitalizations, and mental health providers comprise the main categories. Frequency of psychiatric hospitalization may reveal severity and chronicity of the psychiatric condition. It is important to describe medication dosage, duration, response, side effects, and adherence. Obtaining prior medical records is helpful when developing a differential diagnosis and treatment plan.

FAMILY HISTORY

Psychiatric disorders are based on both genetic and environmental factors. Patients with a family history of a first-degree relative with major depressive disorder, bipolar disorder, substance dependence, or schizophrenia have up to a 10-fold increased chance of having a mental illness (7). Patients who have family members with psychiatric illness often have some understanding of these conditions and may have a better knowledge about treatment and available resources.

SOCIAL HISTORY

The social history lends important information on how the patient functions outside of the clinical setting. Although the information may be detailed and complex, it is most helpful to focus on the patient's level of psychosocial functioning. The social history can be divided into four areas: socioeconomic status, interpersonal relationships, legal history, and developmental history. The four areas with sample questions to prompt dialog in these areas are illustrated on the following page.

Socioeconomic Status

A quick way to determine one's socioeconomic status is to ask the following questions: "How are you doing financially and are you currently employed?" "What is your current living situation and how are things at home?" A patient's ability to secure such basic necessities as food and shelter is an important priority. For a homeless patient, gathering more detail on the factors that led to homelessness often reveals important diagnostic information. Frequent job changes or loss of employment can be clues to occult substance use or mood disorders. A patient who is seeking disability compensation versus one who must return to school or work immediately may have different urgencies about improving his or her situation.

Interpersonal Relationships

In order to explore a patient's ability to initiate and maintain relationships with family, friends, and coworkers, the clinician might ask, "Who are important people in your life and do you rely on them for support?" or "How are these relationships going?" This is also a good time to ask about sexual history. Sexual history includes sexual orientation, sexual identity, current sexual activity, high-risk partners, sexual performance, and the use of contraceptives. Perspectives of the patient's family, friends, and cultural group on mental illness should also be considered, because stigma about treatment and nontraditional approaches may influence treatment attitude and outcomes.

Legal History

Open-ended questions such as "Have you ever had problems with the law?" or "Have you ever been arrested or imprisoned?" are easy ways to broach the topic of legal history. Legal history provides information about psychosocial functioning as well as previous experience with violence and crime. Patients who are recently released from prison and are still on parole or have a felony record may have difficulty finding employment and suffer from stigma. Moreover, those who have been imprisoned for many years often find it difficult to re-assimilate into a less structured lifestyle upon release from prison. These stressors can increase the risk for substance abuse and exacerbate psychiatric symptoms, which can be a cause for nonadherence to medical care.

Developmental History

The developmental history has multiple components and it can be a challenge to obtain in one encounter. Suggested questions include (1) "How would you describe your childhood in one sentence?"; (2) "What was the highest grade you completed in school?"; and (3) "Have you ever been physically, verbally, or sexually abused?" These questions may bring out long-standing stressors and illustrate the patient's most developed (and underdeveloped) coping strategies. Chaotic and unstable childhood development and a history of abuse are often important issues to address as part of a comprehensive psychosocial treatment plan.

Mental Status Examination

The Mental Status Examination (MSE) is an observation and report of the present cognitive, emotional, and behavioral state. Much of the MSE is gathered as the interview unfolds. An accurate and concise description of the MSE also facilitates consultation with mental health professionals. Similar to a comprehensive neurologic exam, an in-depth cognitive assessment is not feasible (or necessary) for most clinical encounters in the primary care setting. The following summarizes high-yield, salient components of the MSE (Table 1.3).

APPEARANCE

Appearance is a description of the overall hygiene, grooming, and dress of the patient. An unkept appearance may indicate a lack of concern with personal hygiene and self-care. For example, there are many ways to interpret the appearance of a 20-year-old depressed college student who is tightly holding onto a large wooden cross and presents with a disheveled appearance; dirty, torn clothes; and pronounced malodor. In addition to depressive symptoms, this presentation would merit evaluation for psychotic symptoms and substance use as well as his or her ability to secure safe housing, food, and clothing. One might also want to consider bipolar disorder, mixed episode as a possible diagnosis.

Table 1.3 Key Features of the Mental Status Examination (MSE)

Appearance	• What is the status of the hygiene and grooming and are there any recent changes in appearance?
Attitude	• How does the patient relate to the clinician? • Is the patient cooperative, guarded, irritable, etc., during the interview?
Speech	• What are the rate, rhythm, and volume of speech?
Mood	• How does the patient describe his or her mood? • This should be reported as described by the patient.
Affect	• Does the patient's facial expressions have full range and reactivity? • How quickly does the affect change (lability)? • Is the affect congruent with the stated mood and is it appropriate to topics under discussion?
Thought process	• *How* is the patient thinking? • Does the patient change subjects quickly or is the train of thought difficult to follow?
Thought content	• *What* is the patient thinking? • What is the main theme or subject matter when the patient talks? • Does the patient have any delusions, obsessions, or compulsions?
Perceptions	• Does the patient have auditory, visual, or tactile hallucinations?
Cognition	• Is the patient alert? • Is the patient oriented to person, place, time, and the purpose of the interview?
Insight	• Does the patient recognize that there is an illness or disorder present? • Is there a clear understanding of the treatment plan and prognosis?
Judgment	• How will the patient secure food, clothing, and shelter in a safe environment? • Is the patient able to make decisions that support a safe and reasonable treatment plan?

ATTITUDE

Attitude is the manner in which the patient responds to or interacts with the interviewer. The attitude can be cooperative in a typical, unimpaired patient; avoidant in a patient who has been traumatized; or guarded and distrustful in a patient who is paranoid. A patient's attitude and level of engagement help in evaluating the reliability of the information given by the patient and may direct the clinician to seek collateral information. Reluctance to provide certain information may suggest avoidant motivations and poor insight.

SPEECH

Speech is described by rate (e.g., slow, rapid, pressured, or uninterruptible), volume, articulation (e.g., dysarthric, garbled), and rhythm (e.g., stuttering, stammering). Dysarthric speech may be due to a cerebral vascular accident, medication side effects, and alcohol or substance intoxication. Rapid or pressured speech may indicate intoxication, corticosteroid-induced mania, anxiety, or bipolar mania. Increased speech latency may point to schizophrenia, dementia, or depression with related psychomotor retardation.

MOOD

Mood is a description of the overall pervasive, subjective, and sustained emotional state and can be assessed by simply asking, "How would you describe your mood?" Mood should be ideally noted in the patient's own words, using quotation marks. Mood generally ranges from *depressed* to *euphoric*, with a normal or *euthymic* mood as the reference point. Other common states include empty, guilty, anxious, angry, and irritable mood.

AFFECT

Affect is the expressed emotional state or degree of emotional responsiveness and is inferred from the patient's collective facial expressions. Components of affect include congruency, range, reactivity, rate of change (lability), and intensity. Under normal circumstances, there should be congruency between the patient's mood and affect. If the affect and mood are incongruent and difficult to reconcile, the clinician should consider an active psychotic disorder, malingering, or factitious disorder. For example, a psychotic patient who is depressed may laugh rather than show a mood-congruent affect. A *restricted* range of affect describes limited expression of emotional states. Reactivity describes the degree of affective change in response to external cues. For example, a depressed patient may have an affect that is restricted to depressive expressions and decreased reactivity to the interviewer. A patient who is manic or intoxicated with a stimulant may exhibit a *labile* and expansive affect. A *blunted* affect is defined as a low-intensity affect with decreased reactivity, often seen in patients who have major depressive disorder. A *flat* affect has little to no emotional or facial expression and is sometimes found in those who have schizophrenia or profound depression.

THOUGHT PROCESS

Thought process describes the organization of thoughts or *how* one thinks. A normal thought process is described as *logical, goal directed,* or *linear,* which means the patient is able to complete a train of thought in reasonable depth. Although no single abnormality of thought process (also referred to as formal thought disorders) is pathognomonic for a specific disorder, this information is critical to the development of an accurate differential diagnosis. A *concrete* thought process may be logical but lacks depth. *Circumstantial* thinking refers to the painstaking movement of thoughts from the origin (point A) to the goal (point B) with excessive focus on insignificant details. A patient who exhibits *tangential* thinking will quickly change the focus of the conversation in a way that ultimately deviates from the main topic (e.g., "I know it is important to take my medications so my schizophrenia can get better. My neighbor is on a medication for his headaches; do you know which one it might be?"). *Derailment* (or looseness of association) is an abrupt change of focus where the thoughts are numerous and disconnected. A *disorganized* thought process refers to disconnected topics or irrelevant answers to questions posed. *Limited* (or *paucity of*) thoughts occur in patients with severe depression, those with profound negative symptoms (e.g., catatonia), or those who are internally preoccupied with delusions or hallucinations.

THOUGHT CONTENT

Thought content is a description of the main themes and preoccupations expressed by the patient. Simply put, the thought content is *what* the patient is thinking. Depressed patients will usually present with themes of poor self-esteem, worthlessness, or hopelessness. Patients with a somatoform disorder often focus almost exclusively on physical symptoms. Substance-dependent patients tend to fixate on specific medications by name. *Obsessions* are ideas, activities, or events that are the focus of constant and nearly involuntary attention, but are by definition nonpsychotic in nature. *Delusions* are fixed, false beliefs and are characterized by a lack of insight. Common delusional themes are paranoid (e.g., "The FBI is trying to kill me."); grandiose (e.g., "I own oil companies and rule five states!"); erotic (e.g., "I know the governor loves me."); and bizarre, reflecting themes that are not physically possible (e.g., "The martians have tattooed me and that is why the police always bother me in the park."). *Illusions* are misinterpretations of sensory information (e.g., mistaking a chair for a person). *Hallucinations* are sensory perceptions in the absence of any stimuli and typically are auditory, visual, or tactile. Hallucinations are found in many psychiatric disorders and are not pathognomonic for any particular disorder, although they are classically associated with schizophrenia. *Command*

CHAPTER 1 Psychiatric Interview

hallucinations (wherein the hallucination directs the patient's behavior) should be evaluated for suicidal or violent content. In addition to documenting major themes of the interview, the key components of thought content include the presence or absence of delusions, perceptual disturbances (hallucinations), suicidal ideation, and homicidal ideation.

COGNITION

Cognitions are higher-order brain functions and include orientation, concentration, calculation, memory, and executive function. Orientation to person, location, date, and purpose should be queried. If the clinician has a high index of suspicion for a cognitive deficit, further assessment can be initiated in the primary care setting. Asking the patient to repeatedly subtract 7 starting from 100 (serial 7's) or spell "world" backward can assess concentration or attention span. Impairment in the level of alertness or consciousness is characteristic of delirium, alternatively termed encephalopathy (by neurologists) or less specifically called altered mental status (by most health professionals). Long- and short-term memory problems may become evident if the patient is unable to provide clear and organized historical data. When obvious deficits are present and when cognitive disorders are suspected, the Mini-Mental State Examination (MMSE), familiar to most primary care providers, should be performed.

INSIGHT

Insight describes the degree by which the patient understands his or her diagnosis, treatment, and prognosis. A patient who denies a problem that clearly exists or minimizes the severity of symptoms has poor insight. Chronic illness and suboptimal insight often lead to poor outcomes. Restoration of insight is usually a key component to the long-term treatment plan.

JUDGMENT

Judgment is the ability to make reasonable decisions that result in safe, desirable, and socially acceptable outcomes. The ability to weigh benefits versus risks and recognize consequences of behavior is a core part of judgment. Examples of questions that assess "real-time" capacity for judgment include "How do you think this antidepressant might affect your life?" and "What do you think you can do to help decrease your cravings for alcohol?"

Physical Examination

The physical examination gives the clinician an opportunity to inquire about historical information that the patient may not have disclosed during the interview. Unexplained tachycardia, diaphoresis, tremors, or hyperreflexia should alert the provider about possible stimulant intoxication or alcohol-sedative withdrawal. A careful inspection of the

NOT TO BE MISSED

- A complete primary care psychiatric assessment should always include the AMPS screening tool as well as direct questions about suicidal ideation and intent.

- The mood and affect should be assessed and recorded as important parts of the mental status exam. Mood is the overall internal emotional state, whereas affect is the expressed emotional state that is manifested by changes in facial expression.

- Disorders of speech and behavior are often found in those with severe mental illness and should be monitored carefully. Thought process describes *how* one thinks and thought content describes *what* one thinks.

- A social history should be obtained on all patients who are being treated for a psychiatric illness. The main components of a primary care psychiatric social history include socioeconomic status, interpersonal relationships, legal history, and developmental history.

extremities and skin revealing tattoos, burns, bruises, scars, or other injuries should be followed up with inquires about their origins. For patients with severe mental illnesses (e.g., schizophrenia) who live under marginal and unsafe circumstances, inspection of hair for parasites, skin for lacerations, and teeth for decay or abscesses is important, because these patients may not have insight into the origin of their physical discomfort and do not readily seek timely medical care. Similarly, a diabetic patient with severe mental illness may not have the insight and cognitive ability to check for infected or injured toes. Therefore, the primary care provider may use the physical exam as another opportunity to gauge an individual's functional status by his or her ability to maintain activities of daily living (ADLs) independently and to manage his or her medical disorders.

Time-Saving Strategies

We recommend the following *time-saving strategies* when completing a primary care psychiatric biopsychosocial assessment.

1. Obtaining the social history is one of the most important pieces of the primary psychiatric interview. There is much to cover and it can certainly be time intensive if not done properly. Although it is not all-encompassing, we suggest the following "starter questions" to help the clinician collect the necessary information for a social history.

   Socioeconomic status
   "How are you doing financially and are you currently employed?"
   "What is your current living situation and how are things at home?"

   Interpersonal relationships
   "Who are the most important people in your life and do you rely on them for support?"
   "How are these relationships going?"

   Legal history
   "Have you ever had problems with the law?"
   "Have you even been arrested or imprisoned?"

   Developmental history
   "How would you describe your childhood in one sentence?"
   "What was the highest grade you completed in school?"
   "Have you ever been physically, verbally, or sexually abused?"

2. If you could only pick three questions during a primary care psychiatry interview, the following are suggested:
   "What is your number one biggest problem that we can work on together?"
   "Currently, how are you dealing with your problem?"
   "Is there someone in your life who you can go to if you need help?"

3. We highly recommend using the Supplemental Psychiatric History form (Figure 1.2) for all new patients or for those who you feel have significant psychiatric symptoms. This form is easy for a patient or clinician to complete and covers the pertinent psychosocial history as well as the AMPS screening questions. The clinician can quickly glance at this form and tailor further assessment accordingly. All "yes" answers should raise concern and prompt further questioning. More in-depth disorder-specific assessments are discussed in the chapters to follow.

Supplemental Psychiatric History Form

Name: _____   Date: _____
Reason for Appointment: _____

Past Psychiatric Diagnoses (circle if applicable): anxiety, depression, bipolar disorder, schizophrenia, schizoaffective disorder, alcohol misuse, drug misuse, borderline personality disorder, other mental diagnosis

Have you ever been treated by a psychiatrist or other mental health provider?	Yes / No
Have you ever been a patient in a psychiatric hospital?	Yes / No
Have you ever tried to hurt or kill yourself?	Yes / No
Have you ever taken a medication for psychiatric reasons?	Yes / No

If yes, please list the most recent medication(s) below:

#1: _____	Did you have any problems with this medication?	Yes / No
#2: _____	Did you have any problems with this medication?	Yes / No
#3: _____	Did you have any problems with this medication?	Yes / No
#4: _____	Did you have any problems with this medication?	Yes / No
#5: _____	Did you have any problems with this medication?	Yes / No

Family Psychiatric History: Did your grandparents, parents, or siblings ever have severe problems with depression, bipolar disorder, anxiety, schizophrenia, or any other emotional problems?   Yes / No

Social and Developmental History:

Socioeconomic Status

Are you currently unemployed?	Yes / No
Are you having any problems at home?	Yes / No

Interpersonal Relationships

Are you having any problems with close personal relationships?	Yes / No

Legal History

Have you ever had problems with the law?	Yes / No

Developmental History

Have you ever been physically, verbally, or sexually abused?	Yes / No
What was the highest grade you completed in school?	_____

Anxiety Symptoms, Mood Symptoms, Psychotic Symptoms, Substance Use

Is anxiety or nervousness a problem for you?	Yes / No

Mood Symptoms

● Have you been feeling depressed, sad, or hopeless over the past two weeks?	Yes / No
● Have you had a decreased interest level in pleasurable activities over the past few weeks?	Yes / No
● Have you ever felt the complete opposite of depressed, *when friends and family were worried about you because you were too happy?*	Yes / No
● Have you ever had excessive amounts of energy running through your body, to the point where you did not need to sleep for days?	Yes / No
● Do you have any thoughts of wanting to hurt or kill yourself or someone else?	Yes / No

Psychotic Symptoms

Do you hear or see things that other people do not hear or see?	Yes / No
Do you have thoughts that people are trying to follow, hurt or spy on you?	Yes / No

Substance Use

How many packs of cigarettes do you smoke per day?	_____
How much alcohol do you drink per day?	_____
Have you ever used cocaine, methamphetamines, heroin, marijuana, PCP, LSD, Ecstacy or other drugs?	Yes / No

Figure 1.2 Supplemental Psychiatric History Form.

Practice Pointers

Case 1: The primary care psychiatric interview

A 55-year-old homeless man with type 2 diabetes and hypertension presents for an initial evaluation with a chief complaint of "pain in my feet." A quick review of the chart shows poor adherence to follow-up appointments. The man is disheveled and poorly groomed. He avoids eye contact and looks downward during the interview. The patient says he is not sure when he first noticed the foot pain and states, "I don't know why I came in this time. I'm so far gone it does not matter anyway."

When the provider asks about his mood, the patient says he feels "depressed." He also conveys hopelessness, anhedonia, a diminished appetite, and decreased energy. When asked about suicidal thoughts, he notes, "Sometimes I wish I was just dead." The AMPS screening questions indicate that he does not have any anxiety symptoms, history of hypomania or mania, perceptual disturbances, delusions, or current substance use.

The patient was put on "some depression medication" a few months ago but stopped after 1 week, stating, "I was still depressed and I didn't think it was working." He is currently sober for 10 years but has recently stopped going to Alcoholics Anonymous meetings. His father was an "alcoholic" and his brother has also received treatment for substance abuse. There is no other mental illness in his family.

During the mental status examination, he initially has poor eye contact but eventually becomes more engaged. His mood is depressed and his affect is restricted and congruent with his mood. His speech is notable for a decreased volume and a slow rate. His thought process is goal oriented and his thought content contains depressive themes with mention of "low self-esteem since childhood." He admitted to suicidal ideation but denies any suicidal intent or plan, and he has no past suicide attempts or access to firearms. He is fully oriented and has no obvious cognitive deficits. Although he has not been fully compliant with office visits in the past, his insight and judgment at this time are fair because he is able to recognize that his depression is getting worse.

Discussion: This case history illustrates a common presentation of depression in the primary care setting. The chronic poor adherence to medical care and homelessness are clues to significant loss of function. Review of past psychiatric history uncovers chronic depression and past alcohol dependence. The AMPS screening tool reveals symptoms consistent with unipolar depression without psychotic features and a remote history of alcohol dependence. Although the patient has vague thoughts of death, he has no prior history of suicide attempts and no current intent or plan to die. Moreover, he has no access to firearms.

The complete biopsychosocial assessment helps the clinician to provide a comprehensive treatment plan. In addition to initiating treatment for his hypertension, diabetes, and foot pain, the use of an antidepressant should be readdressed. The clinician might say, "Many people who take antidepressants think they work like aspirin for a headache (you take it when you need it for immediate relief), but that is not the way these medications work." The patient should also be encouraged to revisit the idea of attending Alcoholics Anonymous meetings, because stress from a worsening depressive episode may lead to use of alcohol. Also, given the frequent thoughts related to poor self-esteem, one may consider a referral for cognitive behavioral therapy. It seems that the patient's lack of housing may be adversely affecting his general medical and psychiatric conditions. The patient should be referred to social services and local shelters that provide meals.

Finally, it is important to understand why he has missed so many appointments in the past and address those specific issues. The therapeutic connection between the patient and the clinician is paramount. In this case, the provider might be compelled to focus exclusively on the medication regimen for his chronic diabetes and hypertension and give less emphasis to the relationship between the patient and the provider. Another approach might be to ask the patient, "What is your number one biggest problem?" and proceed with treatment that addresses the stated issues (in this case it is likely his foot pain and homeless state). Short and somewhat frequent office visits may be indicated over the next few months in order to address his many concerns and maintain a biopsychosocial treatment approach.

Practical Resources

The MacAuthur Inititative on Depression and Primary Care: http://www.depression-primarycare.org/
Substance Abuse and Mental Health Services Administration: http://www.samhsa.gov/index.aspx
American Psychiatric Association Practice Guidelines: http://www.psych.org/MainMenu/PsychiatricPractice/PracticeGuidelines_1.aspx
National Institute of Mental Health: http://www.nimh.nih.gov/health/publications/depression-a-treatable-illness.shtml
National Alliance on Mental Illness: www.nami.org

References

1. Reiger DA, Boyd JH, Burke JD, et al. One month prevalence of mental disorders in the United States. *Arch Gen Psychiatry.* 1988;45:977–986.

2. Onate J. Psychiatric consultation in outpatient primary care settings: should consultation change to collaboration? *Primary Psychiatry.* 2006;13(6):41–45.

3. Kessler RC, Demler O, Frank RG, et al. Prevalence and treatment of mental disorders, 1990 to 2003. *N Engl J Med.* 2005;352(24):2515–2523.

4. Katon W, Roinson P, Von Korff M, et al. A multifaceted intervention to improve treatment of depression in primary care. *Arch Gen Psychiatry.* 1996;53(10):924–932.

5. Vergare MJ, Binder RL, Cook IA, et al. American Psychiatric Association practice guidelines for the psychiatric evaluation of adults second edition. *Am J Psychiatry.* 2006;163(6 Suppl):3–36.

6. Whooley MA, Simon GE. Managing depression in medical outpatients. *N Engl J Med.* 2000;343(26):1942–1950.

7. Hales RE, Yudofsky SC, Gabbard GO. *The American Psychiatric Publishing Textbook of Psychiatry.* 5th ed. Washington, DC: American Psychiatric Association; 2008.

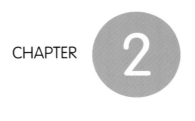

Mood Disorders— Depression

Tonya Fancher, MD, MPH • Robert M. McCarron, DO •
Oladio Kukoyi, MD • James A. Bourgeois, OD, MD

> A 42-year-old woman presents to your office complaining of insomnia. She reports four weeks of insomnia, decreased appetite, weight loss, fatigue, and depressed mood. She continues to work but socializes less than usual. Twenty years ago she had a similar episode and sought a brief course of counseling. Her symptoms improved over several months. She has never been on medications for depression and has no family history of mental illness. She denies suicidal ideation or access to firearms. Her examination is notable for tearfulness and a blunted affect, but is otherwise normal.

Clinical Significance

Up to 10% of patients seen in primary care settings meet the criteria for major depressive disorder (1). The prevalence of major depressive disorder is closer to 30% to 40% among patients with such chronic medical illnesses as coronary artery disease (CAD), cerebrovascular disease, diabetes mellitus, obesity, and human immunodeficiency virus (HIV). Depression is the leading cause of disability and premature death in people aged 18 to 44 years and is associated with worsening medical morbidity and mortality (2, 3). For example, depression in patients with CAD has been consistently demonstrated to be an independent risk factor for increased cardiac mortality (4).

Up to one quarter of adults will have a major depressive episode during their lifetime (5). For the primary care clinician, untreated depression may help explain poor adherence to appointment keeping and prescribed treatments. Women are affected by depression twice as often as men. The lifetime risk of depression increases by 1.5 to 3.0 times in patients with an affected first-degree relative. Onset of depression is most common among patients aged 12 to 24 years and those over 65. The suicide rate is similarly high in both groups.

Diagnosis

Early diagnosis and treatment of depression usually improve a patient's quality of life and health outcomes, and may prevent suicide. Most patients with depression seek care from their primary care provider before presenting to a mental health provider. Increasingly, primary care physicians are managing depression alone or in consultation with

CLINICAL HIGHLIGHTS

• Major depressive disorder is characterized by a depressed mood most of the day nearly every day or a significant loss of interest or pleasure in almost all activities (anhedonia) for a period of 2 weeks or more. Various other specific depressive syndromes are characterized by both duration and number of mood symptoms.

(Continued)

a mental health provider. Major depression is defined by the *Diagnostic and Statistical Manual of Mental Disorders*, 4th edition, text revision (DSM-IV-TR), as the presence of five or more depressive symptoms over a 2-week period (depressed mood or lack of interest in pleasurable activities must be present). The collective symptoms cause significant dysfunction and cannot be due to other illnesses such as anxiety, hypothyroidism, or alcohol- or substance-related disorders (1) (Table 2.1).

Patients who do not meet the criteria for major depression may have a subsyndromal depression such as minor depression or dysthymic disorder. These types of depression are distinguished based on the length and number of symptoms in addition to sad mood and anhedonia, the degree of functional impairment, and the severity of symptoms. Minor depression is characterized by two to four depressive symptoms, including depressed mood or anhedonia, of greater than 2 weeks in duration. Dysthymic disorder is usually described as a chronic feeling of "being down in the dumps" and is characterized by at least 2 years of three or more depressive symptoms, including depressed mood, for more days than not. Also, in order to meet DSM-IV-TR criteria, depressive symptoms will not have been absent for more than 2 months during the 2 or more year-long period of dysthymic disorder.

Major depression can be stratified into three levels of severity: mild, moderate, or severe. A diagnosis of mild depression is indicated when no or few additional symptoms beyond the number required for diagnosis of major depression are present in the setting of minor functional impairment. Moderate depression is diagnosed when more than the required number of symptoms for the diagnosis of major depression are

Table 2.1 DSM-IV-TR Definition of Major Depression
Five or more of the following symptoms have been present during the same 2-week period and represent a change from previous functioning.
• At least one of the symptoms is either *depressed mood* or *loss of interest or pleasure*.
• Depressed mood most of the day, nearly every day, as self-reported or observed by others
• Diminished interest or pleasure in all or almost all activities most of the day, nearly every day
• Significant weight loss when not dieting, or weight gain; or decrease or increase in appetite nearly every day
• Insomnia or hypersomnia nearly every day
• Psychomotor agitation or retardation as described by people who know the patient
• Fatigue or loss of energy nearly every day
• Feelings of worthlessness or excessive or inappropriate guilt nearly every day
• Diminished ability to think or concentrate nearly every day
• Recurrent thoughts of death; recurrent suicidal ideation without a specific plan

From *Diagnosis and Statistical Manual of Mental Disorders*. 4th ed. Washington, DC: American Psychiatric Association; 1994.

(Continued)

CLINICAL HIGHLIGHTS
(*Continued*)

provider within 1 month of their death.

- More than 70% of men and 50% of women who die by suicide used a firearm. Physicians should ask depressed or anxious patients about suicidal ideation and access to firearms at each visit.

present and there is moderate impairment in functioning. Severe depression is suggested by the presence of many more symptoms than required for the diagnosis of major depression and related disabling functional impairment. Psychotic features such as hallucinations or delusions may be present in severe depression. Suicidal ideation may accompany mild, moderate, or severe depression.

IDENTIFYING HIGH-RISK POPULATIONS

There are currently no diagnostic tests or laboratory makers that reliably estimate risk for the development of depression. Moreover, there is much controversy over the actual cause of depression. Although there is strong evidence to support a familial link among first-degree relatives who have depression, there is currently no definitive genetic association with the development of major depressive disorder.

The U.S. Preventive Services Task Force recommends that primary care practices should screen all adults for depression if the practice has systems in place to formally diagnose, treat, and follow patients with depression (6). The following section provides an overview of risk factors for the development of depression. Patients with risk factors should be screened on the initial primary care visit and at least every 1 to 2 years thereafter.

Postpartum Women

Postpartum women often have abrupt hormonal shifts and related short-lived depression commonly referred to as "the blues." Most such subsyndromal, postpartum depressive episodes will subside gradually with supportive care over 1 to 2 weeks after the delivery. In other words, the majority of new mothers will not have the full neurovegetative signs or mood disturbance duration characteristic of a major depressive episode. It is difficult to predict which women will progress to full-spectrum postpartum depression, but women with a previous mood disorder, poor social support, and delivery following an unplanned or unwanted pregnancy are at particularly high risk for postpartum depression. Continued clinical vigilance for up to 1 year after the delivery is indicated for all postpartum women.

Up to 1 in 10 women in the postpartum period will develop major depression (7). Clinicians can screen for postpartum depression using the Edinburgh Postnatal Depression Scale approximately 4 to 6 weeks after delivery. Postpartum depressive episodes are more likely to be complicated by psychotic symptoms, which may lead to poor infant care, infanticide, or suicide.

Personal or Family History of Depression

A personal history of major depression or bipolar disorder is the most significant risk factor for recurrent depression. Major depressive disorder is up to three times more likely among those with first-degree relatives who have either depression or bipolar disorder (1). A family history of depression is also associated with longer depressive episodes, greater risk of recurrence, and persistent thoughts of death and suicide (8).

Advanced Age

Elderly patients with depression can present with apathy, diminished self-care, or severe cognitive deficits. Depression is also common among caregivers of the elderly (9). Elderly depressed patients often have increased primary care utilization for nonspecific physical complaints and may present with significant weight loss and failure to thrive. Depression is also common in patients with dementia.

Neurologic Disorders

The risk of depression is very high in the first year following a stroke. Poststroke depression correlates with failure to regain motor function, more medical complications, and cognitive impairment. Parkinson disease is also frequently complicated by depression. The depression in Parkinson disease may have a greater impact on quality of life than impairment from the associated movement disorder. Patients with chronic neurologic disorders like stroke and Parkinson disease should be watched closely for the emergence of depression or anhedonia.

Comorbid Systemic Physical Illnesses

Patients with diabetes mellitus, cancer, rheumatologic disease, thyroid disease, HIV, myocardial infarction, and obesity have significantly higher rates of depression. At least one quarter of those with cardiac disease or diabetes will develop major depressive disorder. Patients may present atypically with nonadherence, multiple unexplained physical symptoms, or chronic pain syndromes (10–17). Early recognition and treatment of depression can improve morbidity, mortality, and quality of life.

PATIENT ASSESSMENT

The U.S. Preventive Services Task Force encourages routine depression screening for adults in primary care practices that have the resources to treat and follow the identified patients (6, 18). Clinicians with limited resources may consider screening mainly at-risk groups. Clinicians should consider repeated screenings of patients with a history of depression or other psychiatric symptoms, comorbid medical illness, multiple unexplained somatic complaints, high rates of clinical utilization, substance abuse, chronic pain, or nonadherence. Patients should also be asked about the use of recent or current medications that have been associated with depressive symptoms or suicidal ideation (e.g., corticosteroids, interferon, montelukast sodium, varenicline, isotretinoin).

There are no definitive findings of depression on physical examination, although many patients demonstrate a tearful, blunted, or restricted affect. Depressed patients may also have psychomotor retardation or a quiet and slow speech pattern. The physical examination may be useful in helping to rule out common conditions that are often confused with depression (e.g., hypothyroidism, dementia) and in looking for commonly co-occurring illnesses (e.g., obesity, cancer, CAD). When clinical suspicion is high, laboratory testing might include tests for anemia, hypothyroidism, vitamin B_{12} deficiency, and Cushing disease.

Screening Tools and Rating Scales for Depression

The most important first step in the diagnosis of depression is to ask about depressed mood and anhedonia over the past 2 or more weeks. One of the easiest depression screening tools is the two-question Patient Health Questionnaire-2 tool (PHQ-2) (19, 20):

"Over the past 2 weeks have you felt down, depressed, or hopeless?"
"Over the past 2 weeks have you felt little interest or pleasure in doing things?"

A positive response to either question warrants a thorough review of the DSM-IV-TR criteria (or equivalent rating tool) for major depression (Figure 2.1).

An alternative screening tool is the Patient Health Questionnaire-9 (PHQ-9) (Figure 2.2). The PHQ-9 can be used to diagnose depression and to follow the disease over time. It has been validated in primary care settings, is self-administered, and is available in English and Spanish versions (21–23). It is a nine-item self-administered questionnaire that classifies current symptoms on a scale of 0 (no symptoms) to 3 (daily symptoms) (21). Items 1 through 9 are summed to yield a score ranging from 0 to 27. A score of 0 to 4 is considered nondepressed, 5 to 9 mild depression, 10 to 14 moderate depression, 15 to 19 moderately severe depression, and 20 to 27 severe depression. Repeating the PHQ-9 during treatment allows the clinician to objectively monitor response to therapy: a 50% reduction in symptom score suggests an adequate response; a 25% to 50% reduction suggests a partial response, and a reduction by less than 25% suggests a minimal to no response. Patients who fail to respond to initial treatment may warrant an urgent psychiatric referral.

Two items from the PHQ-9 deserve particular attention. Item 9 assesses suicidal ideation. Any positive response should be followed up with direct questioning about suicidal ideation, intent, and planning. Item 10 assesses functional impairment. Like symptom severity, severe functional impairment may suggest the need for psychiatric consultation and consideration for hospitalization (24, 25).

Additional rating instruments for the clinical assessment of depression include the Hamilton Rating Scale for Depression (HAM-D), the Beck Depression Inventory (BDI), and the Zung Self-Rating Depression Scale. The HAM-D is a clinician-administered instrument. Both 17-item and 31-item versions are available, although the 17-item version is more widely used. It relies both on patient-reported symptoms and clinician observation of in-interview behavior (26). Although various cut-off scores have been used to define both syndromal depression and remission from a depressive episode, we use a cut-off of greater than 16 to define a major depression episode and a score of less than 7 to define a remission (27, 28). Because it is clinician administered, the HAM-D has the advantage of including clinician behavioral observations into an overall rating score; however, the length of time required to complete the HAM-D may make it impractical for some clinicians. Like the PHQ-9, the BDI and the Zung are patient self-rating instruments (29, 30). The Zung is a 20-item scale with 10 positively scored items and 10 negatively scored items. Scores of 50 to 59 correlate with mild depression, 60 to 69

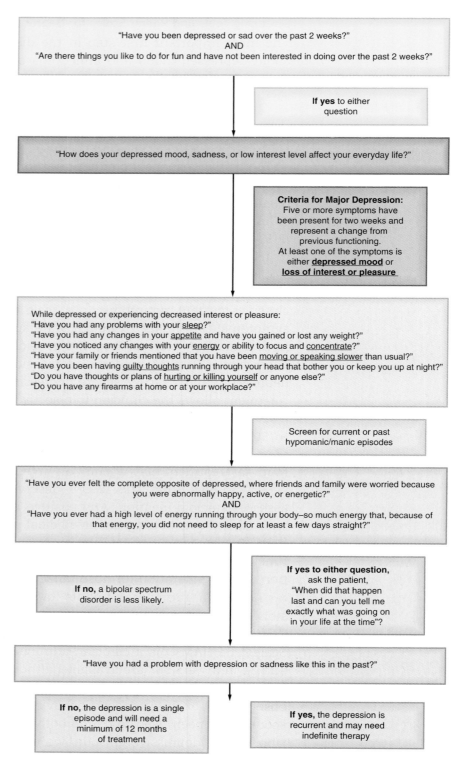

Figure 2.1 Diagnosing depression in the primary care setting.

with moderate to severe depression, and greater than 70 with severe depression. The BDI contains 21 items; scores of 0 to 9 represent minimal symptoms, 10 to 16 mild depression symptoms, 17 to 29 moderate symptoms, and 30 to 63 severe symptoms. Generally, the PHQ-9 is the easiest for the primary care provider to use.

Patient Health Questionnaire (PHQ-9)
Nine Symptom Depression Checklist

Name: _____ Date: _____

Over the *last 2 weeks*, how often have you been bothered by any of the following problems? (Please circle your answer.)

	Not at All	Several Days	More than Half the Days	Nearly Every Day
1. Little interest or pleasure in doing things	0	1	2	3
2. Feeling down, depressed, or hopeless	0	1	2	3
3. Trouble falling or staying asleep, or sleeping too much	0	1	2	3
4. Feeling tired or having little energy	0	1	2	3
5. Poor appetite or overeating	0	1	2	3
6. Feeling bad about yourself—or that you are a failure or have let yourself or your family down	0	1	2	3
7. Trouble concentrating on things, such as reading the newspaper or watching television	0	1	2	3
8. Moving or speaking so slowly that other people could have noticed. Or the opposite—being so fidgety or restless that you have been moving around a lot more than usual	0	1	2	3
9. Thoughts that you would be better off dead or of hurting yourself in some way	0	1	2	3

Add Columns, ☐ + ☐ + ☐

Total Score*, ☐ *Score is for healthcare provider incorporation

10. If you circled *any* problems, how *difficult* have these problems made it for you to do your work, take care of things at home, or get along with other people? (Please circle your answer.)	Not Difficult at All	Somewhat Difficult	Very Difficult	Extremely Difficult

A score of: 0–4 is considered non-depressed; 5–9 mild depression; 10–14 moderate depression; 15–19 moderately severe depression; and 20–27 severe depression.

CHAPTER 2 Depression

Figure 2.2 Patient Health Questionnaire (PHQ-9) nine-symptom depression checklist. (PHQ is adapted from PRIME MD TODAY. PHQ Copyright ©1999 Pfizer Inc. All rights reserved. Reproduced with permission. PRIME MD TODAY is a trademark of Pfizer Inc.)

Suicide Risk Assessment

Clinicians must remain vigilant to the risk of suicide as up to 15% of those with major depressive disorder die by suicide (1). Suicide is consistently a leading cause of death in the United States, accounting for more than 30,000 deaths per year (31). Many patients who die by suicide meet criteria for a depressive disorder and nearly half have seen a primary care physician within a month of their death (32, 33). Clinicians should routinely ask (and document asking) depressed patients if they have had or currently have any thoughts of suicide, of ending their life, or that they would be better off dead. Positive responses should be followed by assessment of the content of suicidal thoughts (including specific plans or actual intent of suicide) and reduction of access to lethal means (especially firearms and medications that may be harmful if taken in large quantities). Clinicians should consult a psychiatrist if there is any uncertainty regarding suicidal risk or need for hospitalization.

Differential Diagnosis

In addition to the systemic illnesses associated with and presenting as depression, many other psychiatric illnesses are associated with depressed mood and other symptoms of depression. "All that is depressive may not be depression" is a useful reminder of this phenomenon. We recommend using the AMPS approach to the psychiatric review of systems when assessing anyone who presents with sadness or anhedonia (see Chapter 1).

Depressive symptoms may be present with psychiatric disorders other than the depressive disorders of major depression, dysthymic disorder, or minor depression. In bipolar disorder, a patient may present with depressive symptoms as part of a depressive or mixed mood episode. Patients with psychotic disorders (e.g., schizophrenia or schizoaffective disorder) may, at some points during their illness, present with prominent symptoms of depression. Anxiety disorders (particularly panic disorder and posttraumatic stress disorder) may coexist with depression or feature prominent depressive symptoms. Dementia and delirium have well-known associations with depressive symptoms; dementia is often associated with comorbid depression, while hypoactive delirium may physically resemble depression. During or following periods of substance abuse, a person may have a substance-induced mood disorder. If depressive symptoms are mild or transient, a person may have an adjustment disorder or bereavement (Table 2.2).

Biopsychosocial Treatment

GENERAL PRINCIPLES

The goals of depression treatment include reducing symptoms of depression, improving daily functioning and quality of life, eliminating suicidal thoughts, minimizing treatment adverse effects, and preventing depression relapse. Medication and psychological therapies are most frequently and successfully used to treat depression. Patients who experience full clinical remission have a better long-term prognosis than patients with only a partial response to therapy (34, 35).

NOT TO BE MISSED

- Suicidal thoughts
- Homicidal thoughts
- Opportunities to reduce access to firearms and medications that may be harmful if taken in large quantities
- Psychotic symptoms
- Illicit drug or alcohol abuse
- Systemic medical causes of depression (e.g., hypothyroidism)
- Bipolar disorder with depressed or mixed episode

Table 2.2 Differential Diagnosis for Major Depressive Disorder

Alcohol abuse/dependence	Can co-occur with depression, mimic depressive symptoms, or actually cause depression. At lease 4 weeks of abstinence is necessary when ruling out depression that is secondary to alcohol use.
Anxiety disorders	Anxiety disorders frequently co-occur with depression. Both generalized anxiety disorder and more episodic, circumstance-specific anxiety disorders (i.e., panic disorder, social phobia, specific phobia, obsessive compulsive disorder, posttraumatic stress disorder, acute stress disorder) should be addressed when present.
Bipolar disorder	Depression is accompanied by a history of one or more manic or mixed episodes. Many patients with bipolar disorder are depressed at the time of initial clinical presentation.
Cobalamin deficiency	Vitamin B_{12} deficiency is associated with macrocytic anemia, paresthesia, numbness, and impaired memory.
Cushing disease	This condition is associated with obesity, dermatologic manifestations, signs of adrenal androgen excess, and proximal muscle wasting.
Dementia	Dementia is characterized by memory changes, mood symptoms, personality changes, psychosis, problematic social behaviors, and changes in day-to-day functioning. Comorbid depression is very common in dementia.
Eating disorders	These disorders are more common in women and sometimes characterized by disturbance in the perception of body weight, size, or shape, and refusal to maintain a healthy body weight in the case of the anorexia nervosa syndrome and impulsive binge eating with compensatory purging behaviors in the bulimia nervosa syndrome. Depression is commonly comorbid in eating disorder patients.
Bereavement	The symptoms of major depression may be transiently present in normal grief. The duration and expression of normal grief vary among racial/ethnic groups. Temporarily hearing the voice of or seeing the deceased person is considered within normal limits of bereavement. Patients with unremitting and significantly impaired function attributable to these mood symptoms should be fully assessed for major depressive disorder.
Hypothyroidism	Associated symptoms include weight gain, constipation, decreased concentration, fatigue, disturbance with sleep, and depressed mood.
Medication adverse effects	Patient should be asked about use of glucocorticoids, interferon, levodopa, and oral contraceptives.
Premenstrual dysphoric disorder (PMDD)	PMDD is characterized by depressed mood, anxiety, and irritability during the week before menses and resolving with menses. PMDD also has prominent pain symptoms.
Psychotic disorders	Patients with major depression may have psychotic symptoms during acute depressive episodes. Mood-congruent hallucinations and delusions are commonly found in patients who have depression with psychotic features. A temporal correlation between increased depressed mood and increased psychotic symptoms is often present with a diagnosis of depression with psychotic features.
Secondary depression	This is depression due to the physiologic consequences of a specific metabolic disturbance, recent drug or substance use, or substance withdrawal. It often remits with treatment of the disorder, removal of the drug or substance, or recovery from withdrawal, but, if persistent, may need specific antidepressant therapy. At least 4 weeks of abstinence is necessary when ruling out depression due to stimulant use.
Adjustment disorder with depressed mood	This is a subsyndromal depression with a clearly identified precipitating event. It usually resolves with resolution of the acute stressor. Although it is not the norm, in some circumstances, a diagnosis of adjustment disorder may justify the short-term use of sedative-hypnotic and antidepressant medications.

CHAPTER 2 Depression

There are several primary care treatment models for the management of depression. One model is that of a physician or other general medical practitioner (e.g., nurse practitioner, physician assistant) as the sole provider of clinical care. In such models, psychiatric or other mental health care must be obtained on a consultation or referral basis from external mental health systems. There is also the same-site consultation model, where a psychiatrist or other mental health professional maintains an office colocated with the primary care provider. This model facilitates comanagement of depression in a combined model often called "collaborative care." Some collaborative care models use nurses in a disease management model for depression where they follow up with patients, by phone or in person, between clinic visits. Finally, with the use of video teleconferencing equipment, primary care clinicians obtain psychiatric consultation from a distance. This model is referred to as "telepsychiatry" and it is often used in rural or underserved areas. The primary care practitioner is advised to avail himself or herself of consultation (and comanagement, where and when available) within the local clinical care models. Cultural consultations are available in some settings to aid in the diagnosis and treatment of depression in culturally diverse populations (36).

PHARMACOTHERAPY

Patients with mild to moderate depression may do equally well with psychotherapy or antidepressant medications (37). Mild depression is often well managed by psychotherapy, attention to health-promoting behaviors, self-help books (e.g., *Feeling Good: The New Mood Therapy* by David D. Burns [38]), or positive changes in social circumstances. Although we do not routinely prescribe St. John's wort, patients with mild depression may request a treatment trial or initiate treatment on their own with over-the-counter preparations (39). Primary care clinicians must remember that St. John's wort acts through a serotonin mechanism, must be discontinued before initiating prescription antidepressants, and has been associated with psychotic symptoms. Combination psychotherapy and medication treatment offer no demonstrated short-term advantage in patients with mild to moderate depression. Patient preference and local psychotherapeutic resources should guide the initial choice of depression therapy.

Severely depressed patients derive the greatest benefit from combined medication management and psychotherapy. Combination medication management and psychotherapy is strongly recommended for those with severe, recurrent, or chronic depression. Primary care–based psychotherapy (e.g., interpersonal or cognitive behavioral therapy) coupled with medication management may also be effective (40). For those patients who prefer only one mode of therapy for severe depression, clinicians usually recommend antidepressant medication over psychotherapy. Whatever treatment is started, close follow-up is essential. Severely depressed patients who harbor suicidal ideation may initially lack the "energy" or initiative to actually kill themselves. As their depression is in early response, they may have increased energy to act on their persisting suicidal thoughts. As detailed above, clinicians must continuously assess all depressed patients for suicidal ideation, intention, and planning.

Fortunately for the busy primary care clinician, there are a variety of pharmacologic options for the treatment of depression (Table 2.3). The most commonly prescribed antidepressants are classified as selective serotonin reuptake inhibitors (SSRIs). Other agents include serotonin norepinephrine reuptake inhibitors (SNRIs), 5-HT2–receptor antagonists, dopamine reuptake inhibitors (DRIs), tricyclic antidepressants (TCAs), and monoamine oxidase inhibitors (MAOIs).

Table 2.3 First-Line Antidepressant Medications

CLASS	INITIAL DOSE (MG/DAY)[a]	THERAPEUTIC DOSE (MG/DAY)	PRACTICAL POINTERS FOR THE PCP[b]
Selective Serotonin Reuptake Inhibitors (SSRIs)			
Sertraline (Zoloft)	50	50–200	Serotonin and dopamine reuptake inhibition Possible early and temporary diarrhea and dyspepsia Relatively low risk for drug interactions
Paroxetine Paroxetine CR (Paxil, Paxil CR)	20 12.5–20	20–60 25–75	High anticholinergic and antihistamine side-effect profile Risk for sedation, weight gain, and dry mouth Short half-life with more risk for discontinuation syndrome High chance for drug interactions Unsafe during pregnancy—class D
Fluoxetine (Prozac)	20	20–60	Long half-life and ideal for intermittently compliant patients Relatively inexpensive High chance for drug interactions
Fluvoxamine (Luvox)	50	50–300	Rarely used due to high side-effect profile
Citalopram (Celexa)	20	20–60	Structurally similar to escitalopram Low risk for drug interactions
Escitalopram (Lexapro)	10	10–20	Structurally similar to citalopram Low risk for drug interactions
Serotonin Norepinephrine Reuptake Inhibitors (SNRIs)			
Venlafaxine XR (Effexor XR)	37.5	75–300	Structurally similar to desvenlafaxine (do not use concurrently) Dual action on serotonin and norepinephrine receptors *Not* consistently "activating" but usually does not cause sedation Sometimes used as an adjunct for chronic pain Not to be used in those with difficult-to-treat hypertension May increase blood pressure and heart rate, especially at higher dosing range (>150 mg/day) Non-XR formulation is rarely used due to side-effect profile and twice-per-day dosing Short half-life with more risk for discontinuation syndrome Reduce dose with renal insufficiency
Desvenlafaxine (Pristiq)	50	50–100	Structurally similar to venlafaxine (do not use concurrently) Dual action on serotonin and norepinephrine receptors *Not* consistently "activating" but usually does not cause sedation Not to be used in those with difficult-to-treat hypertension Short half-life with more risk for discontinuation syndrome Reduce dose with renal insufficiency

(*Continued*)

Table 2.3 First-Line Antidepressant Medications (*Continued*)

CLASS	INITIAL DOSE (MG/DAY)[a]	THERAPEUTIC DOSE (MG/DAY)	PRACTICAL POINTERS FOR THE PCP[b]
Duloxetine (Cymbalta)	30	30–60	Dual action on serotonin and norepinephrine receptors *Not* consistently "activating" but usually does not cause sedation FDA approved for fibromyalgia and diabetic peripheral neuropathic pain Sometimes used for chronic neuropathic pain Short half-life with more risk for discontinuation syndrome Increased risk for drug interactions
Other			
Bupropion	75–150	300–450	
Bupropion SR (Wellbutrin SR)	100	300–400	Given twice per day Likely dual action on dopamine and norepinephrine receptors Contraindicated with seizure and eating disorders
Bupropion XL (Wellbutrin XL)	150	300–450	Increased risk for seizures in those with alcohol withdrawal Not used for anxiety disorders May worsen anxiety associated with depression No serotonin activity and no related sexual side effects XL formulation is supposed to have slower release and lower side-effect profile (permits higher dosing and lower seizure risk) Less frequently used due to side-effect profile
Mirtazapine (Remeron)	15	15–45	Increases central serotonin and norepinephrine activity (possibly through presynaptic α_2-adrenergic receptor inhibition) Decreased frequency of sexual side effects Increased sedation and sleepiness at mainly *lower* doses Although not indicated for anxiety disorders, it may be helpful Remeron Sol tab is orally dissolving for patients who cannot swallow

FDA, Food and Drug Administration; PCP, primary care physician.
[a] Initial dose should be decreased by half when treating an anxiety disorder or an elderly person.
[b] Drug interactions refer to commonly used medications that are principally metabolized by the P450 2D6 pathway.

Medication Management: First-Line Therapy

There are no important clinical differences in response rates among commonly prescribed antidepressants (including SSRIs, SNRIs, bupropion, and mirtazapine). Antidepressant choice must be individualized. Drug selection is based on tolerability, safety, evidence of effectiveness with the patient or first-degree relative, and cost. SSRIs and SNRIs offer similar response rates and can be used as first-line monotherapy. For severe depression, first-line pharmacotherapy should be added to psychotherapy.

Regardless of the drug, medication therapy is effective in the majority of cases (41). Within approximately 6 weeks, half of persons receiving antidepressants have at least a 50% reduction in symptoms (42). In the Sequenced Treatment Alternatives to Relieve Depression (STAR*D) trial, 30% of patients achieved full remission after 12 weeks of treatment with citalopram and 10% to 15% more showed significant improvement (43).

One quarter of patients who failed citalopram responded when switched to sertraline, venlafaxine, or bupropion. A similar number responded when bupropion was added to citalopram.

All first-class antidepressants enhance serotonin, norepinephrine, or dopamine receptor activity. Generally speaking, no single antidepressant is consistently "activating" or sedating. In some cases, symptom profiles may be useful in antidepressant choices. For example, depressed patients with significant weight loss and insomnia may benefit from the sedating and appetite-stimulating properties of low-dose mirtazapine. In contrast, obese patients with excessive fatigue may benefit from a trial of bupropion. Bupropion may also be useful for patients with comorbid nicotine dependence and those concerned about sexual side effects (its relative paucity of serotonergic activity limits the risk of sexual dysfunction). However, bupropion should be avoided in patients with anxiety, seizures, or eating disorders. Side effect profiles vary and clinicians should carefully monitor each patient for any untoward effects.

Medication Management: Second-Line Therapy

In contemporary practice, TCAs have less receptor specificity and are used less often because they may cause intolerable dry mouth, constipation, and dizziness. They are relatively contraindicated in patients with coronary artery disease, congestive heart failure, prostatic hypertrophy, and arrhythmias. When using TCAs to treat depression, the clinician should consult current guidelines for recommended TCA therapeutic range and dose titration. MAOIs are also used infrequently, even by psychiatrists, because of the long list of dietary restrictions, orthostasis, and potential for hypertensive crisis. However, MAOIs may be more effective in patients with atypical depression characterized by hypersomnolence, hyperphagia, and rejection sensitivity. Primary care clinicians should consult with a psychiatrist before considering MAOI therapy. MAOIs should not be prescribed within at least 2 weeks of any serotonergic medication due to the risk of serotonin syndrome.

Other Pharmacotherapeutic Strategies

Before changing medications, the clinician should ensure that the antidepressant is dosed high enough (maximum Food and Drug Administration [FDA]-recommended doses with tolerable side effects) and long enough (at least 6 to 8 weeks) before a medication trial is considered to have failed. If this doesn't work, switching to another antidepressant within the same class or another class leads to a response in many patients. When SSRIs or bupropion fail, using agents with multiple neurotransmitter actions such as mirtazapine, SNRIs, TCAs (all of which act on serotonin and norepinephrine), and sertraline (which is an SSRI with DRI activity) can often provide a benefit.

After medication initiation, symptoms can improve in as little as 1 week (44). After about 6 to 8 weeks of therapy with little response, clinicians can (1) increase the dose of the current medication (if not already done); (2) switch to a different agent from the same or another class; (3) start combination therapy by adding a second antidepressant (e.g., adding bupropion, a TCA, or mirtazapine to an SSRI); or (4) in consult with a psychiatrist, start augmentation with non-antidepressants; (5) add psychotherapy (cognitive behavioral therapy as augmentative therapy is just as effective, albeit with a slower response time, when compared with the addition of a second antidepressant agent [34, 35]); (6) refer to a psychiatrist for medication management. Augmenting agents prescribed in collaboration with a psychiatrist can include lithium, levothyroxine, buspirone (a serotonergic agent that is indicated for generalized anxiety disorder), phototherapy, atypical antipsychotics (e.g., aripiprazole), and dopaminergic agents including stimulants (e.g., methylphenidate) and nonstimulants such as modafinil and atomoxetine. Many of these augmenting agents require expertise in psychopharmacology, and we recommend a psychiatric referral in any case where the primary care clinician feels uncomfortable with the treatment plan and for all patients who require more than one augmenting agent. See Figure 2.3 for guidance in the treatment of depression in the primary care setting.

Medication Side Effects

Side effects from antidepressant medications (Table 2.4) are common. More than 60% of people on antidepressants will experience at least one side effect. It is difficult to predict which drug will cause which side effect for any one person. The most common side effects are constipation, daytime sleepiness, nausea, diarrhea, dizziness, dry mouth, headache, sexual problems, shakiness, trouble sleeping, and weight gain. Many side effects disappear after a few weeks. Clinicians can lessen adverse effects by starting at a low a dose, titrating upward slowly and as tolerated, remaining attentive to the patient's concerns, and thoroughly educating patients and their families about possible side effects.

Sexual side effects are largely due to serotonin or 5-HT2A activation in SSRIs and SNRIs and can be addressed by switching to a different medication with a different mechanism of action (e.g., bupropion or mirtazapine), augmenting with sildenafil (in the absence of contraindications), or augmenting with bupropion. Bupropion is also a good alternative agent for patients who have experienced undesired weight gain but should be avoided in patients with an anxiety, seizure, or eating disorder. If weight gain is a concern, mirtazapine and paroxetine should not be used as first-line agents. Anxiety from an SSRI can be addressed by lowering the dose or switching to another antidepressant. Some clinicians may choose to prescribe a low-dose benzodiazepine (e.g., clonazepam 0.5 mg once nightly) during the SSRI initiation phase. If compliance is a concern, consider using once-weekly fluoxetine.

Some medicines are more likely than others to cause a discontinuation syndrome from serotonin withdrawal. This is characterized by acute headache, dizziness, nausea, insomnia, anxiety, and an electrical "tingling" sensation (often by the ears), and even suicidal ideation. This

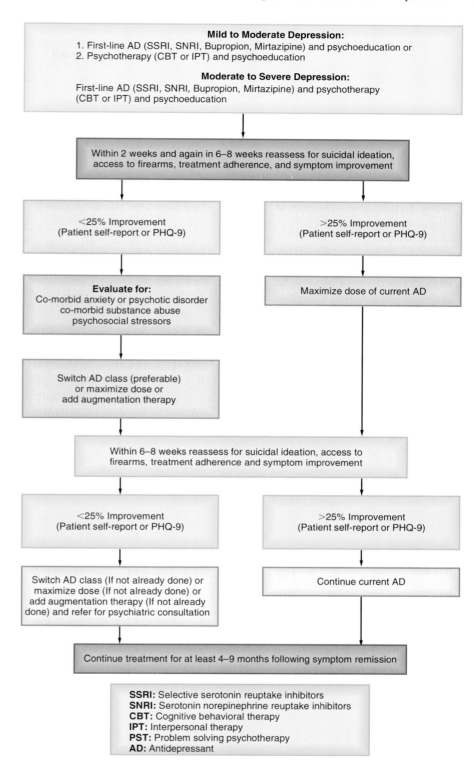

Mild to Moderate Depression:
1. First-line AD (SSRI, SNRI, Bupropion, Mirtazipine) and psychoeducation or
2. Psychotherapy (CBT or IPT) and psychoeducation

Moderate to Severe Depression:
First-line AD (SSRI, SNRI, Bupropion, Mirtazipine) and psychotherapy
(CBT or IPT) and psychoeducation

Within 2 weeks and again in 6–8 weeks reassess for suicidal ideation,
access to firearms, treatment adherence, and symptom improvement

<25% Improvement
(Patient self-report or PHQ-9)

>25% Improvement
(Patient self-report or PHQ-9)

Evaluate for:
Co-morbid anxiety or psychotic disorder
co-morbid substance abuse
psychosocial stressors

Maximize dose of current AD

Switch AD class (preferable)
or maximize dose or
add augmentation therapy

Within 6–8 weeks reassess for suicidal ideation, access to
firearms, treatment adherence and symptom improvement

<25% Improvement
(Patient self-report or PHQ-9)

>25% Improvement
(Patient self-report or PHQ-9)

Switch AD class (If not already done) or
maximize dose (If not already done) or
add augmentation therapy (If not already
done) and refer for psychiatric consultation

Continue current AD

Continue treatment for at least 4–9 months following symptom remission

SSRI: Selective serotonin reuptake inhibitors
SNRI: Serotonin norepinephrine reuptake inhibitors
CBT: Cognitive behavioral therapy
IPT: Interpersonal therapy
PST: Problem solving psychotherapy
AD: Antidepressant

Figure 2.3 Primary care treatment algorithm for depression.

was initially described with the TCAs but is now more commonly associated with missing doses of an antidepressant with a short half-life, like paroxetine or venlafaxine. Fluoxetine is the least likely to cause a discontinuation syndrome because its active metabolite nor fluoxetine increases the effective half-life of fluoxetine.

CHAPTER 2 Depression

Table 2.4 Side-Effects Profile of Antidepressant Classes

	SEXUAL DYSFUNC-TION/DECREASED LIBIDO	WEIGHT GAIN	SEDATION	CARDIAC
SSRIs	+++	+[a]	+/−[a]	0
Venlafaxine	+++	+/−	+/−	+ (↑ BP)
Mirtazapine	+	+++	++	+/−
Bupropion	0	0	0	+/− (↑ BP)
TCAs	++	++	+++	+++ (ECG, BP)

BP, blood pressure; ECG, electrocardiogram abnormalities; SSRIs, selective serotonin reuptake inhibitors; TCA, tricyclic antidepressants.
[a] Paroxetine and fluvoxamine are more likely to cause sedation and weight gain.

Psychotropic drug–drug interactions has been the subject of increasing clinical observation and research (45). Although this topic is broad, there are some important issues to keep in mind in the primary care management of depression. First, MAOIs are absolutely contraindicated with all other antidepressants due to a risk of serotonin syndrome; all other antidepressants must be stopped completely and "washed out" for a period of at least 2 weeks before starting an MAOI. In the case of the longer-acting fluoxetine, it must be stopped 5 weeks before an MAOI can be started. Analogously, MAOIs must be stopped for 2 weeks before any other antidepressant is started. Secondly, paroxetine, duloxetine, fluvoxamine, and fluoxetine can inhibit P450 enzymes in the liver and increase the serum levels of coadministered TCAs, potentially leading to TCA toxicity. Medications that inhibit the P450 2D6 pathway (e.g., paroxetine, duloxetine, fluoxetine) can also dangerously increase serum levels of coadministered beta-blockers. Fortunately, citalopram and escitalopram are less likely to inhibit P450 enzymes and cause drug interactions. Primary care clinicians should show caution when combining TCAs (even in apparently small doses) with SSRIs other than citalopram or escitalopram.

During the first 2 weeks following initiation of antidepressant therapy, patients are more likely to experience side effects than any significant benefit on mood state. The most important possible side effect related to the use of antidepressants is suicidal ideation. The FDA recommends close monitoring of all patients treated with antidepressants, particularly early in the course of treatment. These early encounters should focus on side effects, medication adherence, and suicidal ideation. A warning statement regarding a possible increased risk of suicide has been added to the package insert of many of the commonly prescribed antidepressants and with particular attention to younger age groups.

Duration of Treatment

Depression treatment requires at least 6 to 12 months of close follow-up. Clinicians should follow up with patients 1 to 2 weeks after initiating therapy to help curb the high rate of medication discontinuation during this period. Clinicians should reinforce adherence, address concerns about adverse effects, and monitor for suicidality and emerging psychosocial stressors. Clinical improvement can be quantified with the PHQ-9. Symptom remission and return to normal functioning are the goals of therapy.

In the first episode of depression, patients may require 1 to 6 months of treatment before achieving remission. Once in remission, patients should continue on the effective dose for an additional 12 months.

Recurrence of depression is common. About one third of patients will experience a recurrence within 1 year of discontinuing treatment and about 60% of those with major depressive disorder will have a second episode. Individuals who have had two to three depressive episodes have an 80% to 90% chance of having yet another episode (1). Patients with recurrent depression should be educated about the early signs of depression and be on lifelong antidepressant therapy. Surveillance for recurrence or relapse should continue indefinitely.

ELECTROCONVULSIVE THERAPY

Electroconvulsive therapy (ECT) is usually reserved for patients with medication-refractory or unresponsive depression or when urgent treatment response is critical (e.g., in the severely medically compromised or in patients with psychotic depression). ECT is a safe and effective treatment for severe depression (46). Primary care providers should refer ECT candidates to an experienced psychiatrist (especially one who performs ECT regularly) to address the risks, benefits, and side effect issues of this procedure.

PSYCHOSOCIAL TREATMENT

Although several different types of psychotherapy have been shown to treat depression, cognitive behavioral therapy (CBT) and interpersonal psychotherapy (IPT) provide strong evidence to support their use in patients suffering from depression. Both forms of psychotherapy are brief enough for incorporation into the primary care setting. The following is an overview that is designed to provide an introduction to these two psychotherapies.

Cognitive Behavioral Therapy

The three "R's" can be used to help the patient (recognize, reconstruct, repeat) and the provider (read, refer, review) understand and use CBT in the context of treating and recovering from depressive, anxiety disorders.

Three R's for the patient

Recognize

Patients who are depressed know it. They do not have to contemplate or analyze the "feeling" or "emotion" in order to understand what they are experiencing. The first step with CBT is to simply identify the unhappy emotion or feeling (e.g., "depression" or "sadness"). Patients should also learn to quantify the degree or severity of the emotion by using a Likert scale (e.g., a scale from 1 to 10 can be used, where 10 indicates the most severe depression and 1 indicates no depression).

The next step is the most critical and often the most difficult to initially conceptualize. After labeling and quantifying the emotion, the patient is then encouraged to *recognize* associated dysfunctional thought patterns. One way to teach the patient to do this is to ask, "When you get really depressed, what thoughts run through your head?" Initially, the patient may confuse emotion with thought and answer, "I'm just very depressed." Another way to help the patient recognize dysfunctional thought patterns is to ask, "You mentioned your depression was really bad last night. What thoughts were running through your head when you felt sad?" Common examples of dysfunctional patterns include "Nobody likes me," "I'm a failure at everything I do," "I will never amount to anything," "I will never feel normal again," and "I have always been depressed." The common denominators with these "dysfunctional thoughts" are twofold. First, these thoughts are negative. Second, persistent thoughts are all or none and absolute and therefore usually inaccurate.

Reconstruct

Once the patient learns how to recognize persistent dysfunctional thoughts, he or she can then begin to critically analyze the thoughts by writing them down and *reconstructing* accurate and less absolute or rigid thoughts onto a dysfunctional thought record (DTR). Completion of a DTR requires the patient to write down a specific unhappy and distressing "emotion" or "feeling" followed by the dysfunctional thought that occurs with it. The dysfunctional thought is then analyzed by the patient for accuracy and reconstructed into a more realistic thought. This process is usually completed immediately following or at the time a distressful emotion is experienced. The DTR is usually completed outside of the practitioner's office in the form of CBT "homework." Examples of reconstructed thoughts and a DTR are listed in Tables 2.5 and 2.6, respectively.

Table 2.5 Examples of Dysfunctional Thoughts and Reconstruction Strategies

AUTOMATIC DYSFUNCTIONAL THOUGHTS	RECONSTRUCTED THOUGHTS
"Nobody likes me."	"That can't be true because my wife and kids love me."
"I'm a failure at *everything* I do."	"Maybe I'm just not good in this one area."
"I will *never* amount to *anything*."	"I already have a good job and I might get a promotion next year."
"I will *never* feel normal again."	"Depression can get better with medication and therapy."
"I have *always* been depressed."	"Not true—I was very happy when I got married and graduated from college!"

Table 2.6 Sample Dysfunctional Thought Record (DTR)

EMOTIONS	AUTOMATIC DYSFUNC-TIONAL THOUGHTS	RECONSTRUCTED THOUGHTS	OUTCOME
Specify feeling Rate 1–10 (10 rated as most intense)	"What is running through your head?" (NOT an emotion or feeling)	"Why is the automatic thought inaccurate (be specific)?"	Respecify feeling Rerate feeling using 1–10 scale
"Sad" 9/10	"*No one* will ever really care about me."	"Not true — my parents and wife love me even when I am irritable and unhappy."	"Sad" 3/10
"Depressed" 8/10	"I will never amount to anything."	"I actually have a great job and my kids see me as a great dad.... I think I am just feeling low today."	"Depressed" 2/10
"Really down" 9/10	"I would be much better off dead." "I'm worthless and have no energy."	"Who would take care of my family if I were actually dead?" "The depression makes my energy lower but I can still function." "I feel worthless at this moment but I know my boss relies on me."	"Down" 5/10

Repeat

CBT is a lifelong tool that can be used by patients to recognize early signs of depression and initiate treatment. A DTR should be used indefinitely by all patients who have a history of major depressive disorder. The patient is encouraged to use the DTR during times of worsening depression or stress, and a prethought reconstruction and postthought reconstruction Likert scale should be used to quantify the improvement in mood, as illustrated in Table 2.6.

Three R's for the practitioner

Read

Time constraints and inexperience may prevent primary care practitioners from providing the traditional form of CBT. Abbreviated CBT (ACBT) can be used in the medical setting. This chapter provides only a brief overview of ACBT; interested providers should consult with additional resources in order to become more proficient with this mode of therapy. The first few sections of *Feeling Good: The New Mood Therapy* by Dr. David Burns provides a nice introduction for both the patient and the practitioner (43).

Refer

Patients who have severe depression or suicidal ideation should be immediately referred to a psychiatrist. Patients who lack motivation to complete the CBT homework should be referred to a CBT therapist. Many primary care practitioners may elect to refer depressed patients for regularly scheduled CBT sessions and briefly follow up with them in the medical clinic. Understanding CBT principles will improve communication between primary care providers, CBT providers, and their shared patients.

Review the DTR

Regardless of whether a depressed patient undergoes CBT through self-study or an external therapist, it may be helpful to briefly review the DTR on each visit. Much like the blood glucose log of a diabetic patient, reviewing the DTR can create a "team approach" to the treatment of depression while supplementing the treatment rendered by the psychotherapist.

WHEN TO REFER

Reasons for Routine Psychiatric Referrals

- Primary care provider is uncertain of diagnosis or uncomfortable with managing the treatment plan
- Suboptimal response to commonly prescribed antidepressants
- Repeated adverse effects to medications
- Atypical symptoms (e.g., increased appetite and hypersomnolence)
- Psychotic or manic symptoms
- Comorbid anxiety disorder

Reasons for Urgent Psychiatric Referrals

- Suicidal ideation, intent, or plan
- Homicidal ideation, intent, or plan
- Grave disability due to psychopathology (e.g., unable to provide shelter, food, or clothing)
- Worsening baseline psychotic symptoms
- Need for alcohol or illicit drug detoxification
- Need for ECT

Interpersonal Psychotherapy

Interpersonal psychotherapy is also effective in treating depression but is not readily provided by primary care practitioners. IPT is a brief therapy (lasting about 3 to 4 months) and focuses on examining relationships. During stressful times in a relationship, many depressed patients will deliberately self-isolate due to dysfunctional thought patterns and a related transient drop in self-esteem. The therapist helps the patient discover healthy coping mechanisms to replace the maladaptive interpersonal conflicts. Depressed patients who have interpersonal isolation or numerous conflicts with relationships should be referred for IPT.

Practice Pointers

Case 1: Screening for depression

A 42-year-old woman presents to your office complaining of insomnia. She reports 4 weeks of insomnia, decreased appetite, weight loss, fatigue, and depressed mood. She continues to work but socializes less than usual. Twenty years ago she had a similar episode and sought a brief course of counseling. Her symptoms improved over several months. She has never been on medications for depression and has no family history of mental illness. She denies suicidal ideation or access to firearms. Her examination is notable for tearfulness and a blunted affect, but is otherwise normal. Her PHQ-9 score is 9, consistent with mild to moderate depression.

Discussion: *The clinician should first screen this patient for past or current manic, psychotic, or anxious symptoms. Once the diagnosis of major depressive disorder has been established, she should be asked about her preference for psychotherapy or medications. Should she prefer psychotherapy, the primary care physician should assist with a referral to a local therapist and briefly introduce her to CBT. Should she prefer medication, an SSRI is a reasonable choice to start and the primary care provider should clearly discuss potential side effects. If she tolerates the initial dose well and with minimal side effects, the clinician should repeat her PHQ-9. If she shows a greater than 25% improvement in score, the clinician and patient can discuss the benefits and potential risks of increasing her dose of antidepressant medication. She should be treated for at least 9 to 12 months after symptom remission and her clinician should continue to assess for recurrent depression and suicidal thoughts during subsequent routine primary care visits.*

Case 2: Severe depression and combination therapy

Ms. J is a 29-year-old woman coming to you reporting that her depression has returned. She has struggled with depression and anxiety since she was a teenager and has even spent 3 months in a psychiatric hospital where her treatment included ECT. She recently moved and is hoping to establish care. At times, Ms. J feels "hopeless" and states, "I think I will always be depressed because I have never been anything else." She is not suicidal at this time and does not have access to firearms or prescription medications at home. You decide to refer her to a psychiatrist for management of her depression.

Discussion: *Although recurrent or severe depression is best managed in consultation with a psychiatrist, there are many preventive measures that can be employed. Ideally, given the long-standing history of recurrent depression, Ms. J should have been on lifelong antidepressant therapy. Given her "all or none" dysfunctional thought patterns (e.g., feelings of no hope and persistent depression), she is a good candidate for CBT.*

Ms. J would likely benefit from an antidepressant. Given her history of anxiety, a low-dose SSRI or SNRI might work well. Ms J should be followed closely and monitored for changes in depressive symptoms, medication side effects, and suicidal ideation.

ICD-9

Major Depression	
Single Episode	*296.2x*
Recurrent Episode	*296.3x*
Depressive Disorder NOS	*311*
Dysthymic Disorder	*300.4*
Adjustment Disorder with Depressed Mood	*309.0*
Mood Disorder Due to [General Medical Condition]	*293.83*

x =

0 Unspecified

1 Mild

2 Moderate

3 Severe, without Psychosis

4 Severe, with Psychosis

5 In Partial or Unspecified Remission

6 In Full Remission

Practical Resources

Screening for Depression: U.S. Preventive Services Task Force (USPSTF): http://www.ahrq.gov/clinic/3rduspstf/depression/depressrr.htm
Geriatric Depression Scale: http://www.stanford.edu/~yesavage/GDS.html
Edinburgh Postnatal Depression Scale: http://www.dbpeds.org/media/edinburghscale.pdf
National Alliance on Mental Illness: http://www.nami.org/
National Institute for Mental Health: http://www.nimh.nih.gov/
The MacArthur Foundation on Depression and Primary Care at Dartmouth and Duke: http://www.depression-primarycare.org/
National Institutes of Health (NIH) Medline Plus: www.nlm.nih.gov/medlineplus/depression.html
Agency for Healthcare Research and Quality (AHRQ) review of effective depression treatments: http://effectivehealthcare.ahrq.gov/reports/index.cfm
FDA Drug Safety Guide: http://www.fda.gov/cder/drug/DrugSafety/DrugIndex.htm)

References

1. *Diagnosis and Statistical Manual of Mental Disorders.* 4th ed. Washington, DC: American Psychiatric Association; 1994.

2. Frasure-Smith N. The Montreal Heart Attack Readjustment Trial. *J Cardiopulm Rehabil.* 1995;15:103–106.

3. Gartlehner G, Hansen RA, Thieda P, et al. Comparative effectiveness of second-generation antidepressants in the pharmacologic treatment of adult depression. Comparative effectiveness review no. 7. Bethesda, MD: AHRQ; 2007.

4. Frasure-Smith N, Lesperance F. Reflections on depression as a cardiac risk factor. *Psychosom Med.* 2005;67(Suppl 1):S19–25.

5. Katon W, Schulberg H. Epidemiology of depression in primary care. *Gen Hosp Psychiatry.* 1992;14:237–247.

6. Pignone MP, Gaynes BN, Rushton JL, et al. Screening for depression in adults: a summary of the evidence for the U.S. Preventive Services Task Force. *Ann Intern Med.* 2002;136:765–776.

7. Beck CT. Predictors of postpartum depression: an update. *Nurs Res.* 2001;50:275–285.

8. Kendler KS, Gardner CO, Prescott CA. Clinical characteristics of major depression that predict risk of depression in relatives. *Arch Gen Psychiatry.* 1999;56:322–327.

9. Bergman-Evans B. A health profile of spousal Alzheimer's caregivers. Depression and physical health characteristics. *J Psychosoc Nurs Ment Health Serv.* 1994;32:25–30.

10. Bottomley A. Depression in cancer patients: a literature review. *Eur J Cancer Care.* 1998;7:181–191.

11. Popkin MK, Callies AL, Lentz RD, et al. Prevalence of major depression, simple phobia, and other psychiatric disorders in patients with long-standing type I diabetes mellitus. *Arch Gen Psychiatry*. 1988;45:64–68.

12. Anderson RJ, Freedland KE, Clouse RE, et al. The prevalence of comorbid depression in adults with diabetes: a meta-analysis. *Diabetes Care*. 2001;24:1069–1078.

13. House A, Dennis M, Mogridge L, et al. Mood disorders in the year after first stroke. *Br J Psychiatry*. 1991;158:83–92.

14. Schleifer SJ, Macari-Hinson MM, Coyle DA, et al. The nature and course of depression following myocardial infarction. *Arch Intern Med*. 1989;149:1785–1789.

15. de Maat MM, Hoetelmans RM, Math t RA, et al. Drug interaction between St John's wort and nevirapine. *AIDS*. 2001;15:420–421.

16. Stunkard AJ, Faith MS, Allison KC. Depression and obesity. *Biol Psychiatry*. 2003;54:330–337.

17. Onyike CU, Crum RM, Lee HB, et al. Is obesity associated with major depression? Results from the Third National Health and Nutrition Examination Survey. *Am J Epidemiol*. 2003;158:1139–1147.

18. Screening for depression: recommendations and rationale. *Ann Intern Med*. 2002;136:760–764.

19. Mulrow CD, Williams JW Jr, Gerety MB, et al. Case-finding instruments for depression in primary care settings. *Ann Intern Med*. 1995;122:913–921.

20. Whooley MA, Avins AL, Miranda J, et al. Case-finding instruments for depression: two questions are as good as many. *J Gen Intern Med*. 1997;12:439–445.

21. Lowe B, Unutzer J, Callahan CM, et al. Monitoring depression treatment outcomes with the Patient Health Questionnaire-9. *Med Care*. 2004;42:1194–1201.

22. Spitzer RL, Kroenke K, Williams JB. Validation and utility of a self-report version of PRIME-MD: the PHQ primary care study. Primary Care Evaluation of Mental Disorders. Patient Health Questionnaire. *JAMA*. 1999;282:1737–1744.

23. Brody DS, Hahn SR, Spitzer RL, et al. Identifying patients with depression in the primary care setting: a more efficient method. *Arch Intern Med*. 1998;158:2469–2475.

24. U.S. Department of Health and Human Services Agency for Health Care Policy and Research. *Depression Guideline Panel. Depression in Primary Care. Vol. 2. Treatment of Major Depression. Clinical Practice Guideline No. 5*. Rockville, MD: U.S. Department of Health and Human Services; 1993.

25. U.S. Department of Health and Human Services Agency for Health Care Policy and Research. *Depression Guideline Panel. Depression in Primary Care. Vol. 1. Detection and Diagnosis. Clinical Practice Guideline No. 5*. Rockville, MD: U.S. Department of Health and Human Services; 1993.

26. Hamilton MA. A rating scale for depression. *J Neurol Neurosurg Psychiatry*. 1960;23:56–62.

27. Hawley CJ, Gale TM, Sivakumaran T. How does the threshold score to enter a major depression trial influence the size of the available patient population for study? *J Aff Disord*. 2002;71:181–187.

28. Zimmerman M, Posternak MA, Chelminsk I. Heterogeneity among depressed outpatients considered to be in remission. *Compr Psychiatry*. 2007;48:113–117.

29. Beck AT, Ward CH, Mendelson M, et al. An inventory of measuring depression. *Arch Gen Psychiatry*. 1961;4:53–63.

30. Zung WW. A self-rating depression scale. *Arch Gen Psychiatry*. 1965;12:63–70.

31. WISQARS. National Center for Injury Prevention and Control. WISQARS (Web-based Injury Statistics Query and Reporting System). Available at: http://www.cdc.gov/ncipc/. Accessed May 24, 2007.

32. Carney SS, Rich CL, Burke PA, et al. Suicide over 60: the San Diego study. *J Am Geriatr Soc*. 1994;42:174–180.

33. Luoma JB, Martin CE, Pearson JL. Contact with mental health and primary care providers before suicide: a review of the evidence. *Am J Psychiatry*. 2002;159:909–916.

34. Rush AJ, Trivedi MH, Wisniewski SR, et al. Acute and longer-term outcomes in depressed outpatients requiring one or several treatment steps: a STAR*D report. *Am J Psychiatry*. 2006;163:1905–1917.

35. Thase ME, Friedman ES, Biggs MM, et al. Cognitive therapy versus medication in augmentation and switch strategies as second-step treatments: a STAR*D report. *Am J Psychiatry*. 2007;164:739–752.

36. Kirmayer LJ, Groleau D, Guzder J, et al. Cultural consultation: a model of mental health service for multicultural societies. *Can J Psychiatry*. 2003;48:145–153.

37. Thase ME, Greenhouse JB, Frank E, et al. Treatment of major depression with psychotherapy or psychotherapy–pharmacotherapy combinations. *Arch Gen Psychiatry*. 1997;54:1009–1015.

38. Burns DD. *Feeling Good: The New Mood Therapy*. New York: Avon Books; 1999.

39. Linde K, Mulrow CD, Berner M, et al. St John's wort for depression. *Cochrane Database Syst Rev*. 2005:CD000448.

40. Malt UF, Robak OH, Madsbu HP, et al. The Norwegian naturalistic treatment study of depression in general practice (NORDEP)-I: randomised double blind study. *BMJ.* 1999;318:1180–1184.

41. Schulberg HC, Katon W, Simon GE, et al. Treating major depression in primary care practice: an update of the Agency for Health Care Policy and Research Practice Guidelines. *Arch Gen Psychiatry.* 1998;55:1121–1127.

42. Trivedi MH, Fava M, Wisniewski SR, et al. Medication augmentation after the failure of SSRIs for depression. *N Engl J Med.* 2006;354:1243–1252.

43. Rush AJ, Trivedi MH, Wisniewski SR, et al. Bupropion-SR, sertraline, or venlafaxine-XR after failure of SSRIs for depression. *N Engl J Med.* 2006;354:1231–1242.

44. Taylor MJ, Freemantle N, Geddes JR, et al. Early onset of selective serotonin reuptake inhibitor antidepressant action: systematic review and meta-analysis. *Arch Gen Psychiatry.* 2006;63:1217–1223.

45. Sandson NB, Armstrong SC, Cozza KL. An overview of psychotropic drug-drug interactions. *Psychosomatics.* 2005;46:464–494.

46. Fink M, Taylor MA. Electroconvulsive therapy: evidence and challenges. *JAMA.* 2007;298:330–332.

CHAPTER 3 Mood Disorders— Bipolar Disorder

Donald M. Hilty, MD • Martin H. Leamon, MD • Elizabeth N. Gutierrez, MD • Donald R. Ebersole, MD • Russell F. Lim, MD

A 35-year-old man presents to the outpatient clinic with the following request: "I want to be checked for high blood pressure." During the interview, the patient states, "I was on fluoxetine a few years ago and my wife thinks I need something to take the edge off." Currently he is not feeling depressed, but his wife encouraged him to discuss his episodic irritability at this visit. These episodes appear in waves of weeks, several times per year. He mentioned that his wife took him to the emergency room for a prior "episode."

CLINICAL HIGHLIGHTS

• The "building blocks" for both bipolar spectrum disorders include depressive, hypomanic, manic, and mixed episodes. Patients with bipolar disorder I must have had at least one manic or mixed episode and those with bipolar II must have had at least one depressive and one hypomanic episode. The principle difference between a manic and a hypomanic episode is that the former must result in significant social or occupational dysfunction or need for psychiatric admission.

Clinical Significance

Establishing an accurate diagnosis and appropriate treatment plan for patients with bipolar disorder in the primary medical setting is challenging (1). The lifetime prevalence of bipolar I and bipolar II disorders has been estimated to be 1.0% and 0.8%, respectively (2). Bipolar disorder is a significant source of morbidity and mortality. The World Health Organization (WHO) found bipolar disorder to be the world's sixth leading cause of disability (adjusted life years) for people aged 15 to 44 years. As many as 25% to 50% of bipolar patients attempt suicide during their lifetime and about 15% of inadequately treated bipolar patients die by suicide. Additionally, up to 30% of depressed and anxious patients who present to primary care settings may have an underlying bipolar disorder (3, 4). Therefore, health service utilization rates for patients with bipolar disorder are increasing and many patients are presenting to their primary care providers for treatment.

Diagnosis

The diagnosis of bipolar disorder is often difficult due to its fluctuating course and variable presentation. Patients usually present in a depressed state rather than a manic state. Furthermore, they may not accurately recall previous manic episodes. A misdiagnosis of bipolar depression as unipolar or major depressive disorder can lead to ineffective and possibly adverse treatment outcomes. The National Depressive and Manic-Depressive Association survey of bipolar members showed an average delay of 8 years between the first presentation to mental health professionals and correct diagnosis.

(Continued)

CLINICAL HIGHLIGHTS
(*Continued*)

- Most patients with bipolar disorder present with depression, so it is important to screen for bipolar disorder in all patients who present with depressive symptoms.

- The classic presentation of bipolar mania may be absent in many patients. There is a delay in an accurate diagnosis of bipolar disorder that averages about 8 years after the initial presentation to a mental health professional.

- Up to 30% of depressed and anxious patients who present to primary care settings may have an underlying bipolar disorder.

- Bipolar disorder is a chronic disease with an *episodic*, relapsing-remitting condition that requires long-term treatment.

- Bipolar disorder occurs frequently with substance use disorders and attention deficit hyperactivity disorder (ADHD).

- The contemporary treatment of bipolar acute manic or mixed states involves the use of combination therapy with a mood stabilizer and a second-generation antipsychotic (SGA).

- Treatment options for bipolar depression include lamotrigine, lithium, quetiapine, and an antidepressant combined with a mood stabilizer or SGA. As a general rule, antidepressants should not be used as monotherapy to treat a bipolar spectrum disorder.

The "building blocks" for both bipolar spectrum disorders include manic, hypomanic, mixed, and depressive episodes. The *Diagnostic and Statistical Manual of Mental Disorders,* 4th ed., text revision (DSM-IV-TR), defines a *manic episode* as "a distinct period of abnormally and persistently elevated, expansive, or irritable mood, lasting at least 1 week, or any duration if hospitalization is necessary" (5). During this period of mood disturbance, other manic symptoms also have to be present (Table 3.1). More importantly, the mood disturbance should be sufficiently severe to cause impairment in functioning. The criteria for a *hypomanic episode* are the same for a manic episode, except the duration of the mood disturbance is at least 4 days rather than 1 week, and the disturbance causes less impairment in functioning without the need for psychiatric hospitalization. A *mixed episode* is defined as a period lasting 1 week when the criteria for both a depressive episode and a manic episode are simultaneously met. During this week, the individual may experience mood fluctuation between depression, irritability, unexplained agitation, and euphoria. A *depressive episode* is defined as the presence of either a depressed mood or loss of interest in pleasurable activities for at least 2 weeks. Four other symptoms (e.g., sleep disturbance, weight changes, decreased energy and concentration, guilty thoughts, psychomotor changes, and suicidal ideation) must also be present during this same time period.

The diagnosis of bipolar I disorder is made with the presence (or history) of at least one manic or mixed episode. The diagnosis of bipolar II disorder is indicated with the presence (or history) of at least one major depressive *and* one hypomanic episode. It is important to remember that most bipolar patients spend more time in depressed episodes than manic episodes, but the presence of one or more hypomanic or manic episodes changes the diagnosis from unipolar (i.e., major depressive disorder) to bipolar disorder.

Table 3.1 DSM-IV-TR Criteria for a Manic Episode

A. A distinct period of abnormally and persistently elevated, expansive, or irritable mood, lasting at least 1 week (or any duration if hospitalization is necessary)
B. During the period of mood disturbance, *three* (or more) of the following symptoms have persisted (four if the mood is only irritable) and have been present to a significant degree:
1. Inflated self-esteem or grandiosity
2. Decreased need for sleep
3. More talkative than usual or pressure to keep talking
4. Flight of ideas or subjective experience that thoughts are racing
5. Distractibility
6. Increase in goal-directed activity or psychomotor agitation
7. Excessive involvement in pleasurable activities that have a high potential for painful consequences

From *Diagnosis and Statistical Manual of Mental Disorders.* 4th ed., text revision. Washington DC: American Psychiatric Association; 2002.

Table 3.2 Screening Questions for Manic and Hypomanic Episodes

1. "Have you ever felt the complete opposite of depressed, *where friends and family were worried about you because you were too happy*?"
2. "Have you ever had excessive amounts of energy running through your body, to the point where you did not need to sleep for days?"
   - "How long did these symptoms last?"
   - "During these periods, did you feel like your thoughts were going really fast and it was hard to focus?"
   - "During these periods, did people comment that you were talking really fast?"
   - "During these periods, did you ever make impulsive decisions that you regretted later (e.g., spending too much money or being sexually promiscuous)?"
   - "During any of these periods, did your behaviors get you into trouble at work, at home, or with the law, or cause you to end up in the hospital?"
   - "During these periods, were you using any alcohol or substances?"

PATIENT ASSESSMENT

For patients who do not clearly present in a manic episode, it can be challenging to elicit the history of a previous manic episode. Some sample interview questions designed to increase recognition of a prior manic or hypomanic episode are presented in Table 3.2. Grouping several symptoms together and specifically asking whether they occurred simultaneously can be more revealing when establishing a manic or hypomanic episode. When patients report that their mood episodes last for only a few minutes or hours or less than a day, the differential diagnosis may include a rapid-cycling bipolar disorder, malingering, and personality disorders. *Rapid-cycling bipolar disorder* occurs infrequently and is defined by the presence of four or more discrete mood (depressive or manic) episodes within 12 months.

The Mood Disorder Questionnaire (MDQ) is a validated, self- or clinician-administered questionnaire that takes about 5 minutes to complete and consists of 17 questions (6) (Figure 3.1). The first section contains 13 questions with yes or no answers about possible symptoms. The second section asks whether the symptoms occurred simultaneously, whereas the other questions assess severity, family history, and past diagnosis. A positive screen consists of seven or more affirmative answers to item 1, an affirmative answer to item 2, and at least a "moderate or serious" problem for section 3. The MDQ can identify 7 of 10 patients with bipolar disorder and eliminates 9 of 10 without it. The MDQ has also been validated in the general medical population (7).

In addition to screening for depression and mania, a sleep history should be obtained. Patients with mania or hypomania often report chronic insomnia or episodes of decreased need for sleep. On examination, patients with mania often present with rapid, pressured speech that may be difficult to interrupt. They may be highly distractible or fidgety and have a hard time focusing on the interview. Racing thoughts may explicitly manifest as a flight of ideas (when the interview jumps from one topic to the next) or looseness of association (when multiple disconnected topics are discussed). The content of their thoughts may

THE MOOD DISORDER QUESTIONNAIRE

Instructions: Please answer each question to the best of your ability.

	YES	NO
1. Has there ever been a period of time when you were not your usual self and...		
...you felt so good or so hyper that other people thought you were not your normal self or you were so hyper that you got into trouble?	○	○
...you were so irritable that you shouted at people or started fights or arguments?	○	○
...you felt much more self-confident than usual?	○	○
...you got much less sleep than usual and found you didn't really miss it?	○	○
...you were much more talkative or spoke much faster than usual?	○	○
...thoughts raced through your head or you couldn't slow your mind down?	○	○
...you were so easily distracted by things around you that you had trouble concentrating or staying on track?	○	○
...you had much more energy than usual?	○	○
...you were much more active or did many more things than usual?	○	○
...you were much more social or outgoing than usual, for example, you telephoned friends in the middle of the night?	○	○
...you were much more interested in sex than usual?	○	○
...you did things that were unusual for you or that other people might have thought were excessive, foolish, or risky?	○	○
...spending money got you or your family into trouble?	○	○
2. If you checked YES to more than one of the above, have several of these ever happened during the same period of time?	○	○

3. How much of a problem did any of these cause you—like being unable to work; having family, money, or legal troubles; getting into arguments or fights? *Please circle one response only.*

No Problem   Minor Problem   Moderate Problem   Serious Problem

	YES	NO
4. Have any of your blood relatives (i.e., children, siblings, parents, grandparents, aunts, uncles) had manic-depressive illness or bipolar disorder?	○	○
5. Has a health professional ever told you that you have manic-depressive illness or bipolar disorder?	○	○

If the patient answers:

1. **"Yes"** to 7 or more of the 13 items in question number 1;

AND

2. **"Yes"** to question number 2;

AND

3. **"Moderate"** or **"Serious"** to question number 3;

you have a positive screen. All three of the criteria above should be met. A positive screen should be followed by a comprehensive medical evaluation for bipolar spectrum disorder.

CHAPTER 3 Bipolar Disorder

Figure 3.1. The mood disorder questionnaire (6). (© 2000 by American Psychiatric Publishing, Inc. Reprinted with permission. This instrument is designed for screening purposes only and is not to be used as a diagnostic tool.)

be grandiose or delusional and themes of exaggerated power and achievement are often present.

A review of medical conditions, past psychiatric history, substance use, and current medications are indicated, as well as a physical examination and basic laboratory studies (e.g., thyroid function tests and urine toxicology). Collateral information from significant others, family members, and friends should be obtained whenever possible to remedy any recall errors.

Differential Diagnosis

Manic or depressive symptoms can be indicators of general medical, substance use, mood, or psychotic disorders (Table 3.3). The general approach is to rule out treatable general medical conditions, to identify substance-induced disorders, and then to differentiate among the mood and psychotic disorders. General medical conditions that may mimic manic or depressive symptoms include neurologic, infectious, immunologic, metabolic, and endocrine disorders.

Acute intoxication with stimulants such as methamphetamine or cocaine can mimic a manic episode, whereas withdrawal from these substances can mimic a depressive episode. Chronic use of any substance can also induce chronic mood changes that can be difficult to

Table 3.3 Medications and Medical Conditions Associated with Mood Disturbances

Medications
- Antidepressants
- Corticosteroids
- Dopamine agonists
- Isoniazid
- Interferon
- Opioids
- Sedatives-hypnotics
- Stimulants
- Sympathomimetics

General Medical Conditions
- Adrenal disorders
- CNS infections (e.g., HIV, herpes, syphilis)
- Brain tumor
- Huntington disease
- Multiple sclerosis
- Parkinson disease
- Porphyria
- Seizure disorder
- Stroke
- Systemic lupus erythematosus
- Thyroid disorder
- Traumatic brain injury
- Vasculitis
- Vitamin B_{12} deficiency
- Wilson disease

Substance Conditions
Intoxication
- Alcohol
- Amphetamines
- Cocaine
- Caffeine
- Phencyclidine
- Hallucinogens

Withdrawal
- Alcohol
- Barbiturates
- Benzodiazepines

Other Psychiatric Conditions
- Schizoaffective disorder
- Schizophrenia
- Major depressive disorder
- Attention deficit hyperactivity disorder
- Borderline personality disorder
- Narcissistic personality disorder

CNS, central nervous system; HIV, human immunodeficiency virus.

distinguish from a primary mood disorder. Therefore, it is important to inquire about the existence of any mood disturbances during periods of sobriety.

Among psychiatric disorders, bipolar depression must be distinguished from major depression (by the absence of manic or hypomanic episodes) and less severe forms of depression including adjustment disorder, and dysthymia. Acute manic or mixed episodes may also present with psychotic symptoms, often making it difficult to distinguish from a primary psychotic disorder such as schizophrenia. Psychosis from a manic episode tends to be more grandiose and less bizarre or disorganized than the psychosis related to schizophrenia. Some patients meet the criteria of schizophrenia and a mood disorder (either bipolar disorder or major depressive disorders) and are diagnosed with schizoaffective disorder, depressive or bipolar type. In these patients, the psychosis persists even when the mood symptoms are absent (Figure 3.2).

Other psychiatric disorders may contain symptoms that overlap with bipolar disorder, making the differential diagnosis even more complex. These symptoms include hyperactivity, distractibility, and the impulsivity seen with ADHD and mood lability and impulsivity seen with borderline and cluster B personality disorders (8). Usually, ADHD and personality disorders have a more consistent and chronic course with a preadolescent onset whereas bipolar disorder has an episodic relapsing-remitting course with symptom-free periods in between episodes. In practice, bipolar disorder is often difficult to distinguish from ADHD or borderline personality disorder. These conditions are often highly comorbid and therefore the same patient may have bipolar disorder and ADHD or borderline personality disorder.

Biopsychosocial Treatment

TREATMENT PRINCIPLES

The principles of bipolar disorder management are outlined in Table 3.4 (9). In general, pharmacotherapy is a key component for the treatment of bipolar disorder. The number of medications with Food and Drug Administration (FDA) indications for both bipolar mania and depression has expanded rapidly over the last decade. Nevertheless, a strong, trusting therapeutic relationship is fundamental for enhancing adherence to treatment, detecting recurrence of illness, and addressing psychosocial stressors. Patients require ongoing education regarding the illness, treatment options, medication side effects, and impact of the illness on family and friends, employment, and finances. When needed, families often provide support, living arrangements, and input on treatment adherence. National organizations also offer significant education and social support (see Practical Resources).

PHARMACOTHERAPY

The American Psychiatric Association (APA) treatment guideline for bipolar disorder provides an evidence-based and detailed overview of

NOT TO BE MISSED

- Major depressive disorder (unipolar)
- Substance-induced mood disorders
- Medication-induced mood disorder
- Attention deficit hyperactivity disorder
- Borderline personality disorder
- General medical conditions
- Suicidal ideation

CHAPTER 3 Bipolar Disorder

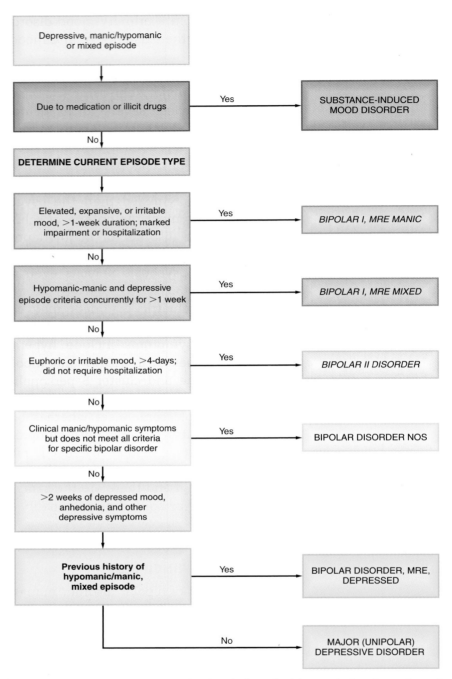

Figure 3.2. Diagnostic algorithm for bipolar disorders. (Adapted with permission from *Diagnosis and Statistical Manual of Mental Disorders*. 4th ed., text revision. Washington DC: American Psychiatric Association; 2002: Appendix A.)

the treatment for bipolar disorder (10). Manic episodes frequently require psychiatric hospitalization. For acute *bipolar mania*, a mood stabilizer (except lamotrigine) is generally indicated in combination with an SGA (11). SGAs have FDA approval for acute bipolar manic and mixed episodes (Table 3.5). For *bipolar depression*, lamotrigine, lithium, quetiapine, and an antidepressant combined with a mood stabilizer or an SGA are possible options. There is currently no FDA-approved medication

Table 3.4 Treatment Principles for Bipolar Disorder

All Patients
- Establish and maintain a positive therapeutic relationship
- Monitor the patient's status to detect recurrence of symptoms early
- Provide education about treatment and risks of relapse
- Promote regular patterns of activity and wakefulness
- Promote understanding of and adaptation to psychosocial stressors
- Discourage the use of tobacco, alcohol, or excessive caffeine
- Engage the patient and family in management decisions
- Collaborate with the psychiatrist as indicated (e.g., management of the high-risk, bipolar patient)
- Communicate with the entire treatment team

Pharmacotherapy
- Bipolar mania: Mood stabilizer and second-generation antipsychotic (SGA)
- Bipolar hypomania: Mood stabilizer or SGA
- Bipolar depression: Lithium, lamotrigine, quetiapine, antidepressants *with* mood stabilizer or SGA
- Bipolar maintenance: Mood stabilizer and/or SGA, lamotrigine

Women of Reproductive Age
- Discuss and document the patient's birth control method
- Discuss and document potential risks for fetal exposure to medication
- Encourage proper nutrition, exercise, and vitamin supplementation
- Inquire about future plans for pregnancy and emphasize pre-pregnancy consultation

The Pregnant Patient
- Discuss and document benefits and risks of treatment options and decisions thoroughly
- Develop a treatment plan to manage mania, depression, and psychosis during pregnancy, with a low threshold for inpatient psychiatric hospitalization

Geriatric and Medically Compromised Patients
- "Start low, go slow"
- Carefully evaluate the risks of reduced liver and renal clearance

CHAPTER 3 Bipolar Disorder

specifically for the treatment of bipolar II disorder, per se. The hypomania of bipolar II may be treated with a mood stabilizer and/or an SGA. The approach to the treatment of depression is similar for both bipolar I and bipolar II disorders. Antidepressants should be used with caution in patients with bipolar disorder (particularly when used as monotherapy) because it carries a small but unpredictable risk of inducing mania and agitation (12).

Bipolar Mania/Hypomania: Mood Stabilizers

Mood stabilizers (Table 3.6) include lithium and the anticonvulsants, divalproex sodium, carbamazepine, and lamotrigine. Lithium, divalproex sodium, and carbamazepine (and its metabolite oxcarbazepine) are the mainstay treatments for acute bipolar mania (usually as part of combination therapy with SGA) and hypomania (as monotherapy). Gabapentin and topiramate have not been demonstrated to be efficacious in randomized placebo-controlled trials and meta-analyses, respectively, and are *not* recommended for routine care.

Lithium is dosed for a therapeutic serum level between 0.6 and 1.2 mEq/mL. It has been demonstrated to reduce suicide risk in large samples of patients, probably because of its antidepressant action, but it is potentially lethal due to its narrow therapeutic window. Common side

Table 3.5 Mood Stabilizers and Antipsychotic Medications with FDA Indications for Bipolar Disorder[a]

INDICATION	LITHIUM	CARBAMAZE-PINE (TEGRETOL)	DIVALPROEX SODIUM (DEPAKOTE/ DEPAKOTE ER)	LAMOTRIGINE (LAMICTAL)	RISPERIDONE (RISPERDAL)	OLANZAPINE (ZYPREXA)	QUETIAPINE (SEROQUEL)	ZIPRASIDONE (GEODON)	ARIPIPRAZOLE (ABILIFY)	OLANZAPINE / FLUOXETINE (SYMBYAX)
Acute mania or mixed	+	+	+	–	+	+	+	+	+	–
Bipolar depression	b	–	–	b	–	–	+	–	–	+
Bipolar maintenance[c]	d	d	d	+	–	+	+	–	–	–

[a] Adapted from American Psychiatric Association. Practice guideline for the treatment of patients with bipolar disorder (revision). *Am J Psychiatry.* 2002;159 (Suppl):1–50; and *Physician Desk Reference* 2008.
[b] Lithium and lamotrigine are commonly used for bipolar depression, although they do not have specific FDA indications for bipolar depression.
[c] In clinical practice, most of the antipsychotics are effective treatments for bipolar maintenance.
[d] Mood stabilizers are commonly used for bipolar maintenance therapy.

Table 3.6 Mood Stabilizers for Bipolar Disorder[a]

	STARTING DOSE[b]	TARGET SERUM LEVEL	TITRATION SCHEDULE	SIDE EFFECTS	MONITORING[b]
Lithium	300 mg BID/TID May be dosed QHS if tolerated	0.6–1.2 mEq/L (acute mania)	Steady-state level reached in 4–5 days Increase by increments of 300–600 mg, as tolerated	Nausea/vomiting, diarrhea, tremor, fatigue, polyuria, acne, worsening psoriasis, diabetes insipidus ECG changes (mainly benign T-wave changes) Hypothyroidism Toxicity (confusion, ataxia, dysarthria, coma) High caution in those with renal insufficiency Potentially lethal due to its narrow therapeutic window Pregnancy category (D)	Check lithium level 5–7 days after each dose change Every 3 months: lithium level, TSH, metabolic panel Lithium toxicity risk increased by: 1. Drugs that decrease glomerular filtration rate, which increase lithium levels (NSAIDs, ACE inhibitors, diuretics) 2. Conditions that cause volume depletion or "dehydration" (e.g., severe vomiting/diarrhea)
Divalproex Sodium (Depakote)	500–1,000 mg BID (25 mg/kg/day for acute mania) Extended release (ER) dosed 500–2,000 mg QHS	85–125 µg/mL (acute mania)	Steady-state level reached in 3–5 days Increase by 500–1,000 mg/day, as tolerated	Sedation Tremor Weight gain Hypersensitivity Thrombocytopenia Transaminitis Hyperammonemia Encephalopathy Pancreatitis Pregnancy category (D)	Baseline, 3-month, 6-month, and annually thereafter: VPA level, CBC, AST, and ALT
Carbamazepine (Tegretol)	ER 200 mg BID	Not established for bipolar disorder	Steady-state level reached in 3–4 days Increase by 200 mg/day (up to 1,600 mg/day), as tolerated	Dizziness Somnolence Stevens-Johnson syndrome Hyponatremia (SIADH) Leukopenia, pancytopenia, thrombocytopenia Hepatitis Drug interactions common Pregnancy category (D)	Baseline, 3-month, 6-month, and annually thereafter: carbamazepine level, CBC, serum chemistry, liver enzymes

(Continued)

Table 3.6 Mood Stabilizers for Bipolar Disorder[a] (Continued)

	STARTING DOSE[b]	TARGET SERUM LEVEL	TITRATION SCHEDULE	SIDE EFFECTS	MONITORING[b]
Oxcarbazepine (Trileptal)	300 mg BID	Not established for bipolar disorder	Increased by 300 mg/day, as tolerated	Fatigue Ataxia Hyponatremia Stevens-Johnson syndrome Pregnancy category (C)	Serum sodium during maintenance treatment (interval not established; consider every 3–4 months)
Lamotrigine (Lamictal)[c]	25 mg/day	Not established for bipolar disorder	25 mg/day for 2 weeks, then 50 mg/day for 2 weeks, then 100 mg/day for 1 week, then 200 mg/day (dose titration pack available), as tolerated[d]	Rash Stevens-Johnson syndrome Hepatitis Anemia, leukopenia, thrombocytopenia Pregnancy category (C)	Signs of rash

ACE, angiotensin-converting enzyme; ALT, alanine transaminase; AST, aspartate transaminase; CBC, complete blood count; ECG, electrocardiogram; NSAIDs, nonsteroidal anti-inflammatory drugs; SIADH, syndrome of inappropriate antidiuretic hormone; TSH, thyroid-stimulating hormone; VPA, valproic acid.
[a] Adapted with permission from Scherk H, Pajonk FG, Leucht S. Second-generation antipsychotic agents in the treatment of acute mania: a systematic review and meta-analysis of randomized controlled trials. *Arch Gen Psychiatry.* 2007;64:442–455; and *Physician Desk Reference* 2008.
[b] Starting dose is for average adult patients. Elderly patients and patients with hepatic and renal disease should have lower starting doses. Frequent monitoring is required for those who have severe symptoms.
[c] For bipolar depression and maintenance, not for acute bipolar mania.
[d] Even slower titration when used with divalproex sodium and hepatic enzyme-inducing drugs (alternate dose titration pack is available).

effects of lithium include gastrointestinal upset, polydipsia, polyuria (usually related to nephrogenic diabetes insipidus), weight gain, cognitive impairment, tremor, leukocytosis, acne, psoriasis, and hypothyroidism. Extended-release forms (Lithobid, Lithium ER, Eskalith) may have fewer gastrointestinal side effects. Laboratory monitoring includes baseline pregnancy test for women of reproductive age, electrolytes, thyroid-stimulating hormone (TSH), and in those older than 45 years of age or with heart disease, baseline electrocardiogram (ECG). A therapeutic level of lithium is usually achieved after 4 to 5 days. Subsequently, lithium level, electrolytes (for renal function), and TSH should be checked every 3 months in the first 6 months, and then every 6 months or as clinically indicated (10). Lithium toxicity should be suspected when a patient presents with acute nausea, dysarthria, lethargy, confusion, or ataxia.

Divalproex sodium for bipolar mania is started at 25 mg/kg to target a serum concentration between 85 and 125 μg/mL. It may also offer broader coverage for irritable, mixed manic episodes and rapid-cycling bipolar disorder. Use of divalproex sodium during pregnancy can cause congenital malformations including neural tube defects. Divalproex sodium should be considered for women of childbearing potential only after the risks have been thoroughly discussed with the patient and weighed against the potential benefits of treatment. Common side effects of divalproex sodium include sedation, tremor, diarrhea, weight gain, and benign elevation of liver transaminases. Rarely leukopenia, thrombocytopenia, pancreatitis, and hepatotoxicity occur. Encephalopathy and hyperammonemia may occur, especially in patients with liver impairment. Risks for hepatic failure include polypharmacy, developmental disability, metabolic disorders, and active or past liver disease; otherwise, the risk for hepatotoxicity is approximately 1 in 500,000 (10). Laboratory monitoring includes valproic acid levels as indicated to ensure adherence and adequate dosing, as well as at baseline and 3 and 6 months into treatment and then annually thereafter. Liver enzymes and a complete blood count (CBC) should be checked annually. A therapeutic level is usually achieved after 4 to 5 days.

Carbamazepine and oxcarbazepine are similar in chemical structure. Carbamazepine induces its own metabolism and that of many other drugs by the liver (e.g., oral contraceptives). Side effects include sedation, nausea, ataxia, and, rarely, leukopenia, hyponatremia (due to syndrome of inappropriate antidiuretic hormone [SIADH]), aplastic anemia, hepatic failure, rash, and exfoliative dermatitis (e.g., Stevens-Johnson syndrome). Oxcarbazepine, a metabolite of carbamazepine, is not FDA approved for bipolar disorder, but may have fewer side effects than carbamazepine and is sometimes used by psychiatrists for the treatment of refractory bipolar disorder. Laboratory monitoring for carbamazepine includes baseline, 3-month, 6-month, and then annual serum sodium, liver enzymes, and CBC. Oxcarbazepine may cause hyponatremia and therefore monitoring of sodium is recommended. Typical doses are 200 to 400 mg BID for carbamazepine and 300 to 600 mg BID for oxcarbazepine.

Bipolar Mania/Hypomania: Second-Generation Antipsychotics

Second-generation antipsychotics are approved for bipolar mania (Table 3.7) and are often used for hypomania or bipolar II disorder. Sedation is a major side effect with olanzapine and quetiapine, and these medications may be selected especially when insomnia is a prominent symptom. There is a small chance of tardive dyskinesia with SGAs. Extrapyramidal side effects (EPS) are most prominent with risperidone. The hyperactivity and agitation of bipolar mania may be difficult to distinguish from the side effect of akathisia. Among the most severe SGA adverse effects is neuroleptic malignant syndrome (NMS), characterized by fever, autonomic arousal, and neuromuscular signs of weakness, tremor, and rigidity. Most of the SGAs may cause significant weight gain and require monitoring of metabolic profiles including body mass index (BMI), fasting glucose, and lipid panel. As a medication class, the SGAs have a black box warning with increased risk of mortality in elderly patients with dementia.

Bipolar Depression

Although mood stabilizers have been best evaluated for the treatment of mania, they may also be useful for bipolar depression (Table 3.5). Lithium and lamotrigine are usually considered best for bipolar depression. Quetiapine also has an FDA indication for bipolar depression. If any of these medications are ineffective, antidepressants may be added with a mood stabilizer or SGA to target depression. However, for the depressive symptoms of bipolar mixed episodes, antidepressants are not generally recommended.

Lamotrigine is approved for bipolar maintenance treatment to prevent the relapse of depressive and manic episodes. Side effects of lamotrigine include dizziness, headache, double vision, somnolence, and rash. In order to reduce the risk of Stevens-Johnson syndrome (1 in 1,000 adults), it must be slowly titrated up to 200 mg/day, over 6 weeks. This is a generalized mucocutaneous (i.e., wet tissue) rash that may be heralded by sore gums, cracked lips, trouble swallowing, and involvement of other moist areas—particularly above the breast line. For nonemergent rash, lamotrigine should be stopped until the patient is examined. Emergent rash may involve airway distress and an emergency evaluation may be necessary. Laboratory monitoring is not required.

Thus far, quetiapine is the only stand-alone SGA approved by the FDA for bipolar depression treatment. There is a combination tablet that includes fluoxetine and olanzapine that is also approved for bipolar depression. Bupropion and the selective serotonin reuptake inhibitors

Table 3.7 Second-Generation Antipsychotics for Bipolar Disorder

	STARTING DOSE	TARGET DOSE (MG/DAY)	PRIMARY CARE TITRATION SCHEDULE	SIDE EFFECTS[a]	MONITORING FOR METABOLIC SYNDROME
Risperidone[b] (Risperdal)	1 mg BID or 2 mg QHS	4–6	Increase up to 2 mg daily, as tolerated	EPS (++) Hyperprolactinemia (+++) Orthostatic hypotension (++) Metabolic abnormalities (++) Sedation (++)	**Initial:** • Baseline weight and BMI, vital signs, fasting plasma glucose, and lipid profile • Consider pregnancy test and substance of abuse drug screen **First 4 weeks:** • BMI, EPS, vital signs, prolactin (if clinical symptoms of hyperprolactinemia) **First 12 weeks:** • BMI, EPS, vital signs, fasting glucose, and lipid profile **Quarterly:** BMI **Annually:** BMI, EPS, fasting glucose **Every 3–5 years:** lipid panel
Olanzapine (Zyprexa)	5 mg BID/QHS	10–20	Increase 5 mg weekly, as tolerated	EPS (+) Orthostatic hypotension (+) Metabolic abnormalities (+++) Sedation (++)	
Quetiapine[c] (Seroquel)	50 mg BID/QHS XR 300 mg QHS	300–800	Increase 50–100 mg every 2 days, as tolerated (monitor for orthostatic hypotension) XR: Increase every 1–2 days, as tolerated	EPS (+/–) Orthostatic hypotension (+++) Metabolic abnormalities (++) Sedation (++)	
Ziprasidone[d] (Geodon)	40 mg BID (with food)	160	Increase every other day to target dose, as tolerated	EPS (+) Orthostatic hypotension (+) Metabolic abnormalities (++) Sedation (++) QTc prolongation (++)	
Aripiprazole (Abilify)	10–15 mg Start QAM	10–30	Increase dose after 2 days, as tolerated	EPS (+) Orthostatic hypotension (+) Metabolic abnormalities (+) Sedation (+)	
Paliperidone[e] (Invega)	3–6 mg QAM	6–12	Increase by increments of 3 mg every 5 days, as tolerated	EPS (+++) Orthostatic hypotension (+) Metabolic abnormalities (++) Sedation (++)	

BMI, body mass index; EPS, extrapyramidal symptoms.

[a] Metabolic effects include hyperglycemia, weight gain, and hyperlipidemia. Common EPS include dystonia, parkinsonism, and akathisia.

[b] Patient may be able to transition to an intramuscular depot formulation of risperidone called Risperdal Consta.

[c] Because of its low potency, quetiapine is ideal for patients who are sensitive to dopamine blockade, particularly patients sensitive to EPS or patients with psychosis in the context of Parkinson disease. The XR formulation has an indication for schizophrenia. Dose is 300 mg QHS for bipolar depression and up to 800 mg/day or as tolerated for bipolar mania.

[d] Contraindications to the use of ziprasidone include persistent QTc >500 msec, history of arrhythmia, recent acute myocardial infarction, and uncompensated heart failure. Ziprasidone should be taken with food to increase gastrointestinal absorption.

[e] Paliperidone is a metabolite of risperidone. Because it is the newest antipsychotic medication, the relative risks for metabolic syndrome and EPS and bipolar disorder efficacy are not fully known.

have a decreased risk for inducing mania or accelerating cycling between episodes when compared with tricyclic antidepressants (TCAs) and venlafaxine. To further reduce this risk, antidepressants are generally used for only 3 to 6 months after the depression remits. One recent study found that patients with bipolar depression may have similar outcomes whether they are on an antidepressant or placebo, as long as they are taking a mood stabilizer (13). This study further highlights the importance of mood stabilizers in the treatment of bipolar disorder.

Bipolar Maintenance Pharmacotherapy

The probability that a bipolar manic, mixed, or depressive episode will recur without treatment is 50% at 1 year and nearly 90% at 5 years. The risk is heightened by the presence of a comorbid psychiatric disorder, psychotic features, or a family history of mania (14). In a 12-year study, patients with bipolar disorder reported higher frequency of depressive (67%) than manic (20%) or mixed (13%) symptoms (15). Although lithium, divalproex sodium, and carbamazepine do not have FDA indications specifically for bipolar maintenance, they are effective and commonly used for bipolar maintenance therapy. Lamotrigine and a few of the SGAs have FDA indications for bipolar maintenance therapy (Table 3.5). For patients who have had more than two severe mood episodes, indefinite maintenance pharmacotherapy is generally indicated. However, long-term medication adherence is sometimes difficult to maintain in the longer run. Therefore, in addition to long-term risk of relapse, patient preference and medication side effects should be taken into consideration when determining the duration of pharmacotherapy.

Treatment Considerations

Several factors commonly influence the selection of medications for bipolar disorder. Providers may take into account target symptoms, side effects, personal or family history of response, ease of adherence (once-per-day dosing is preferable), and access to medications (i.e., cost, formulary restrictions). Other important considerations include the following:

- Rapid-cycling or mixed episodes: A mood stabilizer and antipsychotic combination is preferred. We recommend divalproex sodium (preferably the extended-release formulation).
- Reduced renal clearance: Use lithium with extreme caution in patients who have reduced renal function and those who are volume depleted.
- Insomnia: Olanzapine and quetiapine may be more helpful with acute agitation and insomnia related to bipolar disorder.
- Low energy and motivation: If an antidepressant is needed, bupropion (particularly the SR or XL formulation) may be activating and may have a lower rate of inducing mania. Other medications with dopamine and norepinephrine (e.g., venlafaxine) may have a higher chance of inducing mania or agitation (11).

- Weight issues: Many patients are overweight or obese before treatment. Weight and metabolic profiles needs to be monitored closely because many medications may cause weight gain. Although all of the SGAs have the potential for metabolic abnormalities, olanzapine carries the highest relative risk. These medications can be safely used when proper monitoring is employed (see Table 3.7).
- Drug–drug interactions: Carbamazepine induces hepatic enzymes and may lower the levels of other drugs (e.g., lowers the effectiveness of some oral contraceptives). The serum lithium level may be increased by medications that lower glomerular filtration rate (diuretics, angiotensin-converting enzyme [ACE] inhibitors, nonsteroidal anti-inflammatory drugs [NSAIDs]).
- Pregnancy: Urine pregnancy tests should be obtained when starting mood stabilizers. Lithium and divalproex sodium carry teratogenic risks, especially during the first trimester. In practice, haloperidol and some SGAs may be considered when benefits of treatment outweigh risks. Mood stabilizers may be required in some high-risk patients. It is important to review the risks with the patient and document carefully. If there is any question about the use of a psychotropic medication in a pregnant or nursing patient, consultation with a psychiatrist should be obtained.
- Black-box warnings: Nearly all medications have a black-box warning (e.g., divalproex sodium: hepatotoxicity; lamotrigine: Steven-Johnson syndrome; SGAs: use in patients with dementia-related psychosis). There is also an FDA non–black-box warning against many anticonvulsants and suicide.

PSYCHOSOCIAL TREATMENT

In addition to medication, there are various psychosocial factors that are important for the treatment of bipolar disorder. These include educational groups, peer and family support groups, individual and group psychotherapy, and rehabilitation programs. These interventions greatly reduce rates of nonadherence, support self-efficacy, and decrease the frequency of relapses. Psychoeducation can be helpful in providing a scientific explanation about the course and prognosis of bipolar disorder—thereby instilling hope that bipolar disorder is a "medical" illness that can be effectively treated. Attending groups can reduce the stigmatizing feeling of having a mental illness for patients by normalizing their experience and showing them that they are not the only persons to have the condition. Individual or group psychotherapy with or without family involvement is beneficial to nearly all patients with bipolar disorder. Cognitive behavioral therapy (CBT), family-focused education (also known as behavioral family management), and group psychotherapy have been studied and found to be key components of the treatment plan for bipolar disorder.

The primary care provider can facilitate psychosocial treatments by referring patients and family members to local chapters of the Depressive and Bipolar Support Alliance (DBSA) and the National Alliance for Mental Illness (NAMI). The DBSA is an example of a peer support group that consists of patients who have been diagnosed with bipolar disorder. Local chapters offer monthly or weekly groups where patients can discuss their issues with others who also have the disorder. Higher-functioning patients are more likely to make the best use of the model, but it has applicability to more severely ill patients as well. The DBSA has complete information for patients to help themselves and for family and friends to help a loved one on their recovery to wellness, as well as printable brochures, a blog, chat rooms, and pod casts.

The DBSA is in support of mental health recovery, which is defined as a journey of healing and transformation that enables people with mental health problems to live a meaningful life (as defined by the patients) in a community of their choice while striving to achieve their full potential. We briefly review the Recovery Model because clinicians may hear about this from mental health professionals or from their patients. The Recovery Model has five components: (1) handling the impact of the illness, (2) feeling like life is limited, (3) realizing and believing change is possible, (4) commitment to change, and (5) actions for change (16). These steps help the patient and family cope with the illness, appreciate the accompanying despair that comes with realizing that life will never be the same again, and understand that they can live with a mental illness and still achieve certain life goals.

NAMI provides valuable support for families that have members with bipolar disorder and other mental illnesses. NAMI offers a program called Family-to-Family, a 12-week course that contains current information about the major mental illnesses and their signs, symptoms, and prognoses. It also reviews treatment options, including in-depth presentations on specific medications indicated for psychiatric disorders, their side effects, strategies for treatment adherence, and how family members can support affected love ones in a positive way. The course aims to create empathy in family members by helping them understand the experience of mental illness. Finally, the program teaches skills (such as problem solving, listening and communication, and strategies for handling crises) and helps caregivers find resources and support in the community.

WHEN TO REFER

- Medication unresponsiveness
- Concern about substance use
- Complex comorbid medical or psychiatric conditions
- Uncertainty about diagnosis
- Severe bipolar disorder
- Bipolar disorder and pre-pregnancy planning
- Postpartum depression or psychosis
- Acute or chronic suicidal ideation

Practice Pointers

Case 1: Bipolar Disorder Pharmacology

A 35-year-old man presents to the outpatient clinic with the following request: "I want to be checked for high blood pressure." During the interview, the patient states, "I was on 40 mg of fluoxetine a few years ago and my wife thinks I need something to take the edge off." Currently he is not feeling depressed, but his wife encouraged him to discuss his episodic irritability at this visit. These episodes appear in waves of weeks, several times per year. He mentioned that his wife took him to the emergency room for a prior "episode."

He reports "waves of irritability" while on fluoxetine. He's had recurrent problems with depression for 8 years and has been treated with fluoxetine, sertraline, and bupropion. Other than paroxysms of anxiety, none has had significant side effects, but none has been particularly effective either. While he was on these medications, he would get depressed, gain weight, sleep more than usual, and become much less productive at work. His wife once took him to an emergency room because of morbid suicidal talk; however, he's never been hospitalized or made a suicide attempt. The depressive episodes usually resolve slowly after a month or two. When asked about the irritable periods, he reports feeling tense and anxious, has difficulty sleeping, and notes "problems getting along with other people."

Discussion: *The patient is taking a reasonable dose of fluoxetine. Although the doses of the other antidepressants are unknown, it is concerning that none seemed to have helped the depression. The differential diagnosis includes major depressive disorder, an anxiety disorder, a substance-induced mood disorder, mood disorder due to a general medical condition, and bipolar type I or II.*

Further history: At age 25, he was working on a project that he found both exciting and frustrating. He stayed awake several nights in a row, and although he had plenty of energy and ideas, the end product was uncharacteristically disorganized and grandiose. After a week of hard work with little sleep, he was actually hospitalized at a general hospital for "exhaustion." He remembers frustrating the nurses with his late-night attempts to help them revise procedures to increase efficiency, even though he knew nothing about hospitals. He was prescribed diazepam and slowly began to "feel more normal." He has never had a similar episode since. He does not drink any alcohol or use any recreational drugs.

Discussion: *This patient likely recovered from a bipolar spectrum disorder in which irritability was the main component of the manic episode. Although irritability is usually not the cardinal feature of a manic episode in adults, this somewhat atypical presentation included irritability, insomnia with a related increase in energy and goal-directed activity, and difficulties "getting along with other people." Because the hospitalization was likely tied to his mental state and inability to function at work, his provisional diagnosis is bipolar disorder I, manic episode. If depression or anhedonia were present, one might consider this to be a mixed episode.*

Given the history of depression with suicidal thoughts and his hospitalization, maintenance therapy for his bipolar disorder should include a lifelong mood stabilizer like lithium or divalproex sodium ER (Depakote ER). Alternatively, an SGA can be used as monotherapy or in combination with a mood stabilizer. As a general rule, antidepressants should not be used alone to treat bipolar disorder. This patient should be closely monitored for suicidal ideation, intent, or plan.

Case 2: A Psychiatric Emergency

A worried husband calls you after his 25-year-old wife was awake for 3 days and would not stop cleaning. He states, "She has just been wearing me out. I'm exhausted just staying in the same room with her." In the office, she paces, speaks rapidly, keeps leaving the room, and talks at length with the staff about a fair number of "creative" ideas. The husband confirms she has no substance abuse history and that she has been physically healthy. While being checked in, she "stuck" to the nurse, talking incessantly about a recipe. Oddly, she was not exuberant or irritable. She was asked about delusions and auditory hallucinations. She reported that she receives "information streaming from a satellite" and hears "suggestions" from a voice to "take the cooking industry to another level." After the physical exam, the patient eventually agrees to give a urine sample, which was negative for substances of abuse.

Discussion *It is easy to miss bipolar disorder when patients do not present with euphoria. An expansive mood without euphoria sometimes occurs during a manic episode and generally presents in a way that "wears" others out. The symptoms are episodic and not chronic, which is consistent with bipolar disorder I, most* *recent episode manic. A referral to the local emergency or crisis intervention center is indicated. If the patient only had mania, without psychosis, medications might work well enough to avoid hospitalization, but the determining factor here is the patient's poor insight, lack of decision-making capacity, and impulsivity. Indications for emergent referrals include inability to care for oneself and dangerous behavior toward self or others. Given the severity of illness, combination therapy with a mood stabilizer and an SGA is indicated.*

Case 3: Pregnancy and Bipolar Disorder

A 28-year-old woman presents to the clinic to establish care as a new patient. She recently moved to the area from another state due to her husband's employment. She reports that she has a history of bipolar disorder diagnosed 3 years ago after hospitalization for depression and suicidal ideation. She has been stable on her medication. She reports that prior to treatment, she would go through about three to four major mood episodes a year, usually of euphoric hypomania for a few days followed by depression. She has been taking divalproex sodium (Depakote ER) for the past year. She had been on lithium in the past, but stopped it due to polyuria and tremor. She and her husband have been thinking about starting a family. She wants to know whether she should continue Depakote ER while they try to have a baby and whether to continue after conception.

On mental status examination, she is neatly dressed and groomed. Her speech is somewhat rapid in rate, but is interruptible. She states her mood is "good" and her affect appears bright. Her thoughts are linear. Her physical exam is unremarkable and her BMI is normal.

Discussion: *This patient has a clear history of bipolar disorder. Her mood swings seem relatively well controlled on divalproex sodium, but should she continue it as she tries to conceive? The traditional mood stabilizer treatments for bipolar disorder have been associated with adverse outcomes in the fetus, especially during the first trimester of pregnancy (e.g., lithium with cardiac malformations and anticonvulsants with neural tube defects, and SGAs have a category C designation [Table 3.6]).*

The postpartum period is a high-risk period. About 20% to 50% of bipolar symptoms recur within 2 months (17). The risk of psychosis is also higher in the postpartum period. Resumption of mood stabilizers after delivery can help to prevent mood relapses. In patients with a history of unstable and severe mood swings, continuing medications throughout pregnancy may be a preferable and safer option. Maintaining mood stability during pregnancy and after delivery can promote positive maternal–infant bonding and attachment. Possible fetal defects can be detected by ultrasound screening, echocardiograms, and maternal serum alpha-fetal protein (AFP) screening. Women on anticonvulsants should also be prescribed folate 4 to 5 mg/day, ideally 3 months before conception (18). In some stable patients who wish to stop their medications, a slow and careful taper of medications or a switch to a less teratogenic medication 1 to 2 months before conception can minimize adverse exposure to the fetus.

Primary care providers can provide patients with accurate information about the risks and benefits of the alternatives, often acknowledging the lack of extensive evidence and research in this area. In this case, if the patient decides on taking a medication, other options include the use of haloperidol or SGAs, which are relatively safe compared with lithium and anticonvulsant mood stabilizers, especially during the first trimester. The lowest effective doses should also be prescribed. Ultimately, it is important to support the patient and her husband's decisions. In this case, a psychiatric consultation should be obtained.

ICD9

Bipolar I Disorder

Single Manic Episode	*296*
Most Recent Episode Hypomanic	*296.4*
Most Recent Episode Manic	*296.4x*
Most Recent Episode Mixed	*296.6x*
Most Recent Episode Depressed	*296.5x*
Most Recent Episode Unspecified	*296.7x*

Bipolar II Disorder	*296.89*
Bipolar Disorder NOS	*296.8*
Mood Disorder Due to	*293.83*

[General Medical Condition]

x =

0 Unspecified

1 Mild

2 Moderate

3 Severe, without Psychosis

4 Severe, with Psychosis

5 In Partial or Unspecified Remission

6 In Full Remission

Practical Resources

The Mood Disorder Questionnaire: www.psycheducation.org/depression/MDQ
The Depressive and Bipolar Support Alliance: www.dbsalliance.org
The National Alliance for the Mentally Illness: www.nami.org
The National Institute of Mental Health: www.nimh.nih.gov

REFERENCES

1. Hilty DM, Leamon ML, Lim RF, et al. Diagnosis and treatment of bipolar disorder in the primary care setting. *Primary Psychiatry*. 2006;13(7):77–85.

2. Merikangas KR, Akiskal HS, Angst J. Lifetime and 12-month prevalence of bipolar spectrum disorder in the National Comorbidity Survey replication. *Arch Gen Psychiatry*. 2007;64(5):543–552.

3. Berk M, Dodd S, Berk L. The management of bipolar disorder in primary care: a review of existing and emerging therapies. *Psychiatry Clin Neurosci*. 2005;59(3):229–239.

4. Muzina DJ, Colangelo E, Manning JS. Differentiating bipolar disorder from depression in primary care. *Cleve Clin J Med*. 2007;74(2):89,92,95–99.

5. *Diagnostic and Statistical Manual of Mental Disorders*. 4th ed., text revision. Washington DC: American Psychiatric Association; 2002.

6. Hirschfeld RMA, Williams JBW, Spencer RI, et al. Development and validation of a screening instrument for bipolar spectrum disorder: the Mood Disorder Questionnaire. *Am J Psychiatry*. 2000;15(11):1873–1875.

7. Hirschfeld RM, Holzer C, Calabrese JR, et al. Validity of the mood disorder questionnaire: a general population study. *Am J Psychiatry*. 2003;160(1):178–180.

8. Paris J, Gunderson J, Weingberg I. The interface between borderline personality disorder and bipolar spectrum disorders. *Compr Psychiatry*. 2007;48(2):145–154.

9. Hilty DM, Leamon ML, Lim RF, et al. A review of bipolar disorder in adults. *Psychiatry*. 2006;September:43–55.

10. American Psychiatric Association. Practice guideline for the treatment of patients with bipolar disorder (revision). *Am J Psychiatry*. 2002;159(Suppl):1–50.

11. Scherk H, Pajonk FG, Leucht S. Second-generation antipsychotic agents in the treatment of acute mania: a systematic review and meta-analysis of randomized controlled trials. *Arch Gen Psychiatry.* 2007;64:442–455.

12. Leverich GS, Altshuler LL, Frye MA, et al. Risk of switch in mood polarity to hypomania or mania in patients with bipolar depression during acute and continuation trials of venlafaxine, sertraline, and bupropion as adjuncts to mood stabilizers. *Am J Psychiatry.* 2006;163(2):232–239.

13. Sachs GS, Nierenberg AA, Calabrese JR, Effectiveness of adjunctive antidepressant treatment of bipolar depression. *N Engl J Med.* 2007;356(17):1711–1722.

14. Solomon DA, Keitner GI, Miller IW, et al. Course of illness and maintenance treatment for patients with bipolar disorder. *J Clin Psychiatry.* 1995;56:5–13.

15. Judd LL, Akiskal HS, Schettler PJ, et al. The long-term natural history of the weekly symptomatic status of bipolar I disorder. *Arch Gen Psychiatry.* 2002;58:530–537.

16. The Depressive and Bipolar Support Alliance. www.dbsalliance.org. Accessed December 9, 2007.

17. Viguera AC, Nonacs R, Cohen LS, et al. Risk of recurrence of bipolar disorder in pregnant and non-pregnant women after discontinuing lithium maintenance. *Am J Psychiatry.* 2000;157(2):179–184.

18. Yonkers KA, Wisner KL, Stowe Z, et al. Management of bipolar disorder during pregnancy and the postpartum period. *Am J Psychiatry.* 2004;161:608–620.

CHAPTER 3 Bipolar Disorder

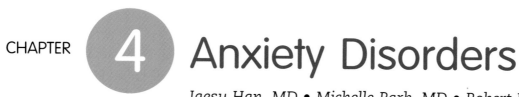

CHAPTER 4 Anxiety Disorders

Jaesu Han, MD • Michelle Park, MD • Robert E. Hales, MD, MBA

A 29-year-old woman presents with her 6-year-old daughter for a well-child check after missing the originally scheduled appointment. She is quiet but informs you that there is an upcoming parent–teacher conference for her daughter. She adds, "I'm just not good with that sort of thing." She apparently showed up late for the last parent–teacher conference, couldn't remember what was said, and "left with a headache."

CLINICAL HIGHLIGHTS

- Screening requires asking about both physical and psychological symptoms of anxiety.

- The somatic presentation of anxiety disorders, where physical symptoms predominate, is common in the primary care setting.

- Specific anxiety disorders are defined and categorized by the presence or absence of specific situational triggers.

(Continued)

Clinical Significance

Anxiety disorders represent the most prevalent group of psychiatric disorders in the general population. This group of conditions accounts for at least $42 billion per year in lost productivity and results in a significantly lower quality of life for the affected patients (1). Data from the 12-year longitudinal, naturalistic Harvard/Brown Anxiety Disorders Research Program showed that, with the exception of panic disorder without agoraphobia, the course of anxiety disorders is both chronic and enduring (2). Twelve years after the original episode, the majority of patients with generalized anxiety disorder, panic disorder with agoraphobia, and social anxiety disorder never achieved recovery, and of those who did recover, nearly half had a recurrence during the follow-up period.

The economic and social costs of these chronic and recurrent disorders are compounded by the persistent underrecognition and undertreatment of anxiety disorders in the primary care setting. One recent study found that nearly one in five patients had at least one clinically significant anxiety disorder and that 41% of these patients were not receiving treatment of any kind (3). Clearly, with knowledge that effective treatment options are readily available for the anxiety disorders, proper screening and diagnosis are critical.

Diagnosis

Anxiety is commonly defined as excessive worrying, nervousness, or feeling "on edge." The prompt and accurate diagnosis of anxiety disorders in the primary care setting can be challenging for several reasons. Anxiety itself is a very normal human emotion and it can be difficult to decide just when it is pathologic. For example, anxiety can be adaptive when it motivates one to complete a task but pathologic when it is excessive and paralyzes one from taking a needed action despite the possible repercussions (or missed opportunities). In order to ensure an accurate diagnosis and effective treatment plan, it is important to document the disability, screen for an anxiety disorder, consider the differential diagnosis, and identify the specific anxiety disorder.

DOCUMENT DISABILITY

Pathologic and clinically relevant anxiety is excessive and persistent and creates disability, often in the form of avoidance behaviors. Essentially, "normal" anxiety helps the patient to maintain order, while "pathologic" anxiety creates disorder. Clinicians should ask questions such as, "What have you given up because of your symptoms?" or "Have your symptoms prevented you from doing something you wanted or needed to do?" In addition to ensuring that the anxiety is clinically significant, the documentation also provides tangible targets for treatment. Diagnosis should include documentation of specific functional impairment, which may include:

- Social impairment: withdrawal from family, friends, and hobbies
- Occupational impairment: job avoidance, inefficiency, lack of promotion, or even disciplinary action
- Impairment with activities of daily living: inability to shop for groceries, take the bus, or drive a car

SCREEN FOR AN ANXIETY DISORDER

The advantage of a screening tool includes the ability to administer and score a validated test prior to seeing the patient. However, unlike tools such as the Patient Health Questionnaire-9 (PHQ-9) for major depression, there is currently no commonly accepted screening tool for all anxiety disorders in clinical practice. One recently studied screening tool is the Generalized Anxiety Disorders Scale (GAD-7), which appears to be sensitive for panic disorder, generalized anxiety disorder, social anxiety disorder, and posttraumatic stress disorder in the primary care setting (Table 4.1) (4). This tool consists of a series of seven questions that incorporates the same *Diagnostic and Statistical Manual of Mental Disorders,* 4th ed. (DSM-IV), diagnostic criteria of generalized anxiety disorder. The first two items (GAD-2 subscale) can be used as an ultra-rapid screening tool. A score of 8 or more on the GAD-7 or 3 or more on the GAD-2 should prompt a more thorough investigation for major anxiety disorders.

The GAD-2 highlights the two key components of anxiety that are present regardless of the specific diagnosis: (1) *psychiatric symptoms:* excessive ruminations or worry, poor concentration, and racing thoughts and (2) *physical symptoms:* muscle tension, sweating, fatigue, restlessness, and tremors. During the screening interview, it is therefore important to inquire about both components. When one component predominates, the clinical presentation may change drastically.

Table 4.1 GAD-7

How often during the past 2 weeks have you felt bothered by:

1. Feeling nervous, anxious, or on edge?	0	1	2	3
2. Not being able to stop or control worrying?	0	1	2	3
3. Worrying too much about different things?	0	1	2	3
4. Trouble relaxing?	0	1	2	3
5. Being so restless that it is hard to sit still?	0	1	2	3
6. Becoming easily annoyed or irritable?	0	1	2	3
7. Feeling afraid as if something awful might happen?	0	1	2	3

Each question is answered on a scale of:
0 = not at all
1 = several days
2 = more than half the days
3 = nearly every day

A score of 8 or more should prompt further diagnostic evaluation for an anxiety disorder.

From Spitzer RL, Kroenke K, Williams JB, et al. A brief measure for assessing generalized anxiety disorder: the GAD-7. *Arch Intern Med.* 2006;166:1092–1097.

When *psychiatric symptoms* (e.g., anxiety) predominate, the patient presents to seek confirmation of an anxiety disorder diagnosis. Sometimes the patient's assessment of a specific anxiety disorder is correct, but at other times the diagnosis may be another psychiatric disorder or even a general medical condition. Although this presentation may be easier for clinicians to recognize because they are "primed" to consider an anxiety disorder, it is also the less common presentation.

When *physical symptoms* predominate, the patient usually does not consider a psychiatric cause. The somatic presentation is more common than the psychiatric presentation in the primary care setting and is more likely to lead to misdiagnosis (5). This may occur when a patient attributes the symptoms to such things as lack of sleep, stress, or poor diet, and the clinician halts further work-up. Alternatively, there may be an extensive work-up in response to multiple medically unexplained physical complaints such as chest pain, dizziness, gastrointestinal symptoms, or dyspnea before an anxiety disorder is considered.

SPECIFIC ANXIETY DISORDERS

The following brief descriptions are intended to distill some salient points that serve to distinguish the disorders from each other. Keep in mind that the symptoms of anxiety often manifest as a waxing and waning "blanket" of symptoms but may also include time-limited "bursts" of symptoms in the form of panic attacks. Panic attacks, sometimes referred to as "anxiety attacks," are in themselves not considered a separate anxiety disorder. These attacks are required for the diagnosis of panic disorder when they occur spontaneously but may occur with other anxiety disorders in response to situational triggers. In a typical panic attack, patients experience a sudden onset of symptoms that typically peak

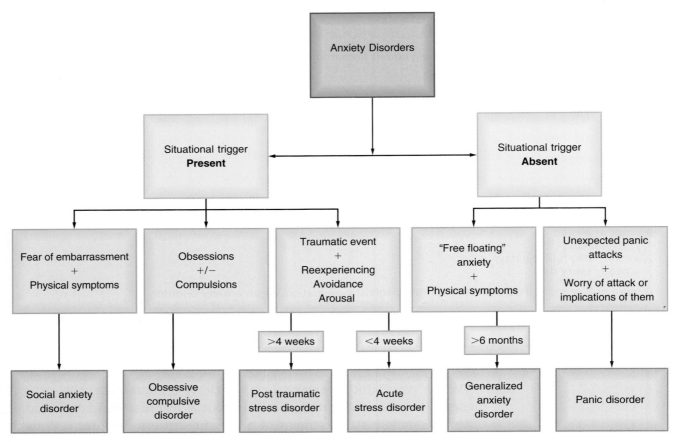

Figure 4.1 Diagnostic algorithm for anxiety disorders.

within 10 minutes and rarely last longer than an hour. During a panic attack, psychological symptoms often include fears of losing control, dying, or "going crazy." Physical symptoms reflecting autonomic activation are equally intense and include a racing heart rate, sweating, shaking, shortness of breath, nausea, dizziness, and chest discomfort.

Differentiating among the anxiety disorders relies on distinguishing if these symptoms, including panic attacks, are precipitated by specific situational triggers or are pervasive and occur with a variety of events (Figure 4.1). The two disorders without specific situational triggers are panic disorder and generalized anxiety disorder. The disorders with specific situational triggers are social phobia, specific phobia, obsessive compulsive disorder, acute stress disorder, and posttraumatic stress disorder. Adjustment disorder with anxiety and anxiety disorder not otherwise specified are quite common and will be discussed separately.

Disorders without a Situational Trigger

Panic Disorder Panic disorder (PD) is characterized by *recurrent panic attacks* that are experienced at least initially as spontaneous and unexpected. Careful review with the patient may reveal benign cues such as emotional stress from an argument or a slightly elevated heart rate from caffeine that is interpreted as a symptom of an impending attack.

Although panic attacks can be terrifying and temporarily disabling, it is the *anticipatory anxiety* of when the next attack will come and the *worry about its implications* that perpetuates the disability. Patients may undergo extensive testing to find the etiology of symptoms, such as chest discomfort or gastrointestinal symptoms, before a diagnosis of PD is made. PD is twice as common in women as in men and onset peaks in late adolescence and the mid-30s. Although the initial panic attack is by definition not caused by an obvious trigger, the majority of patients report some antecedent adverse life event in the year prior to onset of illness.

Over time, agoraphobia may develop when continued apprehension of a panic attack prevents patients from being in places or situations from which they cannot escape, where help is unavailable, or where it would be embarrassing to be seen in the throes of a panic attack. In this respect, panic disorder with agoraphobia can be thought of as an anxiety disorder with a situational trigger. Common avoided places include buses, trains, supermarkets, and traveling away from home. In severe cases, patients may be completely housebound. Those who manage to leave the home usually engage in compensatory behavior such as having a companion around for activities outside the house.

Generalized Anxiety Disorder   Generalized anxiety disorder (GAD) is the other anxiety disorder that does not have a specific situational trigger. In fact, the hallmark of GAD is the lack of a central trigger and the presence of *free-floating* anxiety consisting of ruminations and worries over often trivial matters that are pervasive and excessive. Along with these psychological symptoms are physical symptoms such as muscle tension, restlessness, and fatigue. Symptoms have been present for *at least 6 months*, but many patients will describe themselves as *chronic worriers*. GAD may be relatively common among primary care patients whose main clinical problem is chronic insomnia.

Disorders with a Situational Trigger

Social Phobia   Social phobia, also known as social anxiety disorder (SAD), is sometimes thought of as pathologic shyness. The hallmark is the *fear of embarrassment or humiliation* in front of others. This fear may be relatively mild and circumscribed to a specific situation such as public speaking or more severe and generalized to almost all social situations. Patients may report fears they will be negatively evaluated by others and "say something stupid" or fear that others will notice their *physical symptoms* such as blushing, sweating, or shaking. Panic attacks may occur but are situationally bound to the social trigger. Onset is usually in the early teenage years and patients will often have symptoms for over 10 years before seeking treatment. During this time important social activities may have been missed and job promotions avoided.

Obsessive Compulsive Disorder   The hallmark of obsessive compulsive disorder (OCD) is the presence of obsessions and/or compulsions that serve as triggers for anxiety. **Obsessions** are *recurrent*, unwanted, and *intrusive* ideas, thoughts, impulses, or images. Common themes include contamination, repeated doubts, need for order, horrific thoughts, and sexual imagery. **Compulsions** are *ritualistic behaviors* or mental acts carried out in response to an obsession. Examples include repeated handwashing, checking of locks, and counting.

Those with true compulsions are differentiated from "compulsive" shoppers, gamblers, drinkers, etc., because the latter group derives some pleasure from the activity. These obsessions and compulsions are usually quite distressing for the patient and consume at least 1 hour per day but often many more. In severe cases, patients may not recognize that the obsessions or compulsions are excessive and therefore have OCD "with poor insight." Initially, onset of OCD symptoms usually occurs in the 20s, with a waxing and waning course. The onset of primary OCD after the age of 35 is unusual and should prompt a complete neurologic evaluation. Comorbid tic disorders and compulsive skin picking and hair pulling (trichotillomania) are common in OCD. These comorbid disorders may be the impetus for treatment. The physical stigmata of compulsions (e.g., raw and rough hands from excessive handwashing or hairless patches from hair pulling) may be evident on physical examination.

Posttraumatic Stress Disorder   Exposure to a *highly traumatic event* as a victim or witness in which life or injury was threatened is the situational trigger for posttraumatic stress disorder (PTSD). This traumatic event is followed by symptoms of *re-experiences* (flashbacks, nightmares, intrusive memories of the event), *avoidance/numbing* (avoiding conversations, activities, and people associated with the event or that may trigger experiences of the event), and *increased autonomic arousal* (hypervigilance, restlessness, exaggerated startle). If symptoms resolve within 1 month following the traumatic event, the diagnosis of acute stress disorder (ASD) is made. Patients with symptoms lasting *greater than 1 month* are diagnosed with PTSD.

Groups at risk for PTSD include combat veterans, natural disaster survivors, terrorist attack survivors, victims of childhood abuse, and victims of sexual or physical trauma.

Sometimes the primary care provider will be aware that a traumatic event has occurred, for example, a recent motor vehicle accident or gunshot wound. However, at other times, patients may present with only nonspecific avoidance behaviors and physical symptoms and not mention the traumatic event. Reasons may include not recognizing the impact of the event and fear that they will be seen as damaged or unstable. Therefore, screening patients with these nonspecific symptoms for a recent traumatic event is important. PTSD is more likely to develop in patients with direct exposure to interpersonal trauma (e.g., rape) than indirect exposure and events such as natural disasters.

Other Clinically Relevant Anxiety Disorders

Adjustment Disorder with Anxiety   Adjustment disorder with anxiety is commonly seen in the primary care setting. The hallmark of this disorder is the *close temporal relationship* of the onset of anxiety symptoms to *a stressful event*, usually within days, and *resolution within 6 months* of the termination of the stressor. Although symptoms may initially be quite intense, they are generally short-lived and diminish with the passage of time. There is symptom overlap with other disorders, but the duration and threshold specifiers distinguish adjustment disorder from other anxiety disorders. For example, GAD requires symptoms to be present for at least 6 months and PTSD and ASD require the stressor to be extreme in nature. Unlike the other anxiety disorders, there is an expectation of good outcome with adjustment disorder once the offending stressor is removed. If the stressor persists, anxiety symptoms will be present in a more attenuated form. Treatment is supportive to help the patient resolve or manage the stressor. Pharmacotherapy with antidepressants and benzodiazepines is sometimes utilized, but there is little evidence to support this practice.

Anxiety Disorder Not Otherwise Specified   Many patients in the primary care setting will not initially fit neatly into any of the major anxiety disorders noted above. Assuming the symptoms are causing significant clinical distress, a diagnosis of anxiety disorder not otherwise specified (NOS) can be made. As patients become more comfortable and provide additional history, a specific diagnosis may be more apparent. At other times, a more specific diagnosis is not possible due to confounding general medical conditions. For example, in the case of PD, a reasonable initial diagnosis may be anxiety disorder NOS, to rule out anxiety disorder due to a general medical condition versus panic disorder. Finally, some patients may never manifest the required number of diagnostic criteria for a specific anxiety disorder, yet the symptoms are clinically significant. For example, PTSD without autonomic hyperarousability may be diagnosed as anxiety disorder NOS.

Differential Diagnosis

The two common but different presentations of anxiety disorders highlight the need for a comprehensive patient assessment and differential diagnosis before a definitive diagnosis is made. Patient assessment begins with obtaining the medical history, and particular attention should be paid to the onset of symptoms because anxiety disorders tend to present in late adolescence and early adulthood. For example, new-onset anxiety symptoms in a previously healthy patient beyond the age of 35 years without a recent significant life event or trauma are suspicious for an underlying medical condition. A family history of mood and anxiety disorders increases the likelihood of a primary anxiety disorder. Assessment should also include knowledge of both prescription and over-the-counter medications. The social history is helpful when evaluating relational and occupational factors as well as potential substance abuse. Upon completion of a thorough physical examination, reasonable initial tests for a patient with a possible anxiety disorder include a complete blood count, thyroid-stimulating hormone, and a complete metabolic panel.

Table 4.2 Medical Conditions with Anxiety-Like Symptoms

MEDICAL CONDITION	SUGGESTED BASIC WORK-UP
Cardiovascular: coronary artery disease, congestive heart failure, arrhythmias	ECG (esp. patients >40 years old with palpitations or chest pain)
Pulmonary: asthma, chronic obstructive pulmonary disease	pulmonary function test, CXR
Endocrine: thyroid dysfunction, hyperparathyroidism, hypoglycemia, menopause, Cushing disease, insulinoma, pheochromocytoma	TSH, basic chemistry panel
Hematologic: anemia	CBC
Neurologic: seizure disorders, encephalopathies, essential tremor	EEG, brain MRI
Substance abuse/dependence	Urine or serum toxicology

CXR, chest x-ray; CBC, complete blood count; ECG, electrocardiogram; EEG, electroencephalogram; MRI, magnetic resonance imaging; TSH, thyroid-stimulating hormone.

Common general medical conditions and basic laboratory work-up for symptoms of anxiety are listed in Table 4.2. Many of these conditions will manifest with concurrent non–anxiety-related symptoms and risk factors that will guide the extent of the diagnostic work-up. For example, a nonobese 35-year-old patient who has nonanginal chest pain and no risk factors for coronary disease is unlikely to have an acute coronary syndrome and therefore should not undergo invasive diagnostic cardiac procedures.

Medications may cause anxiety-like symptoms (Table 4.3) (6). For example, patients on antipsychotics may complain of akathisia, which consists of an intense sense of internal restlessness. It can be an extremely anxiety-provoking side effect that resolves after discontinuation of the medication. Stimulants such as methylphenidate used for attention deficit hyperactivity disorder (ADHD) can cause symptoms such as a fine tremor, tachycardia, and irritability that can be confused with anxiety. A general medical condition such as hypothyroidism can be overcorrected with levothyroxine and cause iatrogenic hyperthyroidism with generalized anxiety symptoms.

Other psychiatric disorders commonly coexist with the primary anxiety disorders. More than 70% of patients diagnosed with an anxiety disorder in the primary care setting also have another comorbid Axis I condition. Having an additional anxiety disorder (>60%) is the most common psychiatric comorbid condition followed by major depression (>40%) and substance abuse disorders (14%) (7). Somatoform disorders and personality disorders should also be considered. The importance of identifying comorbid illness is clear, because this will likely lead to quicker recovery and significantly decrease the likelihood of recurrence.

Unrecognized substance abuse and dependence can cause or exacerbate an anxiety disorder. Symptoms may present during the acute intoxication or withdrawal phase of substance use. Any work-up for anxiety disorders must include the nonjudgmental screening for use of

Table 4.3 Medications and Substances That Cause Anxiety-Like Symptoms

Stimulant intoxication	Caffeine, nicotine, cocaine, methamphetamines, phencyclidine (PCP), MDMA (ecstasy)
Sympathomimetics	Pseudoephedrine, methylphenidate, amphetamines, beta-agonists
Dopaminergics	Amantadine, bromocriptine, levodopa, levodopa-carbidopa, metoclopramide
Anticholinergics	Benztropine mesylate, meperidine, oxybutynin, diphenhydramine
Miscellaneous	Anabolic steroids, corticosteroids, indomethacin, ephedra, theophylline
Drug withdrawal	Alcohol, benzodiazepines, opiates

substances in the past month. If abuse or dependence is detected, the longitudinal history is helpful in determining if current symptoms represent a substance-induced state or comorbid substance abuse and anxiety disorder. History suggesting two separate disorders would include (1) onset of symptoms prior to first use of the substance and (2) continued symptoms despite sustained abstinence for at least 1 month. Management of comorbid substance abuse and anxiety disorders include treatment for the anxiety disorder in addition to the substance abuse treatment.

Biopsychosocial Treatment

GENERAL PRINCIPLES

Effective management of an anxiety disorder entails a balanced consideration of other nonspecific but equally crucial steps before actually treating anxiety disorders. These include establishing a trusting, therapeutic relationship and addressing comorbid general medical and psychiatric conditions. Thereafter, specific targeted pharmacotherapy and psychotherapy are added.

Trust

The best plans for medication treatment and referrals to specialists are doomed to fail if a therapeutic alliance is not first established between the patient and provider. The establishment of trust begins with empathy. As noted in Chapter 1, empathy requires the clinician to briefly "become the patient." Key steps include recognizing strong emotions during the interview, pausing to imagine how the patient is feeling, verbalizing what the clinician imagines the patient is feeling and legitimizing it, and offering support and reassurance. Remember that many patients have suffered for many years before finally presenting for treatment and have probably been told that "it's just anxiety." Employing an empathic approach with patients who have pronounced anxiety is both time saving and effective despite unjustified concerns that it will take too much time and be emotionally exhausting to the clinician.

Comorbid Conditions

Comorbid general medical and psychiatric conditions that may contribute to or mimic anxiety symptoms should be treated simultaneously

NOT TO BE MISSED

- Substance intoxication or withdrawal
- Comorbid major depression
- Medication-induced causes
- Systemic medical disorder
- Suicidal ideation or intent

with the anxiety disorder. As noted with the case of PD, it may be tempting to ignore the anxiety disorder and only treat the general medical condition in the hope that the anxiety disorder will resolve spontaneously. Unfortunately, this is not often the case. The same can be said with comorbid substance, personality, and mood disorders, and earlier concurrent treatment of the other conditions should be considered.

PHARMACOTHERAPY

Several classes of medications are used to treat anxiety disorders. Monoamine oxidase inhibitors (MAOIs), tricyclic antidepressants (TCAs), and selective serotonin reuptake inhibitors (SSRIs) are all effective antianxiety medications. More recently the serotonin norepinephrine reuptake inhibitors (SNRIs) have received FDA approval for GAD and panic disorder. All of these medications also function as antidepressants, alter serotonergic neurotransmission, and appear to exert their action by attenuating the physiologic cues associated with anxiety disorders over several weeks. There is a large body of evidence that shows various antidepressant classes have roughly equal efficacy in treating anxiety disorders in both the acute and maintenance phases.

Not all anti-anxiety medications are considered first-line agents. MAOIs have a number of side effects that limit their tolerability and require dietary restrictions to avoid hypertensive crisis. The TCAs require more dosage titration and have significant anticholinergic side effects such as sedation, constipation, and dry mouth. The two classes of medication most often prescribed for anxiety disorders are the SSRIs and SNRIs. Both of these have emerged as the treatment of choice because of their proven efficacy, safety, and ease of use. Additionally, benzodiazepines (BZPs) are still commonly used in current practice. Due to concerns about dependence and potential side effects, benzodiazepines can be used with caution and often adjunctively with other psychotropic medication.

Another drug used to treat anxiety is buspirone. As a 5-HT1A receptor agonist, buspirone has been shown to be effective for GAD but not the other anxiety disorders. While it lacks the abuse potential of the benzodiazepines, the narrow spectrum of efficacy, delay in therapeutic effect of several weeks, and twice-daily dosing tend to limit its popularity.

Serotonin Reuptake Inhibitors

Although SSRIs and SNRIs are more commonly known for the treatment of major depression, they have also been shown to be effective for anxiety disorders. While not every SSRI or SNRI is FDA approved for every anxiety disorder, in clinical practice they are generally used interchangeably. Medication choice is therefore not based on efficacy but rather on the potential side effects and drug–drug interactions. Antidepressants with short half-lives (e.g., paroxetine) have a higher likelihood of causing discontinuation syndrome and related anxiety with abrupt cessation. If a first-degree relative has had a good response to a particular drug or a patient has benefited from prior use of a specific medication, this should be strongly considered when deciding on a treatment

Table 4.4 Selective Serotonin Reuptake Inhibitors (SSRIs) and Serotonin Norepinephrine Reuptake Inhibitors (SNRIs) for Anxiety Disorders

SSRIs	STARTING DOSE (MG/DAY)	THERAPEUTIC DOSE (MG/DAY)	HALF-LIFE	DRUG INTERACTIONS
Fluoxetine (Prozac)	10	20–60	Long[a]	2D6 inhibitor
Sertraline (Zoloft)	25	50–200	Medium[a]	(—)
Citalopram (Celexa)	10	20–60	Short	(—)
Escitalopram (Lexapro)	5	10–30	Short	(—)
Paroxetine (Paxil)	10	20–60	Short	2D6 inhibitor
Paroxetine controlled release (Paxil CR)	12.5	12.5–25	Short	2D6 inhibitor
Fluvoxamine (Luvox)	50	150–300	Short	3A4 and 1A2 inhibitor
SNRIs				
Venlafaxine extended release (Effexor XR)	37.5	75–225	Short[a]	(—)
Duloxetine (Cymbalta)	30	60–120	Short	2D6 inhibitor

[a] Including active metabolites.

plan. Finally, the cost of a medication may be an additional factor. At the time of printing, all the SSRIs are available in generic formulations with the exception of escitalopram (Table 4.4).

Once a medication is chosen, clinical effectiveness depends on the initial information provided to the patient and adherence to treatment. Often, both understanding of the information provided and medication adherence should be explored and clarified in follow-up visits. This information should include expectations of treatment and a discussion of side effects and the need for gradual titration.

Expectations Most patients have heard of antidepressants such as fluoxetine and may have positive or negative expectations that need to be explored. They may also be asking themselves, "Why am I being prescribed an antidepressant when I have anxiety?" or "Why am I not feeling better when I've been taking this drug for over a week?" These questions are better answered at the initial visit rather than 3 months later when the patient continues to suffer from symptoms due to poor medication adherence. Similarly, many patients may take the antidepressant on an as-needed basis once symptoms initially respond, leading to subtherapeutic drug levels and a subsequent relapse.

Side Effects While SSRIs have improved tolerability compared to older antidepressants, there are several side effects common to all SSRIs that warrant discussion:

- Initial activation: While effective for anxiety disorders, some patients may experience increased activation and nervousness after initiation of an antidepressant. This effect is usually dose dependent and time limited to the first

ALWAYS DISCUSS BEFORE PRESCRIBING SSRIs/SNRIs

- **Expectations**
  - **Delayed therapeutic effect**
  - **Not an "as needed" medication**
  - **Long-term treatment is often indicated**
- **Class side effects**
  - **Initial activation**
  - **Sexual side effects**
  - **Gastrointestinal side effects**
- **Slow titration**
  - **Usually start at half the normal starting "antidepressant dose"**
  - **Increase the dose slowly and cautiously in the elderly**

1 to 2 weeks. This is a common cause of noncompliance and can be minimized by preparing the patient for the possibility and using gradual dose titration.

- Gastrointestinal side effects: Transient nausea represents one of the most common effects of SSRIs and a common cause of early medication discontinuation. This may be minimized by a slower titration and patient education.
- Sexual side effects: This occurs to some degree in approximately 30% to 50% of patients and can affect all phases of the sexual cycle but most commonly leads to delayed ejaculation and absent or delayed orgasm (8). While the sexual side effects are dose dependent, they do not appear to improve with time. There is good evidence for adding sildenafil for sexual dysfunction in men and limited evidence for adding bupropion for decreased libido in men and women (9). Patients with premature ejaculation often prefer SSRIs.

Dosage and Slow Titration   The final step to discuss with patients is the need for a slow initial titration. As mentioned above, this slow titration will minimize the dose-dependent side effects of initial activation and nausea. A reasonable strategy would include starting at half the dose normally prescribed for major depression and increased to the initial dose for major depression after the first week. The effective antidepressant dosage is usually similar for major depression and most anxiety disorders. A notable exception is OCD, where higher doses and longer trials are necessary for adequate response.

Benzodiazepines (BZPs)

While antidepressants are considered the first-line choice for patients with anxiety disorders, BZPs continue to serve an adjunctive role or even as monotherapy for some patients. Although there is evidence to support the use of BZPs as monotherapy for panic disorder and generalized anxiety disorder, there are limited data to support use with social phobia and obsessive compulsive disorder (10–12). BZPs alone do not appear to be effective for posttraumatic stress disorder (13).

One advantage that BZPs have over antidepressants is the rapid onset of action. As an adjunct, BZPs can provide immediate relief of symptoms and help mitigate the initial activation or jitteriness when initiating an antidepressant. Evidence for this role is strongest for PD, where this strategy can more rapidly stabilize patients during the initial phase compared to an SSRI alone. While the addition of BZPs does not benefit the patient beyond the initial few weeks over an SSRI alone, patients are able to taper off the benzodiazepine without significant issues of withdrawal. For example, clonazepam (Klonopin) could be initiated 0.5 mg twice daily along with sertraline 25 mg daily. The sertraline could be increased to 50 mg by the end of the first week and increased to 100 mg after another week. At week 4 the clonazepam could be gradually discontinued over the next 2 weeks.

The high-potency BZPs (e.g. alprazolam and clonazepam) are the best studied for anxiety disorders. Generally speaking, the lowest effective dose of BZPs should be prescribed in divided doses. When using

BZPs, the potential benefits must be balanced with the potential drawbacks of use. These drawbacks include:

- Side effects: While generally well tolerated, BZPs can produce sedation as well as impairment in working memory and learning new information. There is an increased risk of falls and confusion with elderly patients.
- Abuse: Patients who use higher doses of BZPs with faster-onset drugs (diazepam, alprazolam) and those with a history of alcohol and drug abuse have a heightened risk of developing benzodiazepine tolerance and withdrawal. As it is often difficult to determine whether a patient has a primary anxiety disorder versus a substance-induced anxiety disorder, BZP use may serve as a trigger for substance misuse and should be used with caution in those who have a substance abuse history.
- Physical dependence and withdrawal: Chronic use can result in a withdrawal syndrome in 40% to 80% of patients upon BZP discontinuation (14). A gradual taper is recommended if used longer than 2 weeks.
- Comorbidity: Monotherapy is not usually indicated and does not address comorbid major depression.

Despite these drawbacks, a short course of BZPs may be preferable to antidepressants in the following circumstances: relatively infrequent symptoms, intolerance to antidepressants, or adjustment disorder with anxiety.

PSYCHOTHERAPY

Over the past 30 years, CBT has emerged as an effective first-line therapy for the treatment of anxiety disorders. Evidence from meta-analysis and large prospective studies has indicated that CBT is at least as effective as medication alone (15, 16). Despite this evidence, CBT continues to be underutilized. In the following section we will discuss the principles of CBT and the role of the primary care clinician.

Cognitive Behavioral Therapy

CBT is a psychotherapeutic technique delivered by trained mental health professionals in a group or individual format. Patients are typically seen weekly and the therapy is time limited (generally 10 to 24 sessions). The therapy is active in that the therapist and patient collaboratively work together to develop and test hypotheses. There is also an expectation that the patient will complete CBT-related "homework" and discuss this work during follow-up sessions.

The general premise of CBT rests on the observation that patients with anxiety disorders hold *distorted beliefs* and expectations about their world, which lead to symptoms and avoidance behaviors. It incorporates symptom management techniques such as progressive muscle relaxation and deep breathing. The cognitive therapy part of CBT is used to identify and address distorted beliefs through a process called cognitive restructuring. During this process, patients are asked to identify and logically evaluate thoughts that affect mood and behavior in a *dysfunctional thought record*. They become aware of cognitive distortions such as mind reading (e.g., "People think I'm a bad parent.") and catastrophizing (e.g., "If I don't leave I'm going to pass out.") and are challenged to replace them with more accurate, reality-based, and adaptive explanations that decrease anxiety symptoms.

Cognitive restructuring is often coupled with exposure interventions to help the patient relearn a sense of safety in previously feared situations. This exposure is performed in a stepwise hierarchical fashion from the least to the most feared (as ranked by the patient). This allows an opportunity to put into practice what has been learned during sessions. For example, the patient with social anxiety might start with simply imagining a brief conversation with a neighbor. Once the patient achieves some mastery over symptoms, the exposure might escalate to a brief conversation with a neighbor. All the while the patient would be working to cognitively restructure his or her thoughts of embarrassment. Ultimately the patient might invite the neighbor over for lunch. Exposure response prevention (ERP) is a component of CBT that is particularly helpful for OCD. In ERP, the patient is repeatedly exposed to a particular trigger that elicits the obsession and refrains from carrying out the compulsion.

The role of the primary care clinician for a patient undergoing CBT is largely supportive, although many providers may wish to learn CBT through formal training. Providers may refer patients for CBT. In such patients, the provider may briefly review the *dysfunctional thought record* with the patient and reinforce what is learned from therapy. Also, reminding the patient that symptoms may actually increase initially as fears are challenged rather than avoided may be helpful in preventing premature discontinuation from therapy. CBT is well tolerated, cost effective, and associated with minimal side effects. Patients routinely experience the benefits of CBT within the same timeframe as antidepressants, as early as the second session.

Social Interventions

As part of the empathic process, the clinician may become aware of obvious social situations exacerbating or complicating a patient's anxiety disorder. While it is often not possible to solve potentially complicated social issues for patients, reasonable interventions may go a long way in developing trust. Interventions may include assessment of safety for a patient in an abusive or unsafe relationship, consideration of short-term disability or time off from work, and consultation with a social worker if available. In cases of adjustment disorder with anxiety, such interventions may be the only treatment required.

Treatment Recommendations (Acute Phase)

With some notable exceptions, the initial treatment for the anxiety disorders is remarkably similar regardless of the specific diagnosis. Options will include some combination of an SSRI, benzodiazepine, and/or psychotherapy. The exact choice will depend on patient preference and to a lesser extent on diagnosis (Table 4.5). For the five major anxiety disorders (PD, GAD, OCD, PTSD, and SAD), starting with either an SSRI or CBT is a reasonable first option as they are equally effective. For OCD, a therapist trained in ERP would also be a reasonable option. Since success is equally likely with either option, choice may depend on factors other

Table 4.5 Acute Treatment for Anxiety Disorders

	SSRI	CBT	CBT + SSRI[a]	BENZODIAZEPINE MONOTHERAPY	BENZODIAZEPINE ADJUNCTIVE
PD	++	++	+	++	+
GAD	++	++	+/−	++	+/−
SP	++	++	+/−	+	+/−
PTSD	++	++	+/−	−	+/−
OCD	++	++[b]	+	+/−	−

CBT, cognitive behavioral therapy; GAD, generalized anxiety disorder; OCD, obsessive compulsive disorder; PD, panic disorder; PTSD, posttraumatic stress disorder; SP, social phobia; SSRI, selective serotonin reuptake inhibitor.
++, good evidence; +, some evidence; +/−, inadequate/mixed evidence; −, no evidence.
[a] Additional combined benefit.
[b] Exposure response prevention.

than efficacy. While many therapists may be familiar with the principles of CBT, this does not always translate to competency in providing CBT. This is important since outcome is influenced by how closely a therapist adheres to the guiding principles and techniques. Even when available, therapists may not accept health insurance. Another potential logistical challenge is the time commitment required from the patient. The weekly visits may not be possible due to required time off from work and need for childcare and consistent transportation.

If the patient chooses to take an SSRI and does not respond within 2 months of adequately dosed treatment, options would include a trial of another SSRI versus switching to an SNRI such as venlafaxine or duloxetine. For patients with a history of inadequate response to a medication in the past, CBT can still be effective. Despite the theoretical appeal of combined treatment with CBT and an SSRI, the current evidence has not consistently shown a substantial benefit over CBT alone except with the possible exceptions of PD and OCD (17, 18). On the other hand, combined treatment was also not associated with diminished effectiveness. Therefore, use of combined medication and psychotherapy may be individually tailored until further information becomes available.

Treatment Recommendations (Maintenance Phase)

The maintenance phase of treatment begins once a patient responds to an antianxiety medication. The goal of maintenance treatment is relapse prevention. Most guidelines suggest a minimum of 6 months to 1 year of treatment. Chances for success with discontinuation of medication treatment may be increased by considering several options: (1) if there is a history of one or more relapses in the past, long-term, indefinite treatment with an antidepressant may be considered; 2) a gradual discontinuation of the antidepressant over several weeks (and BZPs over several weeks) will decrease the likelihood of recurrence as well as prevent the discontinuation syndrome; and (3) consider CBT: A course of CBT in conjunction with the taper from medication can decrease the likelihood of relapse.

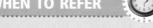

WHEN TO REFER

- Diagnostic uncertainty

- Significant comorbid psychiatric illness: substance abuse, suicidal patients, bipolar disorder, personality disorders

- Severe illness in terms of marked socio-occupational disability

- Prior treatment failure with multiple medications and psychotherapy

- Patient prefers initial trial of psychotherapy

- Close follow-up (e.g., every 2 to 3 weeks) during medication initiation phase is not feasible

- Severe agitation or suicidal ideation

Practice Pointers

Case 1: Afraid of passing out

A 32-year-old woman with a history of Graves disease treated with radioablation therapy 2 years ago complains of "feeling anxious and fearful when leaving the house." Her symptoms prior to the radioablation consisted of a "pounding heart" and "feeling shaky and hot." After radioablation therapy, serial thyroid function values showed that the patient was euthyroid with thyroid hormone replacement. While she does not have daily symptoms, she continues to have sudden and unexpected attacks that she dreads, and states, "I feel like I'm going to pass out." She underwent an extensive cardiac work-up 1 year ago but she is still convinced something was "missed" since "they told me this would all go away and it hasn't." She is becoming hesitant to drive for fear of an attack and stays near an exit in public places "just in case I have to get out of there." She is on thyroid replacement therapy and her thyroid panel has been within normal limits.

Discussion: *This case illustrates an example of PD developing during the course of a general medical condition known to mimic symptoms of anxiety. Initially the attacks occurred without warning, but over time we can see that the early signs of agoraphobia are appearing. The somatic presentation may have delayed early recognition of panic disorder. Treatment should have begun immediately after the negative medical work-up based on risk factors rather than waiting for symptoms to resolve spontaneously. Management at this point first requires improving trust between patient and provider. She is clearly frustrated by the lack of past improvement despite reassurances, and an empathic statement noting such may be a helpful first step. A clear explanation of how her panic attacks are mimicking her previous thyroid disease and are now likely driven by her sympathetic nervous system may find the patient open to a trial of CBT. Alternatively, a slow titration of an SSRI could be considered first depending on patient preference.*

Case 2: Chronic worries

A 27-year-old man with a diagnosis of gastroesophageal reflux disease (GERD) presents with continuing anxiety and worry about his illness despite some mild improvement with a proton pump inhibitor and an unremarkable endoscopic examination earlier in the year. He is concerned from reading articles on the Internet that he may have esophageal cancer or heart disease and worries that his insurance will not cover such a work-up. He wonders if he should change his insurance carrier but continues to be worried despite your assurance that his concerns are premature. He admits that he probably worries too much about things in general and states, "It's the way I've always been." He wishes he could "just relax," but "that's when something will probably go wrong." He has taken zolpidem for several years to help him sleep instead of ruminating on his worries. He describes a brother with similar symptoms who has found some relief with citalopram. He is interested in trying it but worries about side effects and "getting addicted to it."

Discussion: *The presence of multiple, pervasive, and long-term worries without a unifying trigger suggests a diagnosis of GAD. His continuing GERD-like symptoms could represent a somatic manifestation of his anxiety disorder and may be expected to improve with treatment of GAD. Fortunately, he appears willing to accept help, but as we can see from his propensity to worry, it will be important to provide clear information about expectations and potential side effects of treatment options. Initiation of a medication or psychotherapy would be equally reasonable at this point. Because there is a family history of success with citalopram, it may be preferentially considered.*

Case 3: A shy parent

A 29-year-old woman presents with her 6-year-old daughter for a well-child check after missing the originally scheduled appointment. She is quiet but informs you that there is an upcoming parent–teacher conference for her daughter. She adds, "I'm just not good with that sort of thing." She apparently showed up late for the last parent–teacher conference, couldn't remember what was said, and "left with a headache." Further questioning reveals a concern that "the teacher thinks I'm not a good parent" despite lacking the evidence this is true. It is also clear that she has similar concerns with purely social events such as holiday parties or even saying hello to her neighbors.

Discussion: *This case highlights the difficulty many patients have in asking for help due to a sense of shame or embarrassment. Being on the lookout for physical symptoms and the pattern of avoidance is important. Further evaluation should inquire about the extent of triggers. If the triggers are circumscribed around social interactions almost exclusively, social phobia (SP) would be the diagnosis. If the symptoms appear in nearly all activities, including while at home without social triggers, the patient may actually have GAD. Initial management should begin with recognition that the patient has really struggled with symptoms over the years. While medications and psychotherapy are again equally effective with SP, many patients are hesitant about seeing a therapist since by definition they find new social interactions very uncomfortable. If a reasonably strong therapeutic relationship has developed, the patient may be more open to psychotherapy if a trial of a medication was not effective or was only partially effective.*

Case 4: Multiple fears and rituals

A 25-year-old man is a new patient with concerns about holding his job as a substitute teacher. In the past several months he has had intrusive and consuming thoughts that one of his students has been abused. He finds himself repeatedly checking for bruises on his students and finds it very difficult to concentrate on the lesson. He fears that missing a bruise would mean losing his job despite knowing the thoughts are excessive. "I try to resist but I can feel it building up until I think about it." He is now a lesson behind and parents have complained about his "slowness" to the principal. He recently moved to the area to be closer to his girlfriend. As a teenager he had some issues with excessive handwashing and counting in response to obsessions with contamination but denies this is a current issue.

Discussion: *The trigger of an obsession (students are being abused) and the compulsion (checking for bruises) suggest the patient is suffering from OCD. The absence of other triggers and recent traumas would confirm the diagnosis. This case also illustrates the sometimes waxing and waning nature of anxiety disorders, in his case potentially recurring after his recent stressor (the move and new job). Over time, obsessions and compulsions may change, as his obsessions changed from contamination to doubts. The irresistible and time-consuming nature of the obsessions contributes to the disability. Management could include initiation of an SSRI titrated as close to the maximal dose as possible to improve chances of response. Since combining medication with psychotherapy, especially ERP, may have additive value in OCD, this should be considered early. ERP would focus on having the patient imagine the children in the classroom triggering the obsession (students are being abused) and refrain from imagining the search for bruises until the anxiety is minimal (habituation).*

Case 5: A man with acute anxiety

A 42-year-old man presents to his primary care provider for the results of a blood test performed the week before to evaluate jaundice. He is told he has hepatitis C and the provider tries to explain the next step, which includes referral to a liver specialist. However, the patient finds it difficult to listen to the plan as he ruminates on the effect of this illness on his wife and employment. Over the next several days he calls in sick at work due to feeling restless and being unable to concentrate. He pulls out of a planned fishing trip with friends and spends several hours per day on the computer gathering information on hepatitis C. His wife is supportive and during the following week his sleep normalizes and he returns to work. He returns to the clinic several weeks later interested in the referral to the liver specialist and adds, "I'd like to go fishing as long as I can."

Discussion: There is a close temporal relationship with an acute stressor (diagnosis of hepatitis C) and the onset of anxiety symptoms that appear to peak in the first 1 to 2 weeks. However, ASD or PTSD does not result because the stressor is not sufficiently traumatic to produce significant arousal, avoidance, or re-experiencing of the stressor. The symptoms are sufficient to affect function but resolve after he receives support and education. This is a case of adjustment disorder with anxiety.

Case 6: Headaches, insomnia, and flashbacks

A 24-year-old woman presents complaining of headache, difficulty initiating sleep, and fatigue for the past 4 months. She recently withdrew from some community college classes and has avoided going out with friends on weekends, which she previously enjoyed, and admits she has been more irritable. Routine laboratory evaluation reveals normal values. You inquire about any recent stressors besides school and she admits there was an "incident." Apparently a former boyfriend was stalking her and held her at knifepoint 6 months ago before being disarmed by police. He is now in jail but she admits feeling fearful of anyone who looks like her ex-boyfriend and finds herself vividly remembering the events of 6 months ago "as if they're happening now."

Discussion: Despite the potentially lethal nature of her trauma, she did not have any obvious physical sequelae that would have more easily led us to the diagnosis of PTSD. The traumatic event is defined as an event that causes significant fear, horror, or helplessness. The avoidance symptoms are represented by her withdrawal from school and social situations. She is re-experiencing the trauma in the form of flashbacks and the increased arousal is manifesting as irritability. She is clearly disabled by her anxiety disorder and complicating her case is the pending nature of her trauma as the boyfriend is in jail and awaiting trial. Considering the overlap in symptoms and high comorbidity, the patient should also be screened for major depression. Management should include consultation with a social worker to help the patient with counseling and legal resources. A benzodiazepine and/or an SSRI may be used if the anxiety worsens.

ICD 9	
Acute Stress Disorder	*308.3*
Acute Stress Reaction	*308*
Adjustment Disorder (Mixed Anxiety and Depressed Mood)	*309.28*
Agoraphobia without Panic Disorder	*300.22*
Anxiety State, Unspecified	*300*
Generalized Anxiety Disorder	*300.02*
Panic Disorder with Agoraphobia	*300.21*
Panic Disorder without Agoraphobia	*300.01*
Phobia, Specific (Acrophobia, Animal, Claustrophobia, Fear of Crowds)	*300.29*
Phobia, Unspecified	*300.2*
Posttraumatic Stress Disorder	*309.81*
Social Phobia (Social Anxiety Disorder)	*300.23*

Practical Resources

The Anxiety Disorders Association of America: www.adaa.org
Nonprofit organization with information on anxiety disorders and help with finding a therapist
The National Institute of Mental Health: http://www.nimh.nih.gov/healthinformation/anxietymenu.cfm
Information on diagnosis and treatment as well as on how to participate in clinical trials

REFERENCES

1. Greenberg PE, Sisitsky T, Kessler RC, et al. The economic burden of anxiety disorders in the 1990s. *J Clin Psychiatry*. 1999;60:427–435.

2. Bruce SE, Yonkers KA, Otto M, et al. Influence of psychiatric comorbidity on recovery and recurrence in generalized anxiety disorder, social phobia, and panic disorder: a 12-year prospective study. *Am J Psychiatry*. 2005;162:1179–1187.

3. Kroenke K, Spitzer RL, Williams JB, et al. Anxiety disorders in primary care: prevalence, impairment, comorbidity, and detection. *Ann Intern Med*. 2007;146(5):317–325.

4. Spitzer RL, Kroenke K, Williams JB, et al. A brief measure for assessing generalized anxiety disorder: the GAD-7. *Arch Intern Med*. 2006;166:1092–1097.

5. Kirmayer LJ, Robbins JM, Dworkind M, et al. Somatization and the recognition of depression and anxiety in primary care. *Am J Psychiatry*. 1993;150:734–741.

6. Goldberg, RJ. *Practical Guide to the Care of the Psychiatric Patient*. St. Louis: Mosby Year Book; 1995.

7. Rodriguez BF, Weisberg RB, Pagano ME, et al. Frequency and patterns of psychiatric comorbidity in a sample of primary care patients with anxiety disorders. *Compr Psychiatry*. 2004;45(2):129–137.

8. Rosen RC, Lane RM, Menza M. Effects of SSRIs on sexual function: a critical review. *J Clin Psychopharmacol*. 1999;19:67–85.

9. Balon B. SSRI-associated sexual dysfunction. *Am J Psychiatry*. 2006;163:1504–1509.

10. Davidson JRT, Potts N, Richichi E, et al. Treatment of social phobia with clonazepam and placebo. *J Clin Psychopharmacol*. 1993;13:423–428.

11. Hollander E, Kaplan A, Stahl SM. A double-blind, placebo-controlled trial of clonazepam in obsessive-compulsive disorder. *World J Biol Psychiatry*. 2003;4(1):30–34.

12. Crockett BA, Churchill E, Davidson JR. A double-blind combination study of clonazepam with sertraline in obsessive-compulsive disorder. *Ann Clin Psychiatry*. 2004;16(3):127–132.

13. Braun P, Greenberg D, Dasberg H, et al. Core symptoms of posttraumatic stress disorder unimproved by alprazolam treatment. *J Clin Psychiatry*. 1990;51:236–238.

14. Rickels K, Rynn M. Pharmacology of generalized anxiety disorder. *J Clin Psychiatry*. 2002;63(suppl 14): 9–16

15. Gelernter CS, Uhde TW, Cimbolic P, et al. Cognitive-behavioral and pharmacological treatments of social phobia: a controlled study. *Arch Gen Psychiatry*. 1991;48:938–945.

16. Mitte K. A meta-analysis of the efficacy of psycho- and pharmacotherapy in panic disorder with and without agoraphobia. *J Affect Disord*. 2005;88:27–45.

17. Black DW. Efficacy of combined pharmacotherapy and psychotherapy versus monotherapy in the treatment of anxiety disorders [Review]. *CNS Spectr*. 2006 Oct;11(10 Suppl 12):29–33.

18. Furukawa TA, Watanabe N, Churchill R. Psychotherapy plus antidepressant for panic disorder with or without agoraphobia: systematic review [Review]. *Br J Psychiatry*. 2006;188:305–312.

CHAPTER 4 Anxiety Disorders

CHAPTER 5 Psychotic Disorders

Joel Johnson, MD • Malathi Srinivasan, MD • Glen L. Xiong, MD

Susan is a 28-year-old woman who presents with her boyfriend for worsening anxiety and insomnia. During the exam, she is nervous and staring intently at the walls. She states that she is afraid of demons, as they have been asking her to do "weird things." Her boyfriend states that she has not been eating or bathing regularly. Her real estate business has fallen off by 50%, because she can't "close the deal."

CLINICAL HIGHLIGHTS

- Psychosis is a state of disordered thoughts or impairment in reality testing, as manifested by perceptual disturbances (e.g., hallucination) and disorganized speech and behavior.

- Secondary psychotic disorders can be caused by general medical conditions (e.g., dementia or delirium with psychosis), side effects from prescribed medications (e.g., prednisone or potent opioid analgesics), severe mood disorders with psychotic features such as depression and bipolar

Clinical Significance

The lifetime prevalence of psychotic disorders in U.S. residents is about 3%. In a study of over one thousand urban and academic centered primary care patients, roughly 20% reported some type of psychotic symptom, most commonly auditory hallucinations. Those who have psychotic symptoms are much more likely to experience comorbid depression, anxiety, suicidal thinking and alcohol abuse (1).

The ability to accurately diagnose and effectively treat psychotic disorders has become increasingly relevant for primary care providers for several reasons. First, patients with psychotic symptoms, which complicate general medical conditions (e.g., delusions associated with systemic lupus erythematosus), often present in primary care settings. Second, antipsychotic medications used to treat psychosis have significant potential metabolic side effects (i.e., obesity, hyperglycemia, and hyperlipidemia). As a result, more and more patients who chronically take antipsychotic medications and have been traditionally cared for in mental health programs require primary medical care (2). Third, life-prolonging measures for various medical conditions like Parkinson disease have outpaced the treatment of their associated psychiatric disturbances. The resulting increase in such secondary psychotic conditions has caused an increase in the use of antipsychotic medications, particularly in the last decade.

Diagnosis

PRIMARY PSYCHOTIC DISORDERS

Primary psychotic disorders are conditions in which psychosis is a cardinal symptom and not directly caused by another disorder. Currently,

(Continued)

CHAPTER 5 Psychotic Disorders

CLINICAL HIGHLIGHTS
(*Continued*)

- disorder, and illicit substance use.

- Positive psychotic symptoms are outward manifestations of the thought disorder: hallucinations, delusions, and bizarre or disorganized behaviors or speech. Negative psychotic symptoms include affective flattening (decreased expressed emotions), alogia (poverty of thoughts), attention deficits, anhedonia, amotivation, and social withdrawal.

- The American Psychiatric Association recommends indefinite antipsychotic medication treatment against recurring psychosis in patients with primary psychotic disorders, if two or more episodes occur within 5 years.

- Treatment of chronic psychotic disorders, such as schizophrenia, begins with the selection of an appropriate second-generation antipsychotic (SGA) medication and referral for psychosocial services.

- Patients who have schizophrenia are at an increased risk for developing metabolic abnormalities. The addition of any SGA carries an additional risk for weight gain, dyslipidemia, and glucose dysregulation. In addition to obtaining the weight and waist circumference at each visit for all patients who are on an SGA, a fasting glucose must be checked before the SGA is started, at week 12 after it was started, and annually thereafter. A fasting lipid panel should also be monitored before the SGA is started, 12 weeks into treatment, and every 3 to 5 years thereafter.

there are seven defined disorders: schizophrenia, schizophreniform disorder, schizoaffective disorder, brief psychotic disorder, delusional disorder, shared psychotic disorder, and psychotic disorder not otherwise specified (3). Secondary psychotic disorders are clinical conditions in which psychosis is a complicating symptom of a general medical condition or a medication (e.g., encephalitis or the use of high-dose steroids), substance use disorders (e.g., amphetamine- or cocaine-induced psychosis), or mood disorders (e.g., major depression with psychotic features). Patients with relapsing and remitting psychosis usually have a chronic psychotic disorder, representing a primary psychotic disorder. In these cases, symptoms have a high likelihood of recurrence. Patients with untreated psychotic disorders have associated cognitive dysfunction that results in disability, including the inability to work, poor social functioning, poor hygiene, malnutrition, and early death (4). The seven primary psychotic disorders are discussed below.

Schizophrenia

Schizophrenia is the most common primary psychotic disorder in the United States, affecting about 1% of the population. Its economic impact is comparable with that of mood and anxiety disorders, although each of the other two conditions is about 10 times more prevalent than schizophrenia (5). Mortality in those with schizophrenia is about three times that of the general population. About a third of deaths are due to suicide, while a smaller but significant percentage of the deaths are related to violent acts. Approximately 30% of those with schizophrenia attempt suicide and about 10% will die by their attempts (6). Many patients with schizophrenia die of complications of poor lifestyle choices and poor adherence to medical treatments. Half of those who have schizophrenia are obese and have metabolic syndrome, with a resultant increase in cardiac-related mortality (6). Peak symptom onset is late adolescence or early adulthood, although nonspecific symptoms may be present earlier (7).

Schizophrenia has three phases: (1) a nonspecific **prodromal phase,** which is usually recognized in retrospect and characterized by subtle behavioral changes, social withdrawal, and functional decline; (2) an **active phase,** in which psychotic symptoms predominate; and (3) a **residual phase,** which is similar to the prodromal phase but occurs later in the disease process. Active phase symptoms recur in the residual phase. A definitive diagnosis is generally made in the active phase. The diagnostic criteria for schizophrenia are listed in Table 5.1 (8). Patients with schizophrenia may not (and often do not) present with classic hallucinations or delusions. Instead, they may have extremely disordered thoughts or disorganized behaviors. While patients may have various bizarre delusions, paranoid delusions (i.e., of being watched, followed, plotted against, and harmed) are most consistently present. In order to meet the diagnostic criteria for schizophrenia, some continuous sign of disturbance must be present for at least 6 months.

Table 5.1 Diagnostic Criteria for Schizophrenia

1. Two positive or negative symptoms:
   Positive symptoms: hallucinations, delusions, disorganized behavior, and disorganized speech
   Negative symptoms: flat affect, poverty of thought, social withdrawal, and lack of motivation
   These criteria can be fulfilled with only one symptom in three special cases:
   a. A delusional construct that cannot occur in the real world
   b. Two auditory hallucinations, which are in conversation with each other about the patient
   c. An auditory hallucination, which provides a running commentary on the patient's thoughts and/or behaviors

2. Evidence of symptoms for at least 6 months
   The syndrome usually starts with negative symptoms or progressively worsening positive symptoms.

3. Not due to a complication of a systemic medical disorder or other psychiatric disorder
4. Significant decline from previous level of function

Adapted from American Psychiatric Association. *Diagnostic and Statistical Manual of Mental Disorders.* 4th ed., text revision. Washington, DC: American Psychiatric Publishing, Inc.; 2004.

Schizophreniform Disorder

Schizophreniform disorder is often thought of as "early schizophrenia" and is not due to another psychiatric or a general medical disorder. If criteria for schizophrenia are met and symptoms are present for less than 6 months but greater than 1 month, then the diagnosis of schizophreniform disorder is indicated. All patients with schizophreniform disorder should be immediately referred to a psychiatrist with concerns of new-onset psychosis.

Brief Psychotic Disorder

A brief psychotic disorder is also referred to as time-limited schizophrenia. If criteria for schizophrenia are met for more than 1 day but less than 1 month, followed by full clinical recovery, the patient may be diagnosed with a brief psychotic disorder. This diagnosis has a fairly good prognosis and is usually coupled with a significant psychosocial stressor.

Schizoaffective Disorder

Simply put, schizoaffective disorder is schizophrenia with a persistent mood disorder. Someone with schizoaffective disorder simultaneously meets the diagnostic criteria for schizophrenia and either bipolar disorder or major depressive disorder. In order to meet the diagnostic criteria for schizoaffective disorder, there must be evidence that psychotic symptoms are present when the mood disturbance is quiescent for at least a 2-week time period. In general, schizoaffective disorder carries a poor long-term prognosis that is similar to or worse than schizophrenia.

Delusional Disorder

Those who have delusional disorder present with nonbizarre delusions for at least 1 month. Nonbizarre delusions refer to plausible but unlikely events that could happen in real life. For example, a person may believe that his spouse is poisoning his meals for no apparent reason. Those who have one or more nonbizarre delusions should only be diagnosed with delusional disorder when there is related social or occupational dysfunction due solely to the delusion.

Shared Delusional Disorder

Shared delusional disorder (also called "folie á deux") is rare and occurs when two individuals in close proximity share the delusion. Patients with shared delusional disorder should be screened for recent stressors as well as anxiety, mood, and disorders related to substance abuse.

Psychotic Disorder Not Otherwise Specified

Patients with psychotic disorder not otherwise specified (NOS) have clinically significant symptoms that don't meet criteria for a specific psychotic disorder. For example, patients may present with isolated auditory hallucinations, postpartum psychosis in the absence of a mood disorder, or transient stress-induced psychosis. Psychosis NOS often serves as a working diagnosis that may be used while investigating the cause of psychotic symptoms. In order to be diagnosed with psychosis NOS, the symptoms should cause clinically significant distress and not be caused by other general medical or psychiatric illness. For example, an isolated, nondistressing visual hallucination on waking (hypnopompic hallucination) does not merit a psychiatric diagnosis.

PATIENT ASSESSMENT

Patients with psychosis may present in a variety of ways, often with distressing hallucinations or paranoid delusions. More frequently, patients are brought in by family members with a complaint of bizarre behavior, insomnia, or lack of concern for hygiene and grooming. Family members may be concerned over other decline in basic activities of daily living (ADLs) or the patient's failure to keep up with routine social duties. Many patients have little insight into their psychosis although they will often concede that their thinking is impaired. The provider should assess how the psychosis has disrupted the patient's ADLs, interpersonal relationships, school or work performance, and financial well-being. Asking about educational, occupational, and social background will help place the current level of functioning in perspective. Table 5.2 summarizes the evaluation

Table 5.2 Assessment of Patients with Psychotic Symptoms: PSΨCHOSIS Mnemonic

Psychotropis: Ask the patient about past use of antipsychotic and other psychiatric medications; including questions related to efficacy and side effects.

Safety first: When in the room, keep in mind the patient's frame of reference and state of mind. The patient may be scared, paranoid, uncomfortable, potentially violent, angry, or confused. Be prepared to modify your approach as circumstances change in the interview. If the patient seems angry, have a staff member in the room with you, keep the door open, and notify security.

Ψ symptoms: Let the patient know that many other people experience these symptoms and that treatment is available. The clinician can use the following statements to reassure and calm the patient who presents with psychosis: "Many patients in my practice have experienced [symptom]. Is that something that you have experienced as well?" or "I know this is new and may be scary, but I want you to know we can work as a team to make things better."

Caring: Elicit symptoms with a caring, neutral stance, in which you neither challenge nor collude with the patient's symptoms. Often, empathizing with the distress around a symptom without validating the symptom is comforting. For example, you might say, "It must be very frightening to believe the FBI is watching you. Let me know what I can do to make you feel less anxious about this."

Home: Inquire about the living and financial situation, as patients who have a psychotic disorder often struggle with securing safe and stable housing and consistent meals.

Other conditions: Evaluate and treat coexisting general medical, psychiatric, and substance misuse conditions. As with any other medical conditions, assess symptom onset, duration, fluctuation, exacerbating/relieving factors, and associated symptoms.

Suicide: Assess for suicidal and other critical symptoms, such as homicidal thoughts or extreme neglect and inability to care for self. Distinguish between thoughts of death (self or others), plans to harm (self or others), and the degree of development of the plans. All patients who express thoughts of suicide or homicide should be asked about access to a firearm. When indicated, consult with a mental health crisis intervention team or local emergency department.

Impairment: How impaired is the patient because of these symptoms? How have they impacted the patient's family, work, education and relationships?

Substance misuse: People with schizophrenia frequently have comorbid substance abuse or dependence. Moreover, the use of excessive alcohol or illicit drugs dramatically worsens the prognosis of schizophrenia. All patients who have a psychotic disorder should be regularly monitored for a substance misuse disorder.

process of patients who present with psychotic symptoms using the PSΨCHOSIS mnemonic.

Differential Diagnosis

Psychosis is a symptom that, like chest pain, has a broad differential diagnosis. Not all psychotic symptoms are due to schizophrenia! In fact, psychotic symptoms may be due to primary psychosis (e.g., schizophrenia), general medical, other psychiatric, or substance-induced conditions. Figure 5.1 illustrates an approach to patients presenting with psychotic symptoms. In general, *acute, isolated psychotic symptoms* are due to substance use, medication side effects, or a general medical condition since primary psychosis and secondary psychosis due to another psychiatric disorder (e.g., bipolar disorder) tend to have a more *subacute to chronic* course with progressive worsening. When forming a differential diagnosis, we recommend taking the following stepwise approach (9).

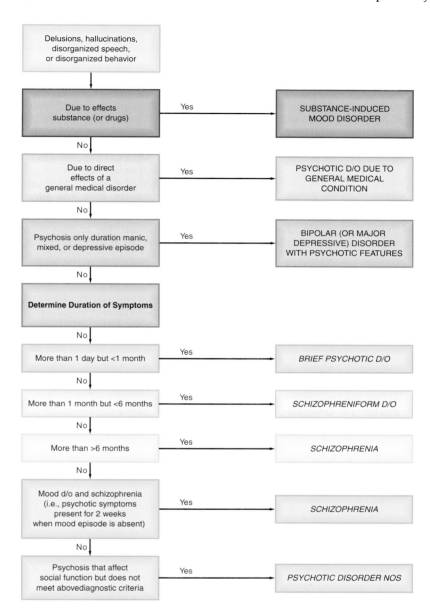

Figure 5.1 Diagnostic algorithm for psychosis. (Adapted with permission from the American Psychiatric Association. *Diagnostic and Statistical Manual of Mental Disorders.* 4th ed., text revision. Washington, DC: American Psychiatric Publishing, Inc.; 2004.)

STEP 1: ELICIT SYMPTOMS

The provider should elicit the course and fluctuation of symptoms and the impact on social functioning. Positive psychotic symptoms are outward manifestations of the psychosis: hallucinations, delusions, and bizarre or disorganized behaviors or speech. Negative psychotic symptoms are the "fall from function" symptoms: flat affect, poverty of thought, social withdrawal, apathy, and lack of motivation. Table 5.3 defines common psychotic symptoms. For acutely psychotic patients, the best way to elicit symptoms is to take a caring, neutral stance in which the provider neither challenges nor colludes with the patient's

Table 5.3 Definition of Psychotic Symptoms

POSITIVE SYMPTOMS	WHAT ARE THEY?	OFTEN CONFUSED WITH...
Hallucinations	• Sensory perception in the absence of sensory stimuli. May occur with any of the senses (visual, auditory, olfactory, skin sensations, etc.)	• Perceptual distortions or illusions: sensory misperception in the presence of stimuli (e.g., mistakenly identifying a chair as a person) • "Mystical experiences," often part of a spiritual belief system • May be due to medical disorders (temporal seizures, migraine auras, uremia, hepatic encephalopathy, etc.)
Delusions	• Fixed belief that is at odds with reality (delusions of persecution, grandeur, parasites, etc.)	• Beliefs due to environmental, social, cultural, or spiritual/religious background (e.g., belief in God's influence over health or destiny, transfer of the soul with blood transfusions, breaking a mirror brings bad luck, etc.)
Bizarre delusions	• Not physically possible (e.g., people walking through walls or traveling back in time)	• Nonbizarre delusions are possible, but untrue—for instance, a patient feeling that "a celebrity is in love with me"
Thought disorder	• Disorders of thought process or *how* one thinks. Patients may have difficulty with logical construction of thoughts (tangential, word salad, flight of ideas, loosening of associations, neologisms, etc.) or expression of their thoughts in unintelligible ways	• Delirium, dementia, aphasia, mania
Bizarre behaviors	• Inability to dress, act, or interact in socially appropriate ways. Behaviors may be crude (cursing, solicitous), offensive, violent, or erratic • Dress in poorly fitting clothing, wear makeup smeared over the face or buttons mismatched and zippers undone • Urinate or defecate in unusual places, even if a bathroom is nearby	• Social trends (intergenerational conflicts), unusual fashions, fads, or social groups with nonconformist behaviors

symptoms. Often, empathizing with the level of distress can be done without challenging or confirming the symptoms. For example, one might say, "It must be frightening and frustrating to believe your co-workers are monitoring your every move while at work and home." Collateral information sources should be obtained to supplement the subjective history whenever possible.

STEP 2: EVALUATE FOR SYSTEMIC MEDICAL CONDITIONS

Psychosis may be caused by illicit or prescribed drugs, infections, vasculitis, autoimmune disorders (e.g., systemic lupus erythematosus), poisoning (e.g., heavy metals), stroke, or dementia. Table 5.4 reviews general medical conditions associated with psychosis and the corresponding work-up. Clinical suspicion should guide diagnostic testing to avoid unnecessary false-positives, inconvenience, and cost. Medical conditions with systemic manifestation (e.g., delirium) often cause acute mental status changes, which often present with acute psychotic symptoms.

Table 5.4 General Medical Causes of Psychosis

CONDITIONS	PRESENTATION	ASSESSMENT	COMMENTS
Neurologic disorders (chronic) (seizure disorder, Parkinson disease, multiple sclerosis, stroke, Huntington disease, traumatic brain injury)	• Acute or progressive development of delusions, hallucinations, disorganized behavior, agitation, and disinhibition • Temporal relationship between the neurologic disorder and the psychotic symptoms • Psychiatric finding may be the only presentation in cases of isolated neurologic lesions (e.g., stroke or occult multiple sclerosis)	• Brain imaging to detect underlying neurologic condition • Lumbar puncture for multiple sclerosis	• Patients with a primary neurologic condition and psychosis should be given a diagnosis of "psychosis due to a general medical condition," rather than be diagnosed with schizophrenia • Pharmacotherapy may be similar to schizophrenia but antipsychotic-associated EPS may be more likely in this patient population
Neurologic disorders (acute) (central nervous system infection or inflammation, e.g., syphilis, herpes encephalitis, HIV, lupus, vasculitides)	• Acute to subacute onset of hallucinations, delusions, agitation, mania, depression, and disorganized behavior • Unless the infection or inflammation also involves other organs, minimal systemic findings may be present in the beginning	• RPR/VDRL • HIV • ANA • ESR/CRP • CBC • Lumbar puncture	• RPR/VDRL and an HIV test should be considered as part of the work-up of psychosis in those who have risk factors (e.g., use of intravenous drugs, unprotected sex with multiple partners, or a history of sex with prostitutes) • Inflammatory markers, ANAs, and more specific antibody tests may also be considered, as clinically indicated
Electrolyte disturbance hypercalcemia, hyponatremia, or uremia)	• Acute to progressive course of lethargy, agitation, disorganization, delirium, or hallucinations	• Basic chemistry panel with calcium and magnesium	• Systemic symptoms are often present • In this case, psychosis is probably a component of delirium
Medication-induced psychosis	• Acute onset of hallucinations, delusions, disorganization, and cognitive deficits following drug ingestion	• Urine drug screen	• Opioids, steroids, stimulants, anticholinergics, dopamine agonists, etc. • Lithium

ANA, antinuclear antibody; CBC, complete blood count; CRP, C-reactive protein; EPS, extrapyramidal symptoms; ESR, erythrocyte sedimentation rate; HIV, human immunodeficiency virus; RPR, rapid plasma reagin; VDRL, Venereal Disease Research Laboratories.

CHAPTER 5 Psychotic Disorders

Patients with delirium frequently have impaired levels of consciousness, such as disorientation and impaired ability to sustain attention. Dementia should be considered as a causative factor for psychotic symptoms as about 30% of patients with dementia have comorbid psychosis. Table 5.5 helps to distinguish between delirium, dementia, and primary psychosis.

STEP 3: ADDRESS MEDICATION- OR SUBSTANCE-INDUCED PSYCHOSIS

Medication-induced psychosis is another potential cause of formal thought disorders and perceptual abnormalities. This typically occurs in the elderly population, although it may also occur in patients who have renal or hepatic impairment with reduced drug clearance. Polypharmacy is another potential precipitant of psychotic symptoms as the risk for drug–drug interactions is elevated. Possible culprits include anticholinergics, sedative-hypnotics, opioid analgesics, anticonvulsants, theophylline, digoxin, and some antidepressants. The most important clue in such cases is the clinical history and timing of symptoms in the susceptible patient.

Psychotic symptoms may occur due to substance intoxication and withdrawal. Psychoactive substances range from phencyclidine (PCP), lysergic acid (LSD), cocaine, methamphetamines, alcohol, and marijuana. Patients with a history of alcoholism may have a related thiamine deficiency and develop Korsakoff psychosis with resultant confabulation, deficits in memory, and diminished ability to perform ADLs. Patients may also develop transient psychotic symptoms in the setting of alcohol withdrawal or delirium tremens. Cocaine and methamphetamine intoxication–related psychosis is very similar to that of the paranoid subtype of schizophrenia. Most substance-induced psychoses resolve over a brief period of time (usually 3 hours to 3 days of detoxification) and therefore would not require prolonged treatment other than counseling about cessation from the offending substance. However, some substances like ecstasy or methylenedioxymethamphetamine (MDMA) may cause persistent psychotic symptoms. The causal association may be difficult to establish and usually requires at least a 3- to 4-week period of sobriety to solidify a diagnosis and treatment plan. Many patients with chronic psychosis are also at high risk for comorbid substance use and should be monitored accordingly.

NOT TO BE MISSED

- Systemic medical conditions
- Delirium
- Dementia
- Mood disorders
- Medication-induced psychosis
- Substance-induced psychosis
- Suicidal and homicidal ideation or intent

STEP 4: ASSESS FOR OTHER PSYCHIATRIC CONDITIONS

Psychiatric causes of psychotic symptoms are summarized in Table 5.6. Mood disorders, such as major depressive disorder and bipolar I disorder, are commonly associated with episodic or temporally associated psychosis. Patients with severe depression may experience nonbizarre delusions associated with contamination, guilt, paranoid thoughts, or auditory hallucinations commanding them to hurt themselves. Patients with psychosis that is directly related to depression will usually report worsening psychosis when the depression is severe. Conversely, when depressive symptoms subside, psychotic symptoms usually improve or disappear entirely. Psychosis in the context of a bipolar manic or mixed episode often presents with expansive, grandiose delusions of infinite wealth or special powers. We recommend all patients with even subtle psychotic symptoms be thoroughly assessed

Table 5.5 Differentiating between Delirium, Dementia, and Primary Psychosis

	DESCRIPTION	PSYCHOPATHO-LOGIC CAUSE	PROTOTYPIC DISEASES	DIFFERENTIATING FACTORS
Delirium	• Fluctuating mental status, with reduced attention, focus, and cognition • Usually reversible	• Global CNS dysfunction that is often from a medical illness or drug side effects • Often in older patients or those with serious medical problems	• Infections (e.g., urinary tract infections, pneumonia) • CNS disorders (e.g., stroke, dementia) • Illicit drugs (e.g., cocaine, methamphetamine, alcohol) • Other serious medical conditions (e.g., end-stage liver disease, untreated renal failure)	• Patients typically present with fluctuations in attention, and may be distractible or disoriented and confused. • Symptoms fluctuate and are often worse at night. • Condition usually corrects once the offending agent is stopped or the illness is treated.
Dementia	• Progressive, chronic cognitive and functional decline • Rarely reversible	• Cortical or subcortical deterioration from various causes. • Vascular dementia is caused by the multitude of conditions associated with cerebral vascular accidents	• Cortical 　○ Alzheimer disease 　○ Frontotemporal disease 　○ Lewy body disease • Subcortical 　○ Parkinson disease 　○ Huntington disease 　○ Wilson disease • Infectious (sometimes reversible) 　○ HIV-associated dementia 　○ Neurosyphilis • Other 　○ Thiamine, niacin, and folate deficiencies 　○ Vascular dementia	• Patients typically present with chronic decline in cognitive function and memory. • In the nonadvanced stages, reality testing is usually initially intact.
Primary psychosis	• Impaired understanding of reality and often accompanied by: 　○ Delusions 　○ Hallucinations 　○ Mood disturbances 　○ Bizarre speech and behaviors 　○ Poor insight 　○ Amotivation with affective flattening	• Although the cause of schizophrenia is not known for certain, positive symptoms are related to dopamine excess in the mesolimbic system of the brain.	• Schizophrenia • Schizoaffective disorder	• Attention and orientation are generally preserved, except if the psychosis occurs in the context of a delirium. • Patients may have delusions or auditory or visual hallucinations and may have difficulty reasoning. • Delusions, hallucinations, or severe negative symptoms may interfere with the ability to function in society. • If symptoms are acute or present after the age of 40, consider a general medical cause (e.g., neurosyphilis, vitamin deficiency, illicit drug use, or a cerebral vascular accident).

CNS, central nervous system; HIV, human immunodeficiency virus.

CHAPTER 5 Psychotic Disorders

Table 5.6 Differentiating Psychiatric Causes of Psychosis

PSYCHOTIC DISORDER	PRESENTATION (SYMPTOMS AND MENTAL STATUS FINDINGS)
Schizophrenia	• One month of active psychosis with evidence of at least 6 months of intermittent or attenuated psychotic symptoms and diminished social or occupational function
Brief psychotic disorder	• Time-limited psychosis directly related to a distressing event in a person's life
Schizophreniform disorder	• The criteria for active phase schizophrenia is present for <6 months
Psychotic disorder not otherwise specified (NOS)	• Transient, clinically significant psychotic symptoms and psychotic symptoms that do not satisfy diagnostic criteria for other psychotic disorders.
Schizoaffective disorder	• Co-occurring psychotic symptoms and mood disturbance that may be difficult to distinguish from mood, psychotic, dissociative, somatic, or personality disorders • Psychotic symptoms are present during periods of normal mood • Categorized as depressed or bipolar type
Delusional disorder	• "Nonbizarre" delusion(s) that may actually occur in the real world
Bipolar disorder	• *Episodic* mood disorder usually characterized by depressive or manic symptoms • Psychotic symptoms may occur during either depressive or manic episodes and usually remit upon treatment of the mood abnormality
Major depressive disorder	• *Episodic* periods of depression and temporally associated psychotic symptoms • Psychotic symptoms may occur during a depressive episode and usually remit upon treatment of the mood abnormality
Posttraumatic stress disorder (PTSD)	• PTSD is often associated with hypervigilance, which can be confused with paranoia, and re-experiencing symptoms in severe form may include outright perceptual disturbances (e.g., auditory or visual hallucinations)
Borderline personality disorder	• Personality disorder characterized by dysregulation of affect and tendency toward brief periods of psychotic symptoms during distress
Dissociative disorders	• Disorders characterized by disruption of a continuous sense of self, including amnestic episodes or transition to altered behaviors and expressions
Substance intoxication or withdrawal	• Illicit drugs like cocaine, methamphetamine, heroin, and even alcohol can cause psychotic symptoms in the context of both intoxication and withdrawal
Malingering	• Intentionally produced symptoms for external gain (e.g., disability insurance or to avoid legal prosecution)

for comorbid psychiatric disorders using the AMPS screening tool (see Chapter 1).

Biopsychosocial Treatment

TREATMENT PRINCIPLES

In general, symptomatic treatment of psychosis should be instituted with an antipsychotic medication concurrently with treatment for the underlying etiology so long as the antipsychotic medication is tolerated.

For example, those who have major depressive disorder with psychotic features should be treated with an antipsychotic and an antidepressant medication until the psychotic depressive episode remits. In most cases, once the psychosis is resolved, treatment with an antidepressant should continue indefinitely. When treating psychosis associated with general medical disorders, treatment of the primary medical problem is critical. For example, masking a patient's psychotic symptoms and behavioral agitation in delirium solely with antipsychotic medication may delay the detection of an impending medical emergency (e.g., septic shock from failure to detect a respiratory infection). For patients with primary, chronic psychotic disorders such as schizophrenia, early diagnosis and treatment are associated with improved outcomes (10). Finally, as patients with chronic psychosis lose the ability to work and their family members suffer from various forms of stigma (e.g., guilt, shame, and isolation), the clinician should consider a comprehensive treatment plan that includes facilitation and referral to psychological support and social services.

PHARMACOTHERAPY

Since their introduction over 50 years ago, antipsychotic or "neuroleptic" medications and their indications have proliferated. In addition to treating psychosis, they are effective and have Food and Drug Administration (FDA) approval for the treatment of movement disorders, mood disorders, and acute agitation.

The first-generation antipsychotics (FGAs) are sometimes referred to as *typical* antipsychotics. They are much more likely to result in immediate and long-term motor problems like tardive dyskinesia (TD). High-potency antipsychotics (e.g., haloperidol) have a high potential for extrapyramidal symptoms (EPS) due to high dopamine-2 receptor (DA-2) blockade per unit dose. Low-potency antipsychotics (e.g., chlorpromazine) have a decreased affinity for the DA-2 receptor and therefore a much lower chance for EPS. The SGAs or *atypical* antipsychotics are less likely to result in EPS but are more expensive and associated with metabolic side effects. Although FGAs and SGAs are both thought to be equally effective treatments for schizophrenia and schizoaffective disorder, we recommend using SGAs as first-line treatment given the lower likelihood for the largely treatment-resistant TD and other EPS.

General Efficacy

Once antipsychotics are administered, psychotic symptom reduction usually occurs within 1 to 2 weeks, although optimal response may take as long as 6 months. For those who adhere to the treatment plan, approximately 50% of patients with schizophrenia respond to an antipsychotic medication, 25% respond partially, and 25% have little to no response (11). Over time the goal is a reduction in *positive* symptoms. An immediate improvement in behavior may be seen because of the tranquilizing effect of antipsychotics. In primary psychotic disorders, negative symptoms and cognitive deficits will generally be more refractory to medication treatment. In fact, the presence of negative symptoms carries a worse long-term prognosis when compared to someone who has predominantly positive symptoms. A patient should be ideally re-evaluated within at least 2 to 4 weeks to assess for side effects, improvement, and further medication dose titration. There should be a low threshold for switching antipsychotics in this initial period if there is insignificant improvement, worsening of symptoms, or emergence of intolerable side effects (12).

For the initial treatment of psychosis, it is reasonable to select one of the agents listed in Table 5.7 and then arrange for psychiatric follow-up. The contemporary first-line treatment for psychotic disorders is to start a SGA medication, except clozapine, which is indicated for treatment resistant schizophrenia. The choice is largely determined by the potential side effects, availability, and cost.

Side Effects

Side effects to antipsychotic medications can be conceptually grouped into short- and long-term side effects (Table 5.7). The short-term side effects usually present within 1 month of starting or increasing the dose of an antipsychotic. These include EPS, anticholinergic effects, orthostatic hypotension, sedation, and a prolonged QT interval on an electrocardiogram. The long-term side effects include irreversible movement disorders, metabolic disorders, and idiosyncratic effects of specific antipsychotics.

EPS are movement symptoms that result from DA-2 blockade of regulatory neurons that modulate descending motor neurons. They include akathisia, dystonic reactions, parkinsonian syndrome, neuroleptic malignant syndrome (NMS), and TD.

Akathisia Akathisia is a subjective, often intolerable, inner restlessness or sensation of the need to move. Patients with akathisia appear hyperkinetic and may anxiously say, "I feel like I want to crawl out of my skin." Fortunately, for most patients, akathisia is a transient reaction that may remit spontaneously over a few weeks. To reduce akathisia, the antipsychotic may be reduced in dose or switched to another agent with a lower potential for EPS. For symptomatic treatment, propranolol may be added at 10 mg BID/TID and rapidly increased as tolerated to up to 20 to 100 mg BID. Benzodiazepines are also effective for the treatment of akathisia.

Dystonia Dystonic reactions usually occur within a few hours to days of starting an antipsychotic and are characterized by painful, uncontrollable tightening of muscles, usually involving the neck, back, or lateral ocular muscles. Intramuscular (IM) injection of anticholinergic medications, such as diphenhydramine (25 mg) or benztropine (2 mg), is a rapid and effective treatment. The emergence of dystonia can be a frightening experience for the patient, and reassurance coupled with education is critical to maintaining a trusting clinician–patient relationship and ongoing adherence with a treatment plan.

Table 5.7 First-Line Antipsychotic Medications for Schizophrenia[a]

	STARTING DOSE	TARGET RANGE[a] (MG/DAY)	PRIMARY CARE TITRATION SCHEDULE	SIDE EFFECTS[b]	MONITORING
Risperidone[c] (Risperdal)	1 mg BID or 2 mg QHS	4–6	Increase up to 2 mg daily, as tolerated	EPS (++) Hyperprolactinemia (+++) Orthostatic hypotension (++) Metabolic abnormalities (++) Sedation (++)	**Initial:** • Baseline weight and body mass index, vital signs, fasting plasma glucose, and lipid profile • Consider doing a pregnancy test and drug toxicology • Brain imaging and a neurologic exam should be done if psychotic symptoms present after the age of 50 • An ECG should be performed on patients who have cardiac disease and start ziprasidone
Olanzapine (Zyprexa)	5–10 mg QHS	10–20	Increase 5 mg every 3–5 days, as tolerated	EPS (+) Orthostatic hypotension (+) Metabolic (+++) Sedation (++)	
Quetiapine[d] (Seroquel)	50–100 mg BID	300–800	Increase 50–100 mg every 2 days, as tolerated (monitor for orthostatic hypotension)	EPS (+/–) Orthostatic hypotension (+++) Metabolic abnormalities (++) Sedation (+++)	**First 4 weeks:** BMI, EPS, vital signs, prolactin (if clinical symptoms of hyperprolactinemia exist) **First 12 weeks:** BMI, EPS, vital signs, fasting glucose, a lipid profile **Quarterly:** BMI **Annually:** BMI, EPS, fasting glucose **Every 3–5 years:** lipid panel
Quetiapine XR (Seroquel XR)	300 mg QHS	400–800	Increase every 1–2 days, as tolerated	EPS (+/–) Orthostatic hypotension (+++) Metabolic abnormalities (++) Sedation (+++)	
Ziprasidone[e] (Geodon)	40 mg BID (with food)[f]	160	Increase every other day to target dose, as tolerated	EPS (+) Orthostatic hypotension (+) Metabolic abnormalities (+) Sedation (++) QTc prolongation (++)	
Aripiprazole (Abilify)	10–15 mg QAM	10–30	Increase dose after 2 days, as tolerated	EPS (+) Orthostatic hypotension (+) Metabolic abnormalities (+) Sedation (+)	
Paliperidone[g] (Invega)	6 mg QAM	6–12	Increase by increments of 3 mg every 5 days, as tolerated	EPS (++) Orthostatic hypotension (+) Metabolic abnormalities (++) Sedation (++)	

BMI, body mass index; ECG, electrocardiogram; EPS, extrapyramidal symptoms.
[a] Dosing information derived from Lehman AF, Lieberman JA, Dixon LB, et al; American Psychiatric Association. Practice guideline for the treatment of patients with schizophrenia, second edition. *Am J Psychiatry.* 2004;161(S2):1–56 and the authors' clinical expert opinion. These doses do not apply to geriatric or pediatric patients.
[b] Metabolic effects include hyperglycemia, weight gain, and hyperlipidemia.
[c] Patient may be able to transition to an intramuscular depot formulation of risperidone.
[d] Because of its low potency, quetiapine is ideal for patients who are sensitive to EPS or patients with psychosis in the context of Parkinson disease.
[e] Contraindications to the use of ziprasidone include persistent QTc >500 msec, recent acute myocardial infarction, and uncompensated heart failure.
[f] Ziprasidone should be taken with food as it increases bioavailability.
[g] Paliperidone is structurally similar to risperidone. Because it is the newest antipsychotic medication, the relative risks for metabolic syndrome and EPS are not fully known.

CHAPTER 5 Psychotic Disorders

Parkinsonian Syndrome Parkinsonian syndrome mimics idiopathic Parkinson disease and may include masked facies, rigidity, bradykinesia, pill-rolling tremor, micrographia, or a shuffling gate with postural instability. Oral anticholinergic medications such as diphenylhydramine (25 to 50 mg TID), trihexyphenidyl (5 to 10 mg bid), or benztropine (1 to 2 mg BID) may be helpful in reducing these symptoms. These medications may also be used for EPS prophylaxis against high-potency antipsychotic medications such as haloperidol. If used for prophylactic treatment, they can generally be tapered and stopped after 10 days. In those who poorly tolerate anticholinergic medications (e.g., patients with dementia), amantadine 100 to 300 mg BID may be used to treat parkinsonian symptoms, although the lowest effective antipsychotic dose should be used.

Neuroleptic Malignant Syndrome Neuroleptic malignant syndrome (NMS) is a rare, life-threatening side effect of FGAs and SGAs. NMS usually occurs immediately following the initiation or increased dose of an antipsychotic medication. It is characterized by muscle rigidity, autonomic dysregulation, fever, leukocytosis, increase in serum creatinine phosphokinase (>300 U/mL), and acute confusion. Gross muscle rigidity may not necessarily occur with NMS from the use of atypical antipsychotics. NMS is difficult to evaluate in the outpatient setting and usually requires emergency medical management.

Tardive Dyskinesia Tardive dyskinesia is a long-term EPS and can develop at a rate of about 3% to 5% per year for FGAs. Nonrhythmic, quick, choreoathetoid movements of the face, trunk, and extremities characterize TD. Examination for writhing of the tongue, hands, or trunk should be checked every 6 to 12 months as this condition is generally permanent with no known treatment. TD can occur with SGAs at a rate of about 0.8% per year. TD risk factors include older age, longer use of antipsychotics, brain damage, diabetes mellitus, and comorbid mood disorder (13).

Common short-term antipsychotic side effects include dry mouth, sedation, and transient orthostatic hypotension. More serious and rare short-term side effects are arrhythmias caused by prolonged QTc and lowered seizure threshold. Long-term antipsychotic side effects are metabolic conditions including weight gain, hyperglycemia, and hyperlipidemia. The potential for metabolic abnormalities exists for all SGAs, but clozapine and olanzapine carry a higher relative risk. The American Diabetes Association and American Psychiatric Association (APA) recommend routine screening and follow-up of metabolic profiles in patients on chronic SGA treatment, as outlined in Table 5.7 (3).

Duration of Pharmacotherapy

For patients with chronic psychotic disorders, the APA recommends at least 1 year of antipsychotic continuation after remission of the psychotic episode. Because relapse rates are so high after a psychotic episode (~80% in 5 years), indefinite treatment with antipsychotics is usually indicated. In 2004, the APA consensus guidelines recommended lifelong antipsychotic treatment in patients with primary psychotic disorders if two psychotic episodes occur within a 5-year period (3).

Special Considerations in Pharmacotherapy

Medication adherence is particularly problematic in those with chronic psychotic disorders because these patients usually have impaired executive functioning. Once-daily medication regimens are optimal. Additionally, injectable depot formulations exist for haloperidol, fluphenazine, and risperidone. Depot formulations provide consistent blood levels and increase patient contact as depot medications are administered every 2 to 4 weeks. From another perspective, patients often struggle with the diagnosis of schizophrenia (and other severe mental illness) and therefore become discouraged about the indefinite need to take antipsychotic medications. In such scenarios, the provider can highlight the possibility of improved functioning, decreased need for hospitalization, achieving independence, and maintaining relationships and employment.

Clozapine is a highly effective antipsychotic that improves both positive and negative psychotic symptoms. Unfortunately, it is not used as a first-line treatment due to its slow titration schedule, the potential for serious side effects, and the need for frequent blood draws. Patients who are on clozapine receive weekly leukocyte monitoring to monitor the development of agranulocytosis for the first 6 months and monitoring frequency is then reduced and continued for the duration of clozapine treatment. Other idiosyncratic side effects include frequent development of sialorrhea and rare occurrence of myocarditis. Due to its anticholinergic, antihistaminic, and anti–alpha-adrenergic effects, clozapine is notorious for its association with delirium in vulnerable populations, sedation, and orthostatic hypotension, respectively. Because of these side effects and the increased chance for seizures, we suggest clozapine be prescribed by a psychiatrist.

PSYCHOSOCIAL TREATMENT

General Considerations

The psychosocial needs of the patients with psychotic disorders depend on the etiology, course, and prognosis of their disorders. This section focuses on the psychosocial treatment options for schizophrenia, although many of the approaches could be considered for most patients who struggle with chronic psychotic symptoms. In general, the severity and persistent course of primary psychotic disorders requires much more psychosocial support than could be provided by traditional primary care medical systems. Since the main cause for morbidity is related to problems with relationships, employment status, cognitive function, and social deficits, treatment involves a multidisciplinary approach.

Patient and Family Education

Much like delivering bad news, clinicians may feel uncomfortable discussing psychotic symptoms and diagnosis with patients and their families. Psychosis itself can be a powerful barrier to the therapeutic alliance, causing misunderstanding or suspicion. Table 5.8 outlines several general points to help facilitate communication with a patient who is experiencing psychotic symptoms. It is important for the clinician to encourage the patient with schizophrenia or schizoaffective disorder to better understand the illness by utilizing available education and support networks (see Practical Resources). Patients and family members typically inquire about the etiology of psychotic symptoms. The provider should inquire about the patients' understanding of psychotic disorders and dispel myths about any wrongdoing on their part. An excess of dopamine via "the dopamine hypothesis" is the most agreed upon cause of primary psychotic disorders, although other neurotransmitters play a role. Schizophrenia is best understood as a multifactorial neurodevelopmental disorder. Concordance rates of schizophrenia in studies of monozygotic twins are only 50%, dramatically illustrating the additional role of environmental and developmental influences in expression of the illness.

It may not be necessary for the patient and family to initially accept the diagnosis of a primary psychotic disorder. Regardless, the patient's goals should be explored. Patients with schizophrenia share common goals compared with the general population, such as achieving independence, maintaining employment, and maintaining interpersonal relationships. The clinician may inquire about how psychotic symptoms are interfering with the patient's goals and explore ways to help the patient achieve these goals.

Both patients and loved ones will ask about the likely duration of their symptoms, the required length of medication treatment, and long-term prognosis. The clinician should avoid providing either an excessively grim or an unrealistic hopeful prognosis. Ultimate functional status varies by individual patients, although medication and psychosocial treatment will optimize long-term prognosis. After a first episode of psychosis due to schizophrenia, risk of a psychotic relapse is up to 80% in the first 5 years (3). Long-term outcomes vary for both symptomatic and functional recovery. Approximately 10% to 15% will be free of further episodes and about the same proportion will be chronically and severely psychotic (3). Patients with schizophrenia who adhere to treatment have a higher likelihood of productive work, advanced education, and independent living.

Family support and vocational rehabilitation appear to increase the likelihood of good outcomes. Family education and support are critical, as this means that the patient will have an advocate, and most frequently a "social safety net" for the provision of basic needs such as food and shelter (14). Family members often struggle with caring for the individual as much as possible without seeking outside help, often due to stigma. While there are advantages to having active caretaker involvement, the patient may struggle with the lack of individual autonomy and overinvolvement from caretakers. Family members often underestimate the possibilities that the patient can achieve due to their own misconceptions about schizophrenia. The provider is encouraged to

Table 5.8 Suggestions for Communicating with Patients who Have Psychosis

GOAL	WHAT YOU MIGHT SAY
Normalize	• "In my practice, many patients have experienced (symptom); have you experienced this as well?" • "Having schizophrenia is very common. In fact, 1% of people in the United States have schizophrenia at some point in their lives."
Empathize, don't collude	• "If it's all right, I would like to learn more about how the voices affect your life."
Ask, don't tell	• "How do you feel when this happens?" or "How do you cope when this happens?" is usually better than "I'd be scared if that happened to me," or "This sounds frightening," unless the patient is indicating a particular emotional state.
Validate, without confirming reality of the patient's symptoms	• *Patient*: "You believe me, don't you, doctor? Can't you see them too?" • *Doctor:* "I believe that these symptoms are very real and troubling to you, and I do not think you are making things up."
Bring up psychotic symptoms in context of more normal experiences	• "The brain is very powerful, and we all have a strong mind–body connection. Have you ever cried or laughed when you watched a movie? Nothing was happening to you when you cried, but you were sad. Your mind lets you experience that sadness, and told you that you were sad. Similarly, your mind has you experiencing voices and visions that others aren't experiencing. Does that make sense?"
Discussing diagnosis: inquiry and biases	• "Have you heard of the term *hallucination* or *delusion*? What does that mean to you? What do you know about people who experience this? What happens to them?"
Preparation of key messages	• For any discussion of diagnosis or prognosis, prepare your key statements in advance. What are the three concise things that you want your patient and their family members to remember? For instance: 1. "You have a disease called schizophrenia." 2. "It is common and has many treatments. Together, we'll find the best treatment for you." 3. "With the right treatment, many people enjoy a good quality of life."

CHAPTER 5 Psychotic Disorders

refer caretakers and family members to support groups and community education programs.

Food, Housing, Income, and Employment

Cognitive deficits and negative symptoms in schizophrenia often lead to an inability to maintain employment and secure food and shelter. Only 10% of those with schizophrenia live in an independent living environment. For those who struggle to secure housing, there are several housing options that are available for patients with severe mental illness. Some patients may live in homeless shelters and charity programs because their income assistance is insufficient for independent housing. Some patients live in low-cost hotels (single-room occupancy) or rooming homes (room and boards). Many patients choose such arrangements because this provides them more autonomy and independence. They are usually savvy about local resources and use free food and clothing programs. Other patients live in board and care facilities, which provide food, activities, and assistance with medication administration.

Patients with primary psychotic disorders may qualify for general public assistance with food and limited monetary support, public housing, social security disability income, and government-sponsored health care insurance. These programs are region specific and administered by different agencies at different levels of government. Therefore, a social work or mental health program referral is indicated for everyone with severe mental illness, as it can be a challenge to navigate "the system."

Evidence-Based Psychosocial Practices

Psychoeducational and CBT are validated interventions for primary psychotic disorders. Both modalities require specialized training. In the United Kingdom, CBT or psychoeducation is provided as standard of care as part of the National Health Service (15). In CBT, patients learn to identify their cognitive distortions and consequent behaviors. For example, a patient will learn to challenge his own paranoia by examining events that support this belief system and evidence that does not. "I think that someone is watching me right now. But, I haven't seen anyone watching me in the past 5 years, even when I've looked around the corner today. Is someone really watching me?" The patient eventually reconciles his delusions as part of schizophrenia rather than reality. The patient may also be encouraged to design "behavioral experiments" to examine the evidence. There is an emerging movement to adopt CBT and other psychiatric rehabilitation programs in many mental health programs throughout the United States. Cognitive remediation therapy via rehearsal of predesigned cognitive tasks is an additional treatment modality that is actively researched for patients early in the course of a psychotic disorder to improve their cognitive capacity.

An intensive model of case management, termed *Assertive Community Treatment* (ACT), involves a multidisciplinary team that will tailor support for the patient to prevent relapse and rehospitalization. The ACT team will typically seek the patient out in the community (including homeless shelters), provide medication and outreach services, and, when necessary, facilitate emergency psychiatric hospitalization (16).

Practice Pointers

WHEN TO REFER

- Suicidal or homicidal ideation
- Grave disability or the inability to care for self due to mental illness
- Persistent psychotic symptoms that are resistant to initial treatment
- Diagnostic uncertainty
- Psychosocial treatments or the need for more intensive case management
- Psychosis in the pregnant or postpartum patient
- Comorbid pathology

Case 1: Initial work-up and treatment of psychotic symptoms

Susan is a 28-year-old woman who presents with her boyfriend for worsening anxiety and insomnia. During the exam, she is nervous and staring intently at the walls. She states that she is afraid of demons, as they have been asking her to do "weird things." Her boyfriend states that she has not been eating or bathing regularly. Her real estate business has fallen off by 50%, because she can't "close the deal."

When asked about the "weird" things, she giggles and says, "I don't know." She first noticed the voices 5 months ago and is unable to determine if they sound like a male or female. The voices do not tell her to hurt herself, or others. She denies any other auditory or visual hallucinations, suicidal ideation, or homicidal ideation. Other symptoms include insomnia, anxiety, uneasy feelings that she might be harmed, and disinterest in her usual leisure or social activities. In fact, the patient has not left her house for the last 4 weeks and has not expressed any concerns about her work. The patient denies substance use and she is currently not taking any medications. She does not know of any medical problems and her appetite has been fair, although she requires frequent prompting from her boyfriend during mealtime.

On exam, her hygiene is fair, although it appears that her clothing and hair are unkempt. She has an intense stare and her affect has decreased reactivity (blunting). Her vitals and physical exam are unremarkable.

Discussion: *Susan reports positive symptoms of hallucinations and paranoid delusions and has negative symptoms of affective blunting and amotivation. Her illness has impaired her ADLs and ability to work for less than 6 months, which makes the diagnosis of schizophreniform disorder likely. Prior to making a primary psychotic disorder diagnosis, secondary psychosis from a general medical disorder or substance misuse should be ruled out.*

Screening lab tests including complete blood count (CBC), metabolic panel, liver enzymes, human immunodeficiency virus (HIV) test, syphilis serology, thyroid-stimulating hormone (TSH), and a urinalysis are all normal. You discuss with the patient your concern that she has a schizophrenia-like illness, which can be helped by medication. You decide to start her on risperidone 2 mg by oral route each night and asked the patient and her boyfriend to call you should she develop galactorrhea or any rigidity in her extremities. You warn them that mild side effects such as dizziness, nausea, or restlessness may occur, and that if mild, they will likely go away over time. She is given reading material about other potential side effects and a referral to psychiatry is initiated.

Susan returns 2 weeks later for a follow-up appointment. She reports that she tolerated the medication well and has been taking her medication diligently. She occasionally hears indistinct voices but notes that they are less frequent and intense. She now confides that she is concerned about being followed, although not as much as before. She has started to take care of her own needs and has started reading some information about schizophrenia and she asks you whether she will be able to return to work in the near future. She again denies command hallucinations or suicidal ideation and has no access to firearms.

Discussion: *Susan has moderate improvement in her symptoms, although residual psychosis persists. She appears to be tolerating the medication well and without significant adverse effects. Her mood and level of interest in pleasurable activities are also improving. It is important to inquire about suicidal ideation during each visit since the recovering period may be associated with an increase in suicidal thoughts, especially if the patient has good premorbid functioning and is having difficulty adjusting to the prognosis of a chronic psychotic disorder. As the patient is tolerating the medication, the provider may increase the risperidone dose to 3 mg by oral route nightly and continue to monitor for treatment adherence, suicidal thoughts, EPS, and other side effects. The provider should offer realistic hope to the patient because her symptoms are improving and inform her that, although uncertain, she may resume her work. Refer to Table 5.6 on communication about diagnosis.*

In this case, the final diagnosis should be made by a psychiatrist. In the future, the provider will communicate with the consulting psychiatrist about continued treatment. Referral to community education, support groups, and social services should be facilitated. Also, if the patient were to continue antipsychotic treatment indefinitely, she will need her weight and blood pressure checked on each visit and a fasting blood glucose drawn at week 12 and annually thereafter. A fasting lipid panel should be checked at week 12 and every 3 to 5 years thereafter (see Table 5.7). The dose of the antipsychotic should be kept at the minimal effective dose possible during the maintenance phase and may need to be switched to another agent if severe side effects develop.

Case 2: Psychosis during a depressive episode
A 34-year-old woman has had treatment-resistant depression for 4 months despite several antidepressant trials. On a follow-up visit, she presents more

melancholic, psychomotor retarded, and sad. Her hair is matted and she clearly has not bathed in recent time. She is malodorous and pale, and has lost 15 pounds over the past 6 months. For the most part, she talks and moves slowly until she anxiously rebuffs your attempt at a cursory physical exam, saying that she is "contaminated" and "contagious."

Concerned, you ask how she is "contaminated." She solemnly informs you that her insides have "putrefied" and that she is "utterly evil." Anything she touches will turn evil, too. She has been a long-term patient of yours who has had several depressive episodes in the past, which have usually responded to increases in her selective serotonin reuptake inhibitor (SSRI) treatment. The course of this episode is particularly severe; you have never noticed such poor hygiene, pronounced psychomotor retardation, and slowed speech from her before. In no other episode had you endorsed a leave of absence from work. She is normally fastidious about keeping appointments but has not shown up for the last three. Her brother had arranged this appointment and escorted the patient here. The family has been worried that she has shut herself in at home and stopped calling them.

Just prior to her coming to the appointment you reviewed the laboratory values from her last visit 2 months ago. There is no evidence of thyroid dysfunction, anemia, or metabolic derangements. She has refused to allow the nurse to take vital signs prior to this appointment. She had a hysterectomy for fibroids and an occasional headache but otherwise has a fairly unremarkable past medical history.

You say that it must be terrible to feel "contaminated." The patient stares blankly at you and mutters, "I must purge it." She refuses to speak again. Concerned about suicide, you call 911 and explain the case to the dispatcher, requesting that the patient be escorted for emergency psychiatric evaluation.

Discussion: *The patient is exhibiting signs of severe depression with psychotic features. As often occurs in such cases, the diagnosis in this patient is suggested by historical information, collateral reports, and her presentation. The course of illness is fairly typical. Often those with psychotic depression will have had previous depressive episodes that become more severe over time, until there is an episode that presents with psychosis. Patients who have severe depression with psychotic features often present with delusions or hallucinations. Moreover, those who have severe depression with psychotic features generally have a full remission of psychosis upon successful treatment of the depression. In this case, the delusion of contamination and contagion are "mood congruent" or consistent with profound depression. Bizarre, incongruent delusions are usually suggestive of bipolar psychosis, schizoaffective disorder, or schizophrenia.*

The patient returns for a follow-up appointment 2 months later. She still seems somewhat sad, but otherwise much improved. She is taking a combination of olanzapine and fluoxetine to control her symptoms. The patient has already seen a psychiatrist, whom she says confirmed the diagnosis of severe depression with psychotic features. She laughs nervously and says, "The belief about contamination felt very real at the time." She expresses concern that she may become "schizophrenic like my uncle."

Discussion: *Treatment of major depressive disorder with psychotic features initially includes a combination of antipsychotic and antidepressant medication. To spare the patient long-term consequences of antipsychotic medication exposure, the antipsychotic may be discontinued with a downward taper after the depressive episode fully remits. An antipsychotic agent should be reinstituted if the psychotic symptoms return. Given the chance of another depressive episode, the antidepressant should remain as prophylaxis against future depressive episodes.*

Psychiatric hospitalization is often a rapid way to connect patients to mental health services, especially in acutely psychotic patients who are gravely disabled (i.e., inability to secure housing, food or clothing). Those patients who have psychotic symptoms during depressive episodes often have an increased chance of developing schizophrenia or schizoaffective disorder. In this case, the patient reports a second-degree relative with schizophrenia. The patient does have a somewhat increased risk of developing schizophrenia, although it will be less and less likely as she gets older without developing full-spectrum schizophrenia. Her overall prognosis will significantly worsen if she starts to use illicit drugs.

Case 3: Antipsychotic medication use with Parkinson disease

An 80-year-old man with Parkinson disease and related dementia as well as frequent urinary tract infections presents with concerns of progressive confusion. He reports that the nursing home staff is abusing him and keeping him away from his family. He also believes that his dead wife has been visiting him regularly. The nursing home caregiver says the patient has been more aggressive and confrontational. He has been leaving the nursing home and wandering into the street.

Discussion: *This patient may have psychosis related to the progression of his Parkinson disease, medications used to treat Parkinson disease, or delirium caused by a urinary tract infection. An antipsychotic must be chosen that will be the least likely to worsen his movement symptoms. Because it is a very-low-potency dopamine antagonist, quetiapine is the most reasonable choice. Given the patient's age, the lowest possible dose of quetiapine (12.5 to 25 mg at night) should be started and then titrated up as tolerated. Particularly problematic side effects of quetiapine in the elderly are its central and peripheral anticholinergic effects, risk of inducing orthostasis, and sedation.*

Dementia with Lewy bodies (DLB) should be considered as part of the differential diagnosis as it can look similar to Parkinson with dementia, where cognitive deficits usually predominate with a fluctuating mental status. Patients with DLB are highly sensitive to the extrapyramidal side effects of antipsychotic medications. It is also important to note that dopaminergic agonists used to treat Parkinson disease may cause or worsen psychotic symptoms. Therefore, the clinician must find a balance between improving the motor symptoms of Parkinson disease and exacerbating or inducing psychosis. If delirium (i.e., altered mental status secondary to a systemic medical condition) is ruled out, the patient would likely need long-term antipsychotic treatment. Antipsychotic medications are associated with an increased risk of mortality in the elderly, and this must be discussed with the caretakers, weighed against the benefit of treating psychosis or agitation, and documented in the medical record.

ICD9	
Schizophrenia	*295.xx*
Paranoid Type	*0.30*
Disorganized Type	*0.10*
Catatonic Type	*0.20*
Undifferentiated Type	*0.90*
Residual	*0.60*
Delusional Disorder	*297.10*
Psychotic Disorder NOS	*298.9*
Psychotic Disorder with Delusions Due to [General Medical Condition]	*293.81*
Psychotic Disorder with Hallucinations Due to [General Medical Condition]	*293.82*
Schizoaffective Disorder	*295.70*
Schizophreniform Disorder	*296.40*
Shared Psychotic Disorder	*297.3*

Practical Resources

National Alliance on Mental Illness: http://www.nami.org/Has complete listings of professional and consumer support with local chapters.
National Institute of Mental Health: http://www.nimh.nih.gov/Has up-to-date information on diagnosis, prevention, and treatment
National Alliance on Research for Schizophrenia and Depression: http://www.narsad.org/Has up-to-date information on research on the etiology, treatment, and prognosis of schizophrenia and depression

References

1. Olfson M, Lewis-Fernandez R, Weissman M, et al. Psychotic symptoms in an urban general medicine practice. *Am J Psychiatry.* 2002;159:1412–1419.

2. Beng-Choon H, Black DW, Andreasen NC. Schizophrenia and other psychotic disorders. In: Hales RE, Yudofsky S, eds. *Essentials of Clinical Psychiatry.* Washington, DC: American Psychiatric Publishing, Inc.; 2004:189–241.

3. Lehman AF, Lieberman JA, Dixon LB, et al; American Psychiatric Association. Practice guideline for the treatment of patients with schizophrenia, second edition. *Am J Psychiatry.* 2004;161(S2):1–56.

4. Green MF. Cognitive impairment and functional outcome in schizophrenia and bipolar disorder. *J Clin Psychiatry.* 2006;67(Suppl 9):3–8; discussion 36–42.

5. Rice DP. The economic impact of schizophrenia. *J Clin Psychiatry.* 1999;60(Suppl 1):4–6; discussion 28–30.

6. Auquier P, Lancon C, Rouillon F, et al. Mortality in schizophrenia. *Pharamcoepidemiol Drug Saf.* 2007;16(12):1308–1312.

7. Addington J, Cadenhead KS, Cannon TD, et al. North American prodrome longitudinal study: a collaborative multisite approach to prodromal schizophrenia research. *Schizophrenia Bull.* 2007;33(3):665–672.

8. American Psychiatric Association. *Diagnostic and Statistical Manual of Mental Disorders.* 4th ed., text revision. Washington, DC: American Psychiatric Publishing, Inc.; 2004.

9. Citrome L. Differential diagnosis of psychosis: a brief guide for the primary care physician. *Postgrad Med.* 1989;85(4):273–274, 279–280.

10. Perkins DO, Gu H, Boteva K, et al. Relationship between duration of untreated psychosis and outcome in first-episode schizophrenia: a critical review and meta-analysis. *Am J Psychiatry.* 2005;162(10):1785–1804.

11. Wilkaitis J, Mulvihill T, Nasrallah HA. Classic Antipsychotic Medications. In: Schatzberg MD, Nemeroff CB, eds. *Textbook of Psychopharmacology.* 3rd ed. Washington, DC: American Psychiatric Publishing, Inc.; 2004:435–441.

12. Lieberman JA, Stroup TS, McEvoy JP, et al. Effectiveness of antipsychotic drugs in patients with chronic schizophrenia. *N Engl J Med.* 2005;353:1209–1223.

13. Correl CU, Leucht S, Kane JM. Lower risk for tardive dyskinesia associated with second-generation antipsychotics: a systemic review of 1-year studies. *Am J Psychiatry.* 2004;161:414–425.

14. Dixon L, McFarlane WR, Lefley H, et al. Evidence-based practices for services to families of people with psychiatric disabilities. *Psychiatric Services.* 2001;52:903–910.

15. Turkington D, Kingdon D, Weiden PJ. Cognitive behavior therapy for schizophrenia. *Am J Psychiatry.* 2006;163:365–373.

16. Phillips SD, Burns BJ, Edgar ER, et al. Moving assertive community treatment into standard practice. *Psychiatric Services.* 2001;52:771–779.

CHAPTER 6

Substance Use Disorders—Stimulants and Opioids

Adrian Palomino, MD • Martin Leamon, MD •
Shelly L. Henderson, PhD

> *Jose is a 22-year-old student presenting with fatigue, dry cough, irritability, and depressed mood. He admits to smoking tobacco and drinking beer "once in a while." When he senses your nonjudgmental approach, he reveals, "I smoke meth only when I need to study."*

CLINICAL HIGHLIGHTS

- Substance use disorders (SUDs) occur in all demographic groups and are common in outpatient settings. Clues from the history and physical exam alert the clinician to their presence.

- A SUD is a chronic medical illness that requires a long-term treatment strategy. The primary care provider's emphasis on longitudinal relationships and preventative care is ideally suited to the management of SUDs.

- Substance users are at increased risk of developing human immunodeficiency virus (HIV), hepatitis B and C, and cardiovascular complications, as well as mood and anxiety disorders.

(Continued)

Clinical Significance

Substance-related disorders (SRDs) are divided into substance use disorders (SUDs) and substance-induced disorders (SIDs). SRDs are ubiquitous, costly, disabling, and potentially lethal. About 10% of Americans will abuse or become dependent on illicit substances such as stimulants (cocaine and methamphetamine) or opioids (heroin and opioid-based pain relievers) within their lifetime (1). In 2006, 4 million adult Americans met the criteria for a stimulant or opioid use disorder. No demographic group is immune: By 2050, SRDs in persons over the age of 65 are expected to double, while 44% of adolescents will have used illicit drugs by age 18. Primary care SRD prevalence estimates range between 10% and 20%. Underdiagnosis remains a common problem. One study found that only one half of clinicians routinely ask their patients about SRDs. Obstacles to clinical intervention include a lack of diagnostic confidence, lack of familiarity with treatment options, and pessimism regarding treatment outcome (2).

Diagnosis

SUDs include *misuse, abuse,* and *dependence* (3). Substance *dependence* is characterized by an overall loss of control over substance use (Table 6.1). Tolerance and withdrawal, reflecting physiologic dependence, are included in the definition, although neither is necessary to make the diagnosis (4). The hallmark of substance *abuse* is persistent use despite at least one profoundly negative interpersonal, legal, behavioral, or social consequence (Table 6.2). If the criteria for substance dependence have ever been met during the patient's lifetime, the diagnosis of abuse is precluded. Substance *misuse* has the potential for or is associated with some negative consequences, but does not meet formal diagnostic criteria. *Addiction* is a term without a formal diagnostic definition that is

Table 6.1 DSM-IV-TR Diagnostic Criteria for Substance Dependence

A maladaptive pattern of substance use, leading to clinically significant impairment or distress, as manifested by three (or more) of the following, occurring at any time in the same 12-month period:

1. Tolerance, as defined by either of the following:
   a. A need for markedly increased amounts of the substance to achieve intoxication or desired effect
   b. Markedly diminished effect with continued use of the same amount of the substance
2. Withdrawal, as manifested by either of the following:
   a. The characteristic withdrawal syndrome for the substance
   b. The same or closely related substance is taken to relieve or avoid withdrawal symptoms
3. The substance is often taken in larger amounts or over a longer period than was intended
4. There is a persistent desire or unsuccessful efforts to cut down or control substance use
5. A great deal of time is spent in activities necessary to obtain the substance, use the substance, or recover from its effects
6. Important social, occupational, or recreational activities are given up or reduced because of substance use
7. Substance use is continued despite knowledge of having a persistent or recurrent physical or psychological problem that is likely to have been caused or exacerbated by the substance

From American Psychiatric Association. *Diagnostic and Statistical Manual for Mental Disorders.* 4th ed., text revision Washington, DC: American Psychiatric Association; 2000.

often used synonymously with *dependence*. The term *substance abuse* is also commonly used in a nondiagnostic fashion for problematic use in general.

Intoxication and *withdrawal* are common SIDs (Table 6.3). *Intoxication* is a reversible syndrome caused by a recent ingestion that results in stereotypical behavioral, psychological, and physical changes. *Withdrawal* is a reversible substance-specific syndrome resulting from a cessation of, or reduction in, substance use.

Table 6.2 DSM-IV-TR Diagnostic Criteria for Substance Abuse

A maladaptive pattern of substance use leading to clinically significant impairment or distress, as manifested by one of more of the following, occurring within a 12-month period:

1. Recurrent substance use resulting in a failure to fulfill major role obligations at work, school, or home
2. Recurrent substance use in situations in which it is physically hazardous
3. Recurrent substance-related legal problems
4. Continued substance use despite persistent or recurrent social or interpersonal problems caused by or exacerbated by the effects of the substance.

The symptoms have never met the criteria for substance dependence in this class of substance.

From American Psychiatric Association. Diagnostic and Statistical Manual for Mental Disorders. 4th ed., text revision. Washington, DC: American Psychiatric Association; 2000.

Table 6.3 Intoxication and Withdrawal

	INTOXICATION	WITHDRAWAL
Stimulants	Time course: 24–48 hours Psychological effects: restlessness, agitation, hyperactivity, irritability, impulsiveness, repetitive behaviors Physiologic effects: hypertension, tachycardia, tachypnea, hyperthermia, pupillary dilation	Time course: peak in 2–4 days, resolution in 1 week Psychological effects: depression, increased risk of suicidality, agitation, paranoia, craving, vivid dreams Physiologic effects: fatigue, increased appetite, insomnia or hypersomnia
Opioids	Time course: 6–24 hours Psychological effects: drowsy/sedated, impaired memory, impaired attention Physiologic effects: pupillary constriction, decreased respiratory rate, decreased bowel sounds, slurred speech	Time course: Short-acting: begins in 6–8 hours, resolves in 7–10 days Long-acting: begins in 1–3 days, resolves in 10–14 days Psychological effects: restlessness, depression, irritability Physiologic effects: myalgias and arthralgias, diarrhea, abdominal cramping, lacrimation, rhinorrhea, piloerection, yawning, insomnia, temperature dysregulation

PATIENT ASSESSMENT

History

Nonspecific complaints of chronic pain, gastrointestinal symptoms, changes in memory, impaired concentration, anxiety, and sleep disturbance should all alert the clinician to a possible SUD. Lost prescriptions or request for refills more frequently than anticipated may be associated with prescription drug abuse. Hepatitis B and C viruses and HIV have strong associations with injection drug use. General life chaos, recent arrests for driving while intoxicated, and unexplained physical trauma all strongly suggest a possible SUD.

Physical Exam

Some patients with an SUD may have a normal physical exam. Chronic stimulant abuse may result in significant short-term weight loss, an emaciated appearance, and with methamphetamine, severe dental problems. Track marks, calluses that follow a subcutaneous vein, are caused by repeated injections into adjacent sites over a vein and are commonly found in accessible areas of the body such as the antecubital fossae, hands, and legs. Abnormal movements and facial gestures are hallmarks of chronic use of both methamphetamine and cocaine (5). Table 6.4 highlights clues for recognizing SUDs from the medical and social histories along with the physical exam.

Screening

All patients should receive a brief substance use screen. Some clinicians choose to incorporate questions into their general history taking, while others prefer a screening tool such as the CAGE Adopted to Include

Table 6.4 Clinical Clues

Commonly associated diseases
  Human immunodeficiency virus (HIV)
  Hepatitis B and C
  Systemic and cutaneous bacterial infections
  Accidents and trauma
  Hypertension

Social history
  Multiple emergency room visits
  Recent arrest for driving while intoxicated
  Poorly explained trauma
  Sudden change in behavior
  Erratic occupational history

Physical exam findings
  Rapid and significant weight loss and/or cachetic appearance
  Severe dental problems
  New-onset heart murmur
  Genital discharge, warts, ulcers, chancres
  Cutaneous track marks and infections
  Abnormal movements and facial gestures
  Cognitive impairment

Drugs (CAGE-AID) (6). The following is a brief overview of the CAGE-AID questions. If two or more answers are affirmative, further assessment is warranted.

- Have you ever felt that you should *Cut* down on your alcohol or drug use?
- Have people *Annoyed* you by criticizing your alcohol or drug use?
- Have you felt *Guilty* about your alcohol or drug use?
- Have you ever had a drink or used drugs first thing in the morning (Eye-opener) to steady your nerves or get rid of a hangover?

Collateral Information

Patients may not be forthcoming with their clinician for several reasons: They may not view substance use as a problem, they may fear social or legal repercussions, or they may not trust the provider. Collateral history is therefore essential. The goal of any collateral interview is to learn whether substance use has caused significant dysfunction with important life roles. Common sources of information include spouse or partner, peers, teachers, and other medical personnel. The need for collateral information must always be viewed in the context of the patient's right to confidentiality of health information.

Laboratory Evaluation

Laboratory tests play a secondary role in the diagnosis of SUDs. Urine testing is widely available, noninvasive, and easy to obtain. It can detect active use, help distinguish intoxication from another co-occurring psychiatric disorder, and detect a second SUD. It does not, however, measure the level of global impairment or routinely detect several opiates (oxycodone, hydrocodone, and fentanyl) that are commonly abused.

Table 6.5 Laboratory Evaluation

- Urine drug screen
- Blood alcohol level (if indicated)
- HIV test
- Liver enzymes
- Hepatitis B: HBsAg and IgM anti-HBc
- Hepatitis C: Anti-HCV
- Tests for sexually transmitted diseases

HBc, hepatitis B core antigen; HBsAg, hepatitis B surface antigen; HCV, hepatitis C virus; HIV, human immunodeficiency virus; IgM, immunoglobulin M.

Given the strong association between substance use and HIV, hepatitis B and C, and other sexually transmitted diseases, these infections should be routinely screened for in those who have an SUD. Suspicion for analgesic abuse should prompt evaluation of liver chemistries given the wide availability of opioid/acetaminophen combinations and the combinations and the hepatotoxicity associated with excessive consumption of acetaminophen. A recommended laboratory evaluation is included in Table 6.5.

Differential Diagnosis

SRDs present two diagnostic challenges. First, induced disorders may mimic nearly every psychiatric disorder. Most, though not all, SIDs are self-limiting and recede soon after cessation of use. Substance-induced depression and anxiety, for example, often resolve within 4 weeks of sobriety. Substance-induced cognitive and sleep disorders may persist for much longer. Second, SRDs commonly co-occur with other psychiatric illness. Nearly 50% of patients with schizophrenia, for example, suffer from alcohol or drug dependence (excluding nicotine), while rates of co-occurrence in patients with bipolar disorder and antisocial personality disorder are 61% and 84%, respectively (7).

While an SRD should prompt evaluation for another co-occurring psychiatric disorder, in practice it may be challenging to differentiate an SID from another psychiatric disorder. An independent, co-occurring psychiatric diagnosis can be made in one of two ways: the clear onset of psychiatric symptoms preceding the SID, or the persistence or worsening of psychiatric symptoms (i.e., depressed mood, anxiety, psychosis, and dementia) after a sufficient period of abstinence. In cases where the diagnosis is unclear, a family history of psychiatric disorders may support a co-occurring psychiatric disorder diagnosis. Conversely, an atypical presentation of a psychiatric disorder (e.g., new-onset mania or psychosis after age 40) suggests an SID. When it is impossible to discriminate an SID from another psychiatric disorder, it is reasonable to diagnose both disorders until time and clinical evidence allow a more definitive answer.

NOT TO BE MISSED

- Use of prescribed medications for inappropriate purposes
- Substance misuse
- Suicidal ideation
- Substance-induced disorder
  - Depression
  - Anxiety
  - Psychosis
  - Bipolar affective disorder
  - Dementia

CHAPTER 6 SUDs—Stimulants and Opioids

Biopsychosocial Treatment

GENERAL PRINCIPLES

When discussing substance use, the ability to relate effectively to the patient may be the clinician's most useful tool, with interview style as important as interview content. An empathic stance by the clinical staff (e.g., "becoming the patient" for a brief moment in time) is associated with positive treatment outcomes. Normalizing SUD questions and beginning with questions about socially accepted substances such as tobacco, caffeine, and alcohol are simple techniques to increase patient comfort and openness. Words such as "illicit" and "illegal" might be viewed as judgmental, may embarrass the patient, and ultimately result in a diminished therapeutic connection, so it is best to ask about the use of specific drugs by name.

GOALS OF TREATMENT

For most substance-dependent patients, the ideal outcome is total cessation of nonmedically supervised substance use. A primary care–oriented conceptualization of treatment goals is a continuum, flanked on one end by initial engagement in treatment and at the other by long-term abstinence. Along this continuum lie intermediate goals that focus on decreasing particular behaviors: decreasing the frequency or quantity of use, the number of substances used, high-risk delivery methods, or high-risk behaviors while intoxicated. The clinician may continue to encourage abstinence as a long-term goal, all the while promoting behaviors that will lessen the psychological, medical, and social consequences of substance use.

ACUTE MEDICATION MANAGEMENT: SUBSTANCE-INDUCED DISORDERS

Stimulant and Opioid Intoxication

Uncomplicated stimulant and opioid intoxication generally require only monitoring and observation until symptoms subside. A quiet environment will lesson agitation and hyperreactivity to external stimuli. Serial vital signs may signal autonomic instability. Increasing agitation may warrant pharmacologic intervention with benzodiazepines such as lorazepam or diazepam. For severe opioid-induced respiratory depression, inpatient admission and administration of the opioid antagonist naloxone should be considered.

Stimulant Withdrawal

Stimulant withdrawal symptoms are less distinctive than those for opioids, are not life threatening, and rarely necessitate pharmacologic intervention. Depressed mood and fatigue are common initial symptoms, and clinicians must be alert to an increased risk of suicidality. For patients recovering from several days of methamphetamine use, symptoms may be more severe, with volatile agitation, paranoia, and hypersomnia. Observation should take place in a quiet, calming environment. If anxiety is acutely problematic, a short course of benzodiazepines may be used.

Opioid Withdrawal

Methadone and Suboxone   Methadone (long-acting opioid agonist) and Suboxone (partial opioid agonist buprenorphine combined with opioid antagonist naloxone) are effective treatments for opioid withdrawal. In the United States, outpatient prescribing of either methadone or Suboxone for the treatment of SRDs requires special licensure, and readers are referred to the Practical Resources section for further information (8, 9).

Methadone or buprenorphine may be used in the inpatient setting without restriction. A common methadone withdrawal protocol begins with a dose of 20 to 30 mg, with upward titration to 40 to 60 mg daily if the patient continues to show objective signs of withdrawal. Once withdrawal symptoms are suppressed, the dose is slowly tapered over time.

Clonidine   Clonidine is an alpha-2-adrenergic receptor agonist that targets the noradrenergic hyperactivity that occurs with opioid withdrawal, and can be used on an outpatient basis. Approved in the United States as an antihypertensive agent, clonidine is widely used to target withdrawal symptoms such as nausea, vomiting, diarrhea, and sweating. It is much less effective at suppressing craving, insomnia, lethargy, restlessness, and myalgias. An initial dose of 0.1 mg given orally three times daily is routinely sufficient to suppress withdrawal symptoms. On days 2 through 4 of sobriety, doses are adjusted upward, to a maximum dose of 0.4 mg three times daily. At higher doses, side effects, including hypotension, dry mouth, and constipation, may be dose limiting. From day 5 to completion, the dose may be reduced by 0.2 mg/day. Clonidine should not be administered if the systolic blood pressure drops below 90 mmHg. A gradual taper is also necessary to avoid rebound hypertension. Treatment of withdrawal from short-acting opioids such as heroin, morphine, or oxycodone usually takes between 4 and 6 days, but longer with opioids such as methadone.

Outpatients should not be given more than a 3-day supply of clonidine, as the dose requires daily titration and overdose may be fatal. Other medications that may be used in conjunction with clonidine for the relief of withdrawal symptoms include muscle relaxants, nonsteroidal anti-inflammatory drugs (NSAIDs), antiemetics, antidiarrheals, and sleeping medications with a low abuse potential.

CHRONIC MEDICATION MANAGEMENT

Opioid Dependence

Methadone and Suboxone   Long-term medication management of opioid dependence, also known as maintenance therapy, entails the substitution of the drug of abuse with a long-acting, less euphorigenic opioid for an indefinite period. Methadone and Suboxone are commonly used for maintenance therapy. Methadone doses are typically in the range of 60 to 100 mg daily, although some patients may require higher doses. Suboxone doses range between 8 mg/2 mg (buprenorphine/naloxone) and 32 mg/8 mg. Unlike methadone, which requires a specially licensed clinic, physicians may obtain a special license to prescribe Suboxone in the outpatient setting. Further advantages of Suboxone include every-other-day dosing, a low risk of toxicity at higher doses, and low abuse potential.

Levomethtadyl acetate (LAAM)   LAAM is a methadone derivative with a longer half-life than methadone that allows for every-other-day dosing. It is, however, no longer approved for use in Europe, and has been withdrawn from the market in the United States, as it may cause potentially fatal QT prolongation and cardiac arrhythmias in vulnerable patients. In settings in which LAAM remains available, candidates should be screened for cardiac risk factors: a prolonged QT interval, the use of QT-prolonging medications, electrolyte imbalances, and structural heart disease. A baseline electrocardiogram (ECG) and periodic ECGs when the dose exceeds the usual upper limit are warranted.

Naltrexone   Naltrexone is an opioid antagonist. If no side effects such as nausea and vomiting are observed on the initial starting dose of 25 mg, 50 mg may be given the next day and daily thereafter. Alternatively, a weekly dose of 350 mg may be taken every other day in three divided doses, two of 100 mg and one of 150 mg. An intramuscular depot formulation that allows for monthly dosing is also available, although in the United States this form has FDA approval only for alcohol dependence. An implantable formulation that remains active for 5 months is also available, although at present it has not been approved in the United States. Naltrexone for opioid dependence may only safely begin with confirmation of complete opioid detoxification, usually necessitating a period of abstinence of 1 to 2 weeks (8). The greatest utility for naltrexone may be found in subgroups of patients who are highly motivated, closely supervised, and under court or professional board order to be opioid-free while in recovery from opioid dependence. Health care professionals, pilots, public safety officers, and incarcerated patients are examples of patient populations in whom naltrexone may be most appropriate. Table 6.6 summarizes medications used to treat opioid dependence.

Stimulant Dependence

More than 40 medications have been evaluated for the treatment of stimulant dependence, and none has been found to have clear-cut efficacy. The result is that neither cocaine nor amphetamine dependence has FDA-approved pharmacotherapies and behavioral strategies remain first-line treatments. In patients who fail to respond to psychosocial interventions, however, a pharmacologic trial may be warranted and consultation with an addiction medicine specialist should be considered.

PSYCHOSOCIAL INTERVENTIONS

Motivational Interviewing

Motivational interviewing (MI) is a "patient-centered," persuasive yet nonjudgmental counseling style meant to elicit behavioral change (10). Based on the Transtheoretical Stages of Change model, it assumes that all patients, even those suffering from long-standing substance dependence,

Table 6.6 Acute and Chronic Pharmacologic Management of Opioid Use Disorders

MEDICATION	ACUTE WITHDRAWAL	CHRONIC MAINTENANCE	CLINICAL INDICATIONS	ADVANTAGES	DISADVANTAGES/ SIDE EFFECTS
Methadone	• Begin: 10–30 mg • Day 2: Same as day 1 • Up-titration: 5–10 mg/day • Peak: 40–60 mg/day • Taper: ↓ 5 mg/day	60–100+ mg/day	• Inpatient withdrawal • Chronic maintenance	• Proven efficacy • Decreases craving • Does not require withdrawal symptoms before initiating	• Highly regulated in the U.S. • Potential for abuse and diversion • Constipation • Urinary retention • Increased sweating • Sexual dysfunction
Suboxone	• Begin: 4/1–8/2 mg/day • Day 2: 8/2–16/4 mg/day • Up-titration: ↑ 4 mg/day • Peak: 8/2–32/8 mg/day Taper: • Rapid: ↓ to 0 in 3 days • Moderate: ↓ 2 mg/day • Extended: ↓ 2 mg every third day	16/4–32/8 mg/day	• Inpatient withdrawal • Outpatient withdrawal and maintenance • Rapid withdrawal	• Minimal sedation • Low abuse potential • Every-other-day dosing	• Requires a special DEA license in the U.S. • Patients must have mild withdrawal before initiating • Side effect profile similar to methadone
Clonidine	• Begin: 0.1 mg TID • Peak: 1.2 mg/day, divided BID or TID	N/A	• Nonopioid treatment of withdrawal • Rapid withdrawal	• Nonaddicting • Does not require withdrawal symptoms before beginning	• Dose-limiting hypotension and bradycardia • Does not limit craving • Limited efficacy against many symptoms
LAAM	N/A	• 80–140 mg every other day	• Outpatient maintenance	• Every-other-day dosing	• Arrhythmias • Not approved in Europe; not available in the U.S.
Naltrexone	N/A	• 50 mg daily; or • 100, 100, 150 mg every other day	• Outpatient maintenance for highly motivated patients who cannot be maintained on opioids	• No addictive or abuse potential • Every-other-day dosing	• Does not limit craving • Initiation requires prior abstinence • Increased risk of overdose if opioid use resumed • Dysphoria • Anxiety • GI discomfort

DEA, Drug Enforcement Agency; GI, gastrointestinal.

CHAPTER 6 SUDs—Stimulants and Opioids

will at some point be capable of change. The key components of MI include reflective listening and objective feedback. Both components are used to highlight the discrepancies between problem behaviors and patient goals, with the specific aim of eliciting self-motivational statements and behavioral change from the patient. In this model, interventions target

Table 6.7 Transtheoretical Stages of Change Model

STAGE	GOALS AND MOTIVATIONAL INTERVIEWING STRATEGIES
Precontemplation	• Help the patient see that change is necessary without increasing patient resistance • Provide education on negative consequences in a nonjudgmental way
Contemplation	• Explore the reluctance or ambivalence to change • Support the patient's self-motivating statements
Preparation	• Provide "menu of options" for change • Set "quit date" or other specific goals
Action	• Praise and reinforce positive gains • Enlist additional support resources as needed
Maintenance	• Help patient acclimate to new healthy lifestyle • Identify potential triggers and develop relapse prevention plan
Relapse	• Explore feelings of hopelessness, guilt, or shame • Encourage patient to re-enter change cycle

Adapted from Prochaska JO, Velicer WF. The Transtheoretical Model of health behavior change. *Am J Health Promot.* 1997;12:38–48.

stage-specific goals that are more effective than nonspecific imposition demanding behavior change (11) (Table 6.7).

The FRAMES approach (Table 6.8) is a practical application of MI (12). Objective feedback to the patient emphasizes the detrimental consequences of substance use, while nonjudgmental advice about options for change highlights alternatives. Simple, motivation-enhancing interventions have been shown to be effective for encouraging patient involvement and compliance with the treatment process. The universality and simplicity of the FRAMES allow for its broad application in a variety of primary care settings.

Cognitive Behavioral Therapy

Many tenets of cognitive behavioral therapy (CBT) are complementary to FRAMES. CBT targets three thought processes or behaviors that are prominent in substance use disorders: dysfunctional thoughts (including the idea that substance use is uncontrollable or inevitable), maladaptive behaviors (e.g., the use of substances to alleviate stress or internal conflict), and relapse. Examining dysfunctional thoughts can assist both clinician and patient to develop effective treatment strategies. For the primary care clinician, even a rudimentary understanding of CBT may facilitate a patient's greater participation in such treatments. We therefore strongly encourage providers to obtain further training in CBT techniques.

Group Therapies

Self-help groups often play vital roles in patients' treatment process, and most patients should be strongly encouraged, although not required, to attend. In general, such groups assist patients to develop substance-free

Table 6.8 FRAMES Guideline to Motivational Interviewing

- *Feedback* is given regarding the negative consequences of substance use behaviors, including future risk
- *Responsibility* for change emphasizes personal choice
- *Advice* is given about behavioral change, from reduction to abstinence
- *Menu* of treatment options reinforces personal responsibility and choice
- *Empathic* and nonjudgmental counseling style
- *Self-efficacy* encourages a sense of optimistic empowerment and positive change

Adapted from Miller WR, Sanchez VC. Motivating young adults for treatment and lifestyle change. In Howard G, ed. *Issues in Alcohol Use and Misuse by Young Adults.* Notre Dame, IN: University of Notre Dame Press; 1994:55–82.

social networks, provide peer support, and motivate personal change. Although best studied in alcohol dependence, regular participation in 12-step groups may also benefit cocaine-dependent users.

Family Involvement

Family members can be active sources of support, education, and collateral information, and their involvement may minimize the chance of relapse. Not all family involvement may be positive, however. Substance use within families is common, and the clinician should evaluate family members for substance use problems or enabling behaviors that may actually encourage the patient's substance use and interfere with treatment goals.

Relapse Prevention

Relapse, the process in which an abstinent patient returns to substance use, is a predictable event in recovery from any SUD. Common precipitants include the use of alcohol, a return to substance-using friends, substance-associated sexual behavior, depression, and craving. Relapse has the potential to spiral out of control, as patients assuage their shame and anxiety over their departure from abstinence with escalating use. Frank discussion about relapse facilitates identification of patient-specific triggers. Contingency measures that specify preplanned responses to relapse (e.g., limiting use and seeking help immediately) are integral components of any relapse prevention strategy. Care must be taken when treating many common medical complaints (13). Cough suppressants containing opioids or dextromethorphan may act as triggers for opioid-dependent patients. Stimulant-containing decongestants should be avoided. Nonpharmacologic pain management strategies such as heat, ice, massage, and physical therapy are preferred, concurrently with nonaddicting medications such as acetaminophen, aspirin, or ibuprofen. If opioids are required, frequent office visits should be the norm, and early refills should not be given. A summary of relapse prevention strategies is listed in Table 6.9.

Treatment of Co-Occurring Psychiatric Disorders

The co-occurrence of substance use and other psychiatric disorders presents a significant clinical challenge. Not only are relapses more

Table 6.9 Relapse Prevention Strategies

- Maintain a supportive patient–clinician relationship
- Educate the patient and family on triggers for and effects of substance use
- Develop a relapse management plan
- Schedule short, frequent primary care visits
- Encourage involvement in 12-step or similar groups
- Manage co-occurring general medical and psychiatric conditions
- Facilitate positive lifestyle changes (e.g., staying away from people and places associated with drug use)

common, but also depressive, anxious, or psychotic symptoms may confound the motivation for behavioral change, interfere with treatment, and be misinterpreted as signs of treatment resistance. Complicating the matter is the lack of integration between primary care and addiction mental health services.

The AMPS screening tool should be used to screen for common disorders. Though any psychiatric disorder may co-occur with any substance use disorder, primary care clinicians should be most familiar with treatment options for depression and anxiety. A substance-using patient with an established major depressive disorder should be treated with a selective serotonin reuptake inhibitor (SSRI) or selective norepinephrine reuptake inhibitor (SNRI) antidepressant while supportive and behavioral psychosocial interventions are delivered. Benzodiazepines have the potential for abuse and dependence, and therefore many clinicians initially prefer to use SSRIs to target anxiety. Insomnia is another frequent complaint and is best addressed by behavioral interventions.

Practice Pointers

WHEN TO REFER
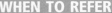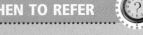

- Pronounced withdrawal symptoms
- Maintenance pharmacotherapy for buprenorphine or methadone
- Need for psychosocial treatments (Narcotics Anonymous, counseling behavioral treatment programs, vocational rehabilitation)
- Suicidal intention
- Repeated failed treatment in primary care or outpatient treatment

Case 1: Amphetamine dependence and psychosocial interventions
Jose is a 22-year-old student presenting with fatigue, dry cough, irritability, and depressed mood. He admits to smoking tobacco and drinking beer "once in a while." When he senses your nonjudgmental approach, he reveals he smokes "meth," but "only to help me study." When asked about his studies, Jose reveals that he used to be a B student, but more recently his grades have slipped. On one hand, he now routinely uses "meth" when studying for finals; on the other, he describes how several times he's done poorly on tests when he's been too "wired" (intoxicated). Once in high school, one of his friends injected him with what he was told was heroin plus methamphetamine (speedball). He's used oxycodone pills twice in the last year, both times to try to relax after using meth to stay up and study. He "parties" most weekends, and often engages in unprotected sex. He seems to understand the importance of safe sex practices, but states, "When I hook up at a party and I'm high, I just don't believe that anything bad will happen." His last meth use was 48 hours ago at a weekend party, and he has not slept since then. Jose is concerned about his insomnia and is asking for a "sleeping pill." His physical exam is notable for hypertension, a 10-pound weight loss, and fine bibasilar crackles. Urine toxicology is positive for methamphetamines. Other studies, including gonorrhea, chlamydia, HIV, and hepatitis B and C, are pending.

Discussion: *Patients with SUDs typically present with nonspecific complaints, and careful history taking is necessary to elucidate any contribution from substance use.*

*Initially asking about socially acceptable substances such as tobacco and alcohol nor-
malizes questions about illicit drugs and is less threatening for many patients. Jose
meets criteria for stimulant dependence. He has mild withdrawal symptoms, gives up
important activities (his studying and other aspects of his role as a student), and continues to use despite knowledge of problems (poor grades, unprotected sex). Clinically, it is unlikely that regular party use plus daily use for 6 months would not lead
to dose escalation and tolerance. Recall that underreporting is the rule in SUDs.*

*The severity of Jose's methamphetamine dependence may be mild-moderate
and seems early in the disease course. For now, the indicated intervention is psychosocial treatment. Jose would benefit from a FRAMES intervention. He is slightly
aware of the likely consequences surrounding his use, and frank, nonjudgmental
feedback would clarify his medical, professional, and legal risks.*

*Advice regarding a variety of treatment options would provide him with tangi-
ble opportunities for change. If Jose is in the "Action Stage" in the Stages of
Change model, a collaborative plan of action (i.e., cessation) should be developed.
While a referral to local drug counseling services or a mental health professional
skilled in CBT could be considered, he may not follow up unless he is motivated to
change. In such cases, further motivational interviewing techniques using the
Stages of Change model and the FRAMES techniques should be utilized (Tables 6.7
and 6.8).*

*Although he described none, if his symptoms suggest a concomitant mood or
anxiety disorder, further exploration of his psychiatric and family history and follow-
up appointments when abstinent would be necessary to evaluate and treat any such
disorder. Methamphetamine withdrawal places him at increased acute risk for suicide, and his potential for self-harm must be evaluated at this visit. His sexual history
and injection use place him at risk for several infectious diseases, and the results of
his pending tests must be closely followed. While his opioid use is minimal, clear recommendations to stop should be incorporated into the FRAMES conversation, and
subsequent use monitored. Close routine follow-up with Jose in the next 1 to 2
weeks would be indicated to monitor his progress.*

Case 2: Management of opiate dependence

Cathy is a 55-year-old attorney who presents as a new patient with 2 days of diffuse joint pain, nonbloody diarrhea, nausea, abdominal pain, and rhinorrhea.
Further questioning reveals insomnia and an irritable, depressed mood over the
same period. As the physical exam is about to begin, Cathy states, "I don't think
I have the flu. What I need is something for my back. It's this back pain that is
making me miserable." Cathy relates that 2 years ago, she suffered injury to her
lumbar spine, and has been using Vicodin ever since for symptomatic relief.
When pressed, Cathy admits to taking 8 to 10 Vicodin daily, obtained from several doctors. She has made many unsuccessful attempts to reduce her usage, but
when she does she feels "much worse." A more focused symptom history suggests that her back pain is better. Physical exam is notable for a moist forehead,
clear nares, benign abdomen, and normal musculoskeletal evaluation.

Discussion: *Arthralgias, diarrhea, abdominal pain, rhinorrhea, sweating, insomnia,
and an irritable depression all point toward an opioid withdrawal syndrome (particularly when relieved by more Vicodin). Clonidine, 0.1 mg three times daily, may be
given for symptomatic relief, along with an NSAID, antiemetic, antidiarrheal, and
sleeping medication with a low abuse potential. Due to its potential for lethality in
overdose and the need for closer monitoring, no more than a 3-day's supply of clonidine should be given. Cathy's withdrawal syndrome, her multiple attempts to
reduce her usage, and her persistent use despite the resolution of her back pain
supports a diagnosis of opioid dependence. Prescription-opioid dependence commonly begins with a legitimate physiologic complaint (in this case back pain), and a
careful history and physical exam are necessary to determine if untreated physical
pain is contributing to her illness. Cathy may be an appropriate candidate for*

office-based Suboxone therapy, and an urgent referral to a Suboxone provider should be considered. Alternatively, naltrexone may be efficacious with certain highly motivated individuals and its use may be considered once her withdrawal symptoms have abated. Motivational interviewing, CBT, and group and family therapy will all be vital components in a well-rounded treatment strategy. Finally, liver enzymes must be evaluated given the potential hepatic toxicity of the acetaminophen in Vicodin.

ICD9

Amphetamine Abuse	305.70
Amphetamine Dependence	304.40
Cocaine Abuse	305.60
Cocaine Dependence	304.20
Hallucinogen Dependence	304.50
Hallucinogen Abuse	305.30
Opioid Abuse	305.60
Opioid Dependence	304.00
Other Substance Abuse	305.90
Other Substance Dependence	304.90
Other Substance-Induced Delirium	292.81
Phencyclidine (PCP) Abuse	305.90
Phencyclidine (PCP) Dependence	304.90
Polysubstance Dependence	304.90
Sedative, Hypnotic, or Anxiolytic Abuse	305.40
Sedative, Hypnotic, or Anxiolytic Dependence	304.10
Substance-Induced Anxiety Disorder	292.89
Substance-Induced Mood Disorder	292.84

Practical Resources

Substance Abuse and Mental Health Services Administration: http://www.samhsa.gov
Treatment Improvement Protocols: http://www.ncbi.nlm.nih.gov/books/bv.fcgi?rid=hstat5.part.22441
Buprenorphine prescribing information: www.buprenorphine.samhsa.gov
Directory of substance abuse treatment centers: http://www.findtreatment.samhsa.gov
National Institute on Drug Abuse: http://www.drugabuse.gov
American Society of Addiction Medicine: http://www.asam.org

12-Step Programs:
Narcotics Anonymous: http://www.na.org
Cocaine Anonymous: http://www.ca.org
Nar-Anon: http://nar-anon.org
Al-Anon: http://www.al-anon.alateen.org/

References

1. Compton WM, Thomas YF, Stinson, FS, et al. Prevalence, correlates, disability, and comorbidity of DSM-IV drug abuse and dependence in the United States. *Arch Gen Psychiatry.* 2007;64:566–576.

2. Nace EP, Tinsley JA. *Patients with Substance Abuse Problems: Effective Identification, Diagnosis, and Treatment.* New York: W.W. Norton and Company; 2007.

3. Kleber HD, Weiss RD. Treatment of patients with substance use disorders, 2nd edition. *Am J Psychiatry.* 2007;164(4 Suppl):1–130.

4. American Psychiatric Association. *Diagnostic and Statistical Manual of Mental Disorders.* 4th ed. Washington, DC: American Psychiatric Association; 2000.

5. Center for Substance Abuse Treatment. *Treatment for Stimulant Use Disorders.* Treatment Improvement Protocol (TIP) Series 33. Rockville, MD: Substance Abuse and Mental Health Services Administration; 1999.

6. Brown RL, Leonard T, Saunders LA, et al. The prevalence and detection of substance use disorders among inpatients ages 18 to 49: an opportunity for prevention. *Prev Med.* 1998;27:101–10.

7. O'Brien D, Charney L, Lewis J, et al. Priority actions to improve the care of persons with co-occurring substance abuse and other mental disorders: a call to action. *Biol Psychiatry.* 2004;56:703–713.

8. Center for Substance Abuse Treatment. *Medication-Assisted Treatment for Opioid Addiction in Opioid Treatment Programs.* Treatment Improvement Protocol (TIP) Series 43. Rockville, MD: Substance Abuse and Mental Health Services Administration; 2005.

9. Center for Substance Abuse Treatment. *Clinical Guidelines for the Use of Buprenorphine in the Treatment of Opioid Addiction.* Treatment Improvement Protocol (TIP) Series 40. Rockville, MD: Substance Abuse and Mental Health Services Administration; 2004.

10. Miller WR, Rollnick S. *Motivational Interviewing: Preparing People for Change.* 2nd ed. New York: The Guilford Press; 2002.

11. Prochaska, JO, Velicer WF. The Transtheoretical Model of health behavior change. *Am J Health Promot.* 1997;12:38–48.

12. Miller WR, Sanchez VC. Motivating young adults for treatment and lifestyle change. In: Howard G, ed. *Issues in Alcohol Use and Misuse by Young Adults.* Notre Dame, IN: University of Notre Dame Press; 1994:55–82.

13. Jones EM, Knutson D, Haines D. Common problems in patients recovering from chemical dependency. *Am Fam Physician.* 2003;68:1971–1978.

CHAPTER 6 SUDs—Stimulants and Opioids

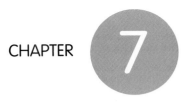
CHAPTER 7 Substance Use Disorders—Alcohol

L. Joby Morrow, MD • Craig R. Keenan, MD • Glen L. Xiong, MD

Mary is a 43-year-old woman with a history of hepatitis C and hypertension who presents with depressed mood and insomnia. She denies any suicidal thoughts but states, "Life just doesn't seem to be heading in the right direction." On this visit, she is most concerned about her persistently elevated blood pressure and insomnia. She reluctantly reports losing her job and apartment 3 months ago and now lives with her sister. She divorced 1 year ago and has one adult son who is estranged from her. She reports a history of intravenous heroin use more than 8 years ago, smokes two packs of cigarettes per day, and drinks three to four beers each evening. Her physical exam is unremarkable except for a blood pressure of 165/95 mmHg, heart rate of 108 beats per minute, moderate bilateral hand tremor, and inability to perform tandem gait.

CLINICAL HIGHLIGHTS

- Problematic alcohol use is widespread, costly, and underrecognized by primary care providers.

- Screening tools such as the CAGE and AUDIT-C questionnaires should be used in the primary care setting as they are highly effective in identifying patients at risk for alcohol use disorders (AUDs).

- Management strategies of AUDs share similarities with those of other chronic illnesses, and

(Continued)

Clinical Significance

The primary care community cannot afford to ignore the economic, social, medical, and personal impact of AUDs. Alcohol-related disorders are chronic, relapsing problems that have a prevalence of up to 20% in the primary care patient population, a rate similar to other primary care conditions like hypertension and diabetes mellitus (1). However, they are identified and treated by clinicians at one fourth the rate of similarly prevalent illnesses. On average, alcohol use is responsible for about 100,000 deaths and nearly $200 billion in direct and indirect costs each year (2).

Benzodiazepines (BZPs) are among the most widely prescribed drugs in the world. Like alcohol, BZPs act as central nervous system depressants by their agonist effects on the gamma-aminobutyric acid A ($GABA_A$) receptor. The relatively new class of non-BZP hypnotics (e.g., zolpidem and zaleplon) has been increasingly used for the treatment of insomnia. They are chemically similar to BZPs and potential for misuse and dependence still exists. Like BZPs, non-BZP hypnotics are potentiated by alcohol and concomitant use can cause severe, potentially fatal respiratory depression. Although sedative-hypnotic use disorders are not addressed in this chapter, we caution providers on the judicious use of BZPs and non-BZP hypnotics and the potential for abuse, dependence, and cross-addiction with alcohol.

Diagnosis

Alcohol use can be characterized along a spectrum from nonproblematic use, misuse, abuse, to dependence. For simplicity, the rest of the chapter will describe AUDs to include alcohol abuse and alcohol dependence, unless otherwise specified. The unit of alcohol consumption is the standard drink (1.5 oz of liquor, 12 oz of beer, or 5 oz of table wine), which contains 12 to 14 grams of ethanol and raises the blood ethanol level to about 0.08 g/dL in a 150-pound man. Alcohol use or "moderate drinking," by consensus, is no more than one to two drinks per day for men and no more than one drink per day for women. The National Institute on Alcohol Abuse and Alcoholism (NIAAA) considers "at-risk drinking" to be more than 14 standard drinks weekly (or more than four drinks per occasion) for men and more than seven drinks weekly (or three drinks per occasion) for women and anyone of either sex over age 65 (3).

ALCOHOL ABUSE

The core feature of the *Diagnostic and Statistical Manual of Mental Disorders,* 4th edition, text revision (DSM-IV-TR), diagnostic criteria for alcohol abuse (Table 7.1) is the recurring use of alcohol despite a person's inability to fulfill social role obligations and despite hazardous, legal, and interpersonal problems (4). One or more of these problems must be present for more than 1 year in order to diagnose alcohol abuse. In order to meet the diagnostic criteria for alcohol abuse, alcohol dependence must be ruled out first. Therefore, when insufficient information is available, alcohol dependence should be considered first.

ALCOHOL DEPENDENCE

The diagnosis of alcohol dependence (Table 7.2) requires abuse of alcohol plus physical, psychological, and social consequences of the excessive use: physical tolerance and withdrawal, unsuccessful attempts to stop or reduce alcohol use, excessive time spent in alcohol-related

---

Table 7.1 DSM-IV-TR Diagnostic Criteria for Alcohol Abuse

A maladaptive pattern of alcohol use leading to clinically significant impairment or distress, as manifested by one (or more) of the following, occurring within a 12-month period:

1. Recurrent alcohol use resulting in a failure to fulfill major role obligations at work, school, or home (e.g., repeated absences or poor work performance related to alcohol use; alcohol-related absences, suspensions, or expulsions from school; neglect of children or household)
2. Recurrent alcohol use in situations in which it is physically hazardous (e.g., driving an automobile or operating a machine when impaired by alcohol use)
3. Recurrent alcohol-related legal problems (e.g., arrests for alcohol-related disorderly conduct)
4. Continued alcohol use despite having persistent or recurrent social or interpersonal problems caused or exacerbated by the effects of alcohol (e.g., arguments with spouse about consequences of intoxication, physical fights)
5. The symptoms have never met the criteria for alcohol dependence.

From American Psychiatric Association. *Diagnostic and Statistical Manual of Mental Disorders.* 4th ed., text revision. Washington, DC: American Psychiatric Association; 2000.

Table 7.2 DSM-IV-TR Diagnostic Criteria for Alcohol Dependence

A maladaptive pattern of alcohol use, leading to clinically significant impairment or distress, as manifested by three (or more) of the following, occurring at any time in the same 12-month period:

1. Tolerance, as defined by either of the following:
   - A need for markedly increased amounts of the substance to achieve intoxication or desired effect
   - Markedly diminished effect with continued use of the same amount of alcohol
2. Withdrawal, as manifested by either of the following:
   - The characteristic withdrawal syndrome
   - Alcohol (or a closely related substance like a benzodiazepine) is taken to relieve or avoid withdrawal symptoms
3. Alcohol is often taken in larger amounts or over a longer period than was intended
4. There is a persistent desire or unsuccessful efforts to cut down or control alcohol use
5. A great deal of time is spent in activities to obtain alcohol, use the alcohol, or recover from its effects
6. Important social, occupational, or recreational activities are given up or reduced because of alcohol use
7. The alcohol use is continued despite knowledge of having a persistent or recurrent physical or psychological problem that is likely to have been caused or exacerbated by the substance (e.g., continued drinking despite recognition that an ulcer was made worse by alcohol consumption)

From American Psychiatric Association. *Diagnostic and Statistical Manual of Mental Disorders.* 4th ed., text revision. Washington, DC: American Psychiatric Association; 2000.

activities, impairment in interpersonal and social functioning, and continued use despite physical or psychological consequences. Alcohol dependence is diagnosed when three of these criteria have been met for more than 1 year (4).

ALCOHOL WITHDRAWAL

Alcohol withdrawal is often part of the diagnosis of alcohol dependence. The symptoms of alcohol withdrawal stem from unregulated excitatory neuronal activity, and may include diaphoresis, tachycardia, increased blood pressure, peripheral tremor, anxiety, insomnia, nausea, vomiting, and restlessness. The symptoms begin anywhere from 4 hours to 3 days after the last use of alcohol. Potentially dangerous endpoints for the alcohol withdrawal syndrome include seizures and delirium tremens. These complications of severe alcohol withdrawal can have fatal consequences if left untreated.

ALCOHOL WITHDRAWAL SEIZURES

Alcohol withdrawal seizures are generally tonic-clonic seizures and, other than the temporal relationship to the discontinuation of alcohol, are clinically indistinguishable from other seizure disorders. They generally appear 2 to 48 hours after the last drink, and are also caused by central neuronal hyperactivity. Patients typically have a single seizure, but they can have multiple seizures in a row, and up to 3% of patients develop status epilepticus. Recurrent or prolonged seizures during withdrawal should prompt an investigation for other potential causes of the seizures. The risk of developing alcohol withdrawal seizures is proportionally increased by the number of times a patient has required detoxification.

ALCOHOLIC HALLUCINOSIS

In alcoholic hallucinosis, hallucinations develop within 12 to 24 hours of abstinence and resolve within 24 to 48 hours. These are typically visual hallucinations, but tactile and auditory hallucinations can occur. *Formication,* or tactile hallucinations, occurs classically in patients who describe a feeling of bugs crawling on their skin. The patient's sensorium is otherwise clear, which differentiates hallucinosis from delirium tremens (DTs), where hallucinations also occur but concomitantly with global clouding of the sensorium. Delirium tremens does not usually begin until *after* 24 to 48 hours of abstinence.

DELIRIUM TREMENS

Delirium tremens occur in about 5% of all cases of alcohol withdrawal and can be life threatening with a mortality rate of up to 5% (5). DTs are characterized by acute altered consciousness that includes disorientation, confusion, agitation, hallucinations, and signs of severe autonomic instability (including tremor, hypertension, diaphoresis, tachycardia, and fever). Symptoms may appear within 2 weeks of abstinence, but usually 48 to 96 hours after the last drink. Risk factors for DTs include concurrent acute medical illness, daily heavy alcohol use, a previous history of delirium tremens or withdrawal seizures, age over 30, and at least 3 days since the last drink (6). Patients at high risk for alcohol withdrawal seizures or DTs require immediate evaluation at a medical emergency room. Those with DTs need close monitoring, fluid and electrolyte replacement, and high-dose intravenous benzodiazepines in an intensive care unit.

SCREENING AND ASSESSMENT

Patients in the primary care setting who have alcohol dependence receive proper assessment and treatment for AUDs only about 10% of the time. The U.S. Preventive Services Task Force recommends that primary care practitioners screen all patients for AUDs, with an increased focus on those who are at high risk of alcohol abuse or dependence (i.e., family or personal history of substance misuse, recent stressors, or comorbid mood, anxiety, or psychotic disorders) (7). A number of user-friendly screening instruments have been validated to facilitate screening and diagnosis of AUDs. The most popular instrument is the 4-item CAGE questionnaire (Table 7.3), which has a sensitivity of up to 94% and specificity of 70% to 97% for detecting current abuse or dependence disorders in the primary care setting (8). One affirmative answer should lead to a more detailed evaluation (9).

The Alcohol Use Disorders Identification Test (AUDIT) is a 10-item questionnaire available from the World Health Organization (WHO). Despite the fact that the AUDIT can be given verbally or via written questionnaire in less than 3 minutes, its use in busy practices is reduced

Table 7.3 Brief Screening Instruments for Alcohol Use Disorders

CAGE Questionnaire[a,b]

1. Have you ever felt that you should **C**ut down on your alcohol use?
2. Have people **A**nnoyed you by asking about or criticizing your alcohol use?
3. Have you ever felt **G**uilty about your alcohol use?
4. Have you ever used alcohol as an **E**ye-opener first thing in the morning to avoid unpleasant feelings?

Alcohol Use Disorder Identification Test-Consumption (AUDIT-C)[c,d]

1. How often do you have a drink containing alcohol?

Never	0
Monthly or less	1
2–4 times a month	2
2–3 times a week	3
4 or more times a week	4

2. How many drinks containing alcohol do you have on a typical day when you are drinking?

1 or 2	0
3 or 4	1
5 or 6	2
7 to 9	3
10 or more	4

3. How often do you have six or more drinks on one occasion?

Never	0
Less than monthly	1
Monthly	2
Weekly	3
Daily or almost daily	4

[a] One affirmative answer should prompt further questioning about alcohol use and two or more affirmative answers increase the chance of alcohol use disorders.
[b] From U.S. Preventive Services Task Force. Screening and behavioral counseling interventions in primary care to reduce alcohol misuse: recommendation statement. *Ann Intern Med.* 2004;140(7):554–556.
[c] A score of 4 or more most likely indicates alcohol abuse or dependence and warrants further investigation.
[d] From Fiellin DA, Reid MC, O'Connor PG. Screening for alcohol problems in primary care: a systematic review. *Arch Intern Med.* 2000;160:1977–1989.

by its length. A quicker modification, called AUDIT-C, includes only the first three questions of AUDIT that quantify alcohol intake (Table 7.3). A score greater than 4 has a sensitivity of 86% and specificity of 72% for heavy drinking or abuse (10). Once a screening tool is positive, further assessment should assess the following: (1) quantity, frequency, and pattern of consumption; (2) alcohol-related problems; (3) use of other illicit or prescription drugs; (4) severity of dependence (e.g., history of withdrawal and symptoms with prior attempts to quit); (5) comorbid medical or psychiatric conditions; and (6) patient recognition of the problem and readiness to change. We recommend using either the CAGE or AUDIT-C screening tools as a means to determine the need for a more extensive substance abuse evaluation.

Without using screening tools, AUDs are often overlooked in the clinical settings, and detection requires a high index of suspicion. Certain clinical conditions and findings should raise this suspicion (Table 7.4). Typical clues may include comorbid psychiatric symptoms such as

Table 7.4 Clinical Clues for Alcohol Dependence

Commonly associated conditions	Dilated cardiomyopathy Erectile dysfunction Fetal alcohol syndrome Alcohol-related hepatitis Hepatic encephalopathy Hepatitis B and C HIV/AIDS Hypertension Malnutrition states Neuropathy Pancreatitis Pneumonia (often due to aspiration) Tuberculosis Sexually transmitted infections Unintended pregnancy
Social history	Multiple traumatic injuries Recent arrest for driving while intoxicated Arrests for property damage Sudden change in behavior Erratic occupational history Domestic violence
Physical exam findings	Weight changes with muscle atrophy Shrunken, firm liver Genital discharge, warts, ulcers, chancres Jaundice Scleral icterus Ascites Asterixis Hemorrhoids Cognitive impairment

AIDS, acquired immunodeficiency virus; HIV, human immunodeficiency virus.

anxiety, depression, irritability, panic attacks, impaired concentration, and persistent insomnia. Physical symptoms may include malaise, fatigue, headaches, loss of consciousness, amnesia, heartburn, hematemesis, jaundice, erectile dysfunction, hemorrhoids, and paresthesias or neuropathic pain from peripheral neuropathy. Several medical conditions are commonly associated with alcohol use: gastroesophageal reflux disease (GERD), peripheral neuropathy, hypertension, and pancreatitis. Alcohol use is also implicated as a factor in a large percentage of sexually transmitted infections and unintended pregnancies.

Asking about how a patient deals with life stressors or psychological symptoms may reveal the use of alcohol as a maladaptive coping mechanism. Unstable interpersonal relationships and work history are common manifestations of AUDs. Difficulties with managing a patient's medical conditions or unexplained medication nonadherence should alert the provider to screen for occult alcohol use. Skillful interviewing is required to normalize questions about alcohol use. Confidence, empathy, and a nonjudgmental stance are equally important in soliciting honest and complete information from the patient. The clinician may want to ask about the role or function of alcohol in the patient's life (e.g., "How has alcohol benefited or harmed you?" or "Has alcohol

Table 7.5 Laboratory Evaluation for Alcohol Use Disorders

TEST	SENSITIVITY	SPECIFICITY	RELATIVE COST
ALT	50%	86%	$
AST	50%	82%	$
AST:ALT >2	19%	96%	$
MCV	52%	85%	$
GGT	67% men 44% women	74% men 90% women	$$
CDT	60% men 29% women	92% men 92% women	$$$
CDT and GGT	86% men 61% women	68% men 81% women	$$$

ALT, alanine aminotransferase; AST, aspartate aminotransferase; CDT, carbohydrate-deficient transferrin; GGT, gamma-glutamyltransferase; MCV, mean corpuscular volume.

Data adapted from Bell H, Tallaksen CM, Try K, et al. Carbohydrate-deficient transferring and other markers of high alcohol consumption: a study of 502 patients admitted consecutively to a medical department. *Alcohol Clin Exp Res.* 1994;18(5):1103–1108; and Miller PM, Anton RF. Biochemical alcohol screening in primary care. *Addict Behav.* 2004;29:1427–1437.

affected your relationships with family and close friends?"). The rest of the social history that details a patient's support system and occupational history can be utilized in screening, diagnosis, and later in the treatment process. The mental status exam of someone who is suspected of having an AUD may reveal anxious, depressed, or irritable moods; psychomotor changes; slurred speech; cognitive slowing; clouded sensorium; paranoia; and impaired insight and judgment.

In addition to the history and physical exam, laboratory studies may suggest an AUD but are usually not diagnostic due to lack of specificity (Table 7.5). The sensitivity and specificity for the alcohol-related biomarkers vary by gender (11). Carbohydrate-deficient transferrin (CDT) and gamma-glutamyltransferase (GGT) may be used to monitor occult alcohol use but are relatively more expensive. GGT is limited by specificity, as it can be elevated in many other common conditions, including biliary disease, nonalcoholic liver disease, obesity, and ingestion of certain medications. Using a combination of CDT and GGT elevation raises the sensitivity, but lowers specificity. A 30% decrease in GGT or CDT is indicative of a significant decrease in alcohol intake or abstinence, and thus these tests can be useful adjuncts to monitor occult alcohol use in a treatment program (12).

Differential Diagnosis

As with all substance use problems, diagnosing an alcohol use disorder can be difficult. The symptoms of alcohol use may mimic mood or anxiety disorders and those of alcohol withdrawal may resemble anxiety or psychotic disorders. While alcohol use is far more common than illicit drug use, there is a high rate of co-occurring use, and identifying the

....

NOT TO BE MISSED

- Substance-induced psychiatric disorder
  - Mood disorders (major depressive disorder or bipolar disorder)
  - Anxiety disorders
  - Psychotic disorders
  - Cognitive disorders (dementia, delirium, or Wernicke-Korsakoff syndrome)
- Delirium tremens
- Alcohol withdrawal seizures
- Abuse or dependence of other substances

symptoms of problematic use of one substance versus another can be clinically challenging. Moreover, co-occurring substance use and other psychiatric disorders are so common as to be considered "the rule rather than the exception." After adjustment for sociodemographic variables, the National Epidemiological Survey found that alcohol dependence is most highly associated with bipolar spectrum disorder, major depressive disorder, panic disorder, and antisocial and histrionic personality disorders (13). Alcohol use, however, can cause mood and anxiety symptoms that mimic other psychiatric disorders and cessation of alcohol may lead to resolution of these symptoms in as little as 3 to 4 weeks (14). An independent, co-occurring psychiatric diagnosis requires serial observations of mood and behavior after cessation of use. According to consensus opinion among addiction specialists, if psychiatric symptoms persist 4 weeks after alcohol or substance cessation, or if the symptoms of the disorder clearly antedate alcohol, the patient can be diagnosed with the psychiatric disorder (15).

Biopsychosocial Treatment

Alcohol use disorders are often conceptualized as chronic medical disorders and a biopsychosocial treatment approach should be utilized. Biologic treatment focuses on acute detoxification of patients who are at high risk for moderate to severe withdrawal symptoms. Subsequently, pharmacologic agents may be added for maintenance treatment and relapse prevention, as an adjunct to psychosocial treatment. Psychosocial interventions include a combination of 12-step programs, supportive therapy, brief intervention, CBT, motivation-based treatments, family therapy, and residential or vocational rehabilitation.

PHARMACOTHERAPY

Acute Detoxification and Management of Withdrawal

Pharmacologic detoxification can be used to reduce withdrawal symptoms from alcohol and is often used in patients with physiologic dependence to prevent withdrawal seizures or DTs. A long-acting benzodiazepine such as chlordiazepoxide or diazepam is substituted for the substance of abuse and the dosage is gradually tapered. The longeracting agents are preferred due to a smoother withdrawal course. Shorter-acting agents such as lorazepam, oxazepam, or temazepam may be particularly useful for patients with advanced liver disease as there is less risk of serum accumulation and resultant sedation or delirium. For patients receiving inpatient treatment, the revised Clinical Institute Withdrawal Assessment for Alcohol (CIWA-A), a validated assessment instrument, may be used. Provider and staff training are required to ensure proper use of the instrument, and the scale is generally used by the nursing staff to guide benzodiazepine dosing (16). A typical regimen may be chlordiazepoxide 25 mg four times (day 1), 15 mg four times (day 2), 10 mg four times (day 3), 5 mg four times (day 4), and 5 mg twice (day 5) (17). For patients with liver disease, lorazepam at roughly 2 mg may be substituted for each 25 mg of chlordiazepoxide. However, there is no standard universal guideline for the frequency of administration, dosage strength, or length of administration of BZPs in treating alcohol withdrawal (18). The dose and duration of the benzodiazepine required to prevent complications typically correlate with a patient's tolerance to alcohol.

For a patient with a history of withdrawal seizure or underling seizure diathesis, use of anticonvulsants such as phenytoin, carbamazepine, or divalproex sodium may be added. Beta-blockers and the central alpha-agonist clonidine are also helpful *adjuncts* in treating the hyperadrenergic symptoms of alcohol withdrawal. They both may decrease withdrawal symptoms, while beta-blockers may also reduce cravings (18). All patients with heavy alcohol use should be closely monitored for volume and electrolyte abnormalities and given multivitamin, thiamine, and folate supplements.

Stable, motivated patients with mild to moderate withdrawal symptoms can be managed in the outpatient setting as long as there is available support at home to monitor progress and the patient has no history of severe alcohol withdrawal or seizures. Complicated cases of alcohol withdrawal that involve progressively worsening symptoms must be treated in an inpatient hospital or detoxification facility equipped to manage severe complications.

Maintenance Therapy

Maintenance medication to prevent relapse should always be used adjunctively with psychosocial interventions. Drugs approved by the FDA for alcohol dependence include the opioid antagonist naltrexone, the glutamate and N-methyl-D-aspartate (NMDA) receptor antagonist acamprosate, and the acetaldehyde dehydrogenase inhibitor disulfiram (Table 7.6). Naltrexone is available in an oral form (ReVia) and a long-acting injectable form (Vivitrol). Disulfiram, which causes severe discomfort (e.g., nausea, vomiting, flushing, hypotension, and tachycardia) when used with alcohol, must be used with caution as it can be hazardous in patients with cardiovascular or liver diseases.

Naltrexone and acamprosate, which work by decreasing craving, are much safer to use and are supplanting the use of disulfiram. In several clinical trials, both naltrexone and acamprosate have shown modest efficacy for maintaining abstinence or reducing heavy drinking, but their effectiveness is more variable when translated into clinical practice (19). In 2006, a large trial of nearly 1,400 patients compared naltrexone and acamprosate, alone or in combination, in conjunction with specialist behavioral treatments and against specialist behavioral treatments alone. In this study, naltrexone monotherapy and behavioral monotherapy were shown to have the most robust success in achieving abstinence at 16 weeks, and were equivalent to combined naltrexone and specialist behavioral therapy (20). At 1 year, however, even the best treatment had an over 75% rate of return to heavy drinking. Surprisingly, acamprosate, with or without behavioral therapy,

Table 7.6 FDA-Approved Pharmacologic Treatment of Alcohol Dependence

MEDICATION	DOSAGE	SIDE EFFECTS/CAUTION
Naltrexone (ReVia, Vivitrol)	• Start first dose at 25 mg given the possibility of precipitating withdrawal symptoms. If tolerated, subsequent doses may be given at 50 mg • 380 mg IM every 4 weeks	• Must be opioid-free for 7–10 days; otherwise, severe opioid withdrawal may occur • Contraindicated in active opioid users • Caution in patients with depression, suicidal ideation, thrombocytopenia, or liver disease • Pregnancy class C
Acamprosate (Campral)	• 666 mg TID	• May be continued despite alcohol relapse • Requires dose adjustment in renal failure • Caution in patients with depression, anxiety, and suicidal ideation • Pregnancy class C
Disulfiram (Antabuse)	• 250–500 mg/day; start at 125 mg	• Must be abstinent from alcohol for >12 hours prior to use • Toxic reaction of headache, nausea, malaise, and generalized distress when used with alcohol • Severe pharmacokinetic and additive drug–drug interactions are possible with isoniazid and metronidazole • Pregnancy class C

was not effective in this trial. Subsequently, a smaller head-to-head comparison found that naltrexone was superior to acamprosate (21). Therefore, although both medications are indicated for the treatment of alcohol dependence, naltrexone may be superior to acamprosate in certain patient populations. Naltrexone and acamprosate should be used with caution in those who have liver and kidney impairment, respectively.

Antidepressants, anticonvulsants, and antipsychotics have also been studied for the prevention of alcohol relapse in patients with and without comorbid psychiatric disorders. Most recently, topiramate titrated to 300 mg/day has been shown to be effective in reducing alcohol relapse (as measured by percentage of heavy drinking days and serum GGT) in a randomized, placebo-controlled, multicenter study involving 371 subjects over 14 weeks (22). Although promising, these findings need to be replicated before recommending topiramate routinely.

Medication adherence is a major obstacle to the efficacy of pharmacologic treatment. In addition, limited access to and experience with these medications by primary care providers have precluded their widespread use. Although most patients with alcohol use disorders that succeed in cessation do not receive any targeted addiction treatment, it is prudent to use an FDA-approved medication to reduce alcohol relapse. We recommend naltrexone or acamprosate as the first-line treatment for alcohol dependence, due to their evidence base, safety profile, and efficacy. The injectable form of naltrexone can be considered in patients with problems adhering to daily oral medications. Finally, psychosocial treatments are widely regarded as the foundational method for long-term relapse prevention. Therefore, even with provision of medication, the primary care provider should encourage and facilitate a patient's participation in psychosocial treatment.

PSYCHOSOCIAL TREATMENT

Brief Intervention

Advice and counseling approaches to the treatment of AUDs closely parallel other strategies used by primary care providers to treat other chronic conditions. The most effective model is the use of brief intervention, which has been systematically studied to be helpful for treatment of problem drinking in primary care settings in four 15-minute weekly sessions (Table 7-7) (23). The key elements of brief intervention

Table 7.7 Brief Intervention for Alcohol Use Disorders

STEPS	COMMENTS	SAMPLE STATEMENTS
1. Assessment and direct feedback	Ask about alcohol use (CAGE, AUDIT-C) Provide education and feedback about the connection between alcohol use and legal, occupational, or relationship problems	"Your liver disease is likely to be related to alcohol use. Would you like me to give you some information about your hepatitis and alcohol use?" "I am very concerned about your drinking and how it is affecting your health."
2. Goal setting	Individually tailored goals based on collaboration between the patient and the provider Goals may change depending on readiness for change Goals should be realistic and include psychotherapy, social support, and use of medications when indicated	"What are your thoughts about alcohol use?" "Although I would advise complete alcohol cessation, how realistic is that for you?" "Although the use of medications is important in your recovery, it is critical to attend AA and monitor for triggers that may lead to relapse."
3. Behavioral modification	Identify situational triggers, finding other enjoyable activities and adaptive coping skills Includes relapse prevention	"What causes you to start drinking?" "What else can you do when you feel alone, stressed, or frustrated?" "Who can you talk to when you feel that you have failed to cut down on drinking?"
4. Self-help	Encourage self-discipline and increased self-awareness about alcohol use disorder	"Would you like an information booklet about alcohol addiction?" "Do you know where you can get help for your drinking problem?"
5. Follow-up and reinforcement	Often considered the most important aspect of the treatment plan Provide praise, reassurance, and encouragement during periods of sobriety Returning to appointment is a sign of patient motivation and efforts, even if relapse occurs	"I'm very glad to see you come back to talk more about your alcohol use." "How did your plan to stop or reduce your drinking work?"

Modified from Bertholet N, Daeppen JB, Wietlisbach V, et al. Reduction of alcohol consumption by brief alcohol intervention in primary care: systematic review and meta-analysis. *Arch Intern Med.* 2005;165:986–995.

include nonjudgmental discussion and the provision of ongoing education and feedback. Once the goals are identified (e.g., cession or reduction of drinking), then the provider may help the patient identify a plan of action (e.g., seeking behavioral counseling, group support, use of medications for detoxification and maintenance therapy, treatment of comorbid conditions, and use of self-help programs). Further feedback and refinement of goals and action plans are then continually addressed on follow-up, usually as early as possible, depending on the particular action plan (24).

Motivational Interventions

Motivational interventions are adapted from motivational interviewing, a caring, nonconfrontational, persuasive counseling style that elicits long-standing behavioral change. The basic assumption is that most people are ambivalent about behavioral change (i.e., continuing vs. stopping alcohol use). Therefore, providers should attempt to identify an individual's ambivalence and explore rationales for and against continued alcohol use. For example, rather than arguing incessantly about why the person should stop drinking, it may be more productive to explore the patient's motivation for alcohol cessation in a nonjudgmental way. Action plans and goals may then be tailored according to the patient's "readiness to change" (see Table 6.7 or see Chapter 6). Motivational enhancement therapy (MET) is a systematic psychological intervention that can also be used in the primary care setting to address AUDs. MET aims to improve patients' motivation for alcohol cessation and has been shown to be as efficacious for most patients as compared to other classic approaches, including CBT and 12-step programs (25).

Self-Help and 12-Step Programs

A variety of self-help, patient-initiated programs employ learning, acceptance, change, and support when combating alcohol and substance dependence with the eventual goal of achieving abstinence. The oldest and most well-known of these programs is Alcoholics Anonymous (AA). AA is a fellowship of men and women where the primary purpose is for members to help other members stay sober. The only requirement for membership is "the desire to stay sober." AA is based on a step-by-step approach and encourages total abstinence. In the first step, members admit that they are "powerless over alcohol" and that their lives have become "unmanageable." Subsequent steps include acquiring mentorship and support from a "sponsor," making amends to past mistakes, and admitting to new mistakes when they occur. The 12th step encourages members to pass on lessons learned to other individuals who have AUDs (26). Traditional 12-step programs have not been studied due to the organization's reluctance to participate in formal research. Twelve-Step Facilitation (TSF) is a formal program that incorporates AA principles. In a large multisite study involving 1,700 patients, Project MATCH found that there was no difference in the efficacy of CBT, MET, and TSF during the year following treatment.

However, TSF was most effective in persons from heavy drinking social environments (27).

Family and Community Programs

Social stability, such as full-time employment and supportive networks of friends and family, is associated with good overall outcomes in those who are alcohol dependent. With the patient's consent, family and friends can help facilitate access to community resources and act as chaperones or "sponsors" to which the patient must be accountable. Moreover, family and friends often serve as the key sources of support and motivation to maintain sobriety and will usually prompt their loved one to consider treatment after a relapse. When maladaptive family dynamics precede or contribute to AUDs, couple's and family therapy should be considered to address issues of anger, guilt, and shame that often interfere with sobriety. Family and loved ones often struggle alone and would benefit from involvement in support groups such as Al-Anon. For a patient who is unemployed or has minimal psychosocial support, it is reasonable to encourage participation in a therapeutic community or a substance abuse treatment program that provides a supportive environment, housing, and vocational rehabilitation.

OTHER TREATMENT CONSIDERATIONS

Preventing and Addressing Relapse

Although feared and misunderstood by patients and support networks alike, relapse of alcohol use after cessation is an expected event in long-term management. Common precipitants of relapse include use of a secondary substance, a return to substance-using friends, substance-associated sexual behavior, depression, anxiety, and craving for alcohol. These triggers need to be discussed openly and frankly with patients as an early part of their treatment program. Ideally, the clinician and patient collaboratively identify patient-specific triggers and create a prevention plan to address such situations when they arise. The plan may encourage the patient to use proactive strategies such as self-imposed alcohol reduction or cessation while in a supportive environment, calling a "sponsor" or similarly knowledgeable and supportive person, acknowledging relapse in the treatment setting, and staying away from people, places, and things that have been tied to past alcohol use. If a relapse does occur, patients should be encouraged to use it as an opportunity for self-evaluation of treatment goals, evaluation of the efficacy of treatment, identification and recognition of triggers associated with misuse, and reassessment of comorbid medical and psychiatric disorders.

Treatment of Comorbid Psychiatric Disorders (Dual Diagnosis)

Studies have shown that primary psychiatric disorders (those not related to substance use) frequently co-occur with alcohol and substance use disorders and are more chronic than the primary psychiatric disorders alone. Dual diagnosis, loosely defined as the co-occurrence of a primary psychiatric disorder and a substance use disorder, can create

<table>
<tr><td>

WHEN TO REFER

- Continued alcohol use despite a reasonable primary care intervention (e.g., failure to respond in 3 to 4 months)

- Need for specific psychosocial treatments (AA, CBT, MET, support groups, couple's and family therapy, or a therapeutic community)

- Use medications that could potentially be addictive or trigger alcohol use

- Diagnosis and treatment of complex comorbid psychiatric disorders

- Suicidal intent or worsening psychiatric symptoms

</td></tr>
</table>

serious morbidities and complications for treatment. Most of the studies that showed that psychotropic medications were effective for the prevention of alcohol relapse were in patients with comorbid psychiatric disorders such as bipolar disorder or schizophrenia. For patients with comorbid psychiatric disorders, it is recommended to treat the primary psychiatric disorder concurrently with the alcohol use disorder (15). Treatment of the primary psychiatric disorder should not be delayed due to concerns about therapeutic futility. In more difficult cases where diagnostic uncertainty is high, consultation with a psychiatrist or an addiction medicine specialist should be considered.

Practice Pointers

Case 1: Occult alcohol dependence

Mary is a 43-year-old woman with a history of hepatitis C and hypertension who presents with depressed mood and insomnia. She denies any suicidal thoughts but states, "Life just doesn't seem to be heading in the right direction." On this visit, she is most concerned about her persistently elevated blood pressure and insomnia. She reluctantly reports losing her job and apartment 3 months ago and she now lives with her sister. She divorced 1 year ago and has one adult son who is estranged from her. She reports a history of intravenous heroin use more than 8 years ago, smokes two packs of cigarettes per day, and drinks three to four beers each evening. Her physical exam is unremarkable except for a blood pressure of 165/95 mmHg, heart rate of 108 beats per minute, moderate bilateral hand tremor, and inability to perform tandem gait.

Discussion: *Mary has subtle physical findings (e.g., tremor, ataxia, and tachycardia), which, in the context of excessive daily alcohol intake, are consistent with occult alcohol dependence. Note that many patients do not disclose the full degree of alcohol use, especially in the first visit. The clinician should use the CAGE questions to screen further for alcohol misuse. If the screen is positive, further questions must determine the degree of use, abuse, or dependence. Specific questions relating to DSM criteria for abuse and dependence should be asked (Tables 7.1 and 7.2). The clinician should also inquire about a history of legal problems (e.g., DUI charges), past withdrawal symptoms or seizures, and reasons for divorce and estrangement from her son.*

If Mary is suspected to have an AUD, it is important to determine her feelings about alcohol use. In addition to providing education and feedback about continued alcohol use, brief intervention as outlined in Table 7.7 may be initiated. The patient should also be screened further for depression and anxiety disorders, although her symptoms are most likely secondary to a substance-induced mood or anxiety disorder. As she is quite concerned about her blood pressure, it would be important to let her know that in order to adequately treat her hypertension and insomnia, alcohol cessation would be important. If she agrees with alcohol reduction or cessation, her goals and plan of action should be reviewed. It would also be helpful to understand how Mary was able to stop injection drug use and employ a similar action plan. If the patient is ready to attempt cessation and is deemed to be medically stable, with adequate home support and minimal risk for severe alcohol withdrawal (i.e., no history of seizures or severe withdrawal syndromes in the past), a beta-blocker could be started for the treatment of hypertension and withdrawal symptoms, and a detoxification regimen may not be needed. If this is done, close daily follow-up to assess withdrawal symptoms must occur. The patient should also be referred for available psychosocial treatment programs such as AA or other 12-step programs. Eliciting family support from her sister would also be beneficial. The patient could also be prescribed naltrexone to prevent relapse. If she meets the criteria for anxiety or depression, pharmacologic therapy and psychotherapy should be started. The patient will need follow-up appointments for further treatment of her hypertension, any persistent psychiatric disorders, and review of laboratory studies. Future office visits should focus on how Mary is following her treatment plan (e.g., adherence with prescribed medications, avoidance of triggers associated with alcohol use, and attendance of AA meetings and psychotherapy for existing mood disorders) and addressing relapse if it occurs.

> **Case 2: Alcohol-induced mood disorder versus major depression**
>
> James is a 58-year-old accountant with a long history of heavy alcohol use resulting in poor performance at work and a recent arrest for driving while under the influence of alcohol. He used to drink five to seven 20-oz beers per night (heavier over the last 5 years) and started to drink in the morning before going to work. He is very shameful of his drinking and started to attend AA groups as suggested by the court. He presents to his primary care provider for treatment of depression. Over the past 15 days, he has noticed increased depressed mood, low energy and poor concentration at work, restlessness, insomnia, and increasing anxiety without any provocations. He denies any suicidal ideation. He reports that his relationships with his wife and three children are improving as they are very glad and supportive of his resolution to stop drinking. He was able to tell his boss, who was similarly supportive.
>
> The AMPS screening tool for psychiatric symptoms is negative for any history of hypomania, mania, psychotic symptoms, or anxiety. He smokes about 1.5 packs per day of tobacco and notices that his smoking habit may be getting worse since he has stopped drinking. There is no history of past psychiatric treatment or family psychiatric history except for alcohol dependence in his father and older brother. His vitals are normal and there is no evidence of alcohol withdrawal. His mental status exam is notable for a depressed mood and a fully reactive affect.

Discussion: *This patient presents with symptoms that meet the diagnostic criteria for major depressive disorder. However, he has recently just stopped drinking successfully without any medical treatment. At the moment, the most suitable diagnosis is substance-induced mood disorder. The American Psychiatric Association (APA) suggests allowing at least 3 to 4 weeks of monitored abstinence in order to definitively diagnose a primary mood disorder and initiate antidepressant medication management (15). However, a few exceptions apply: (1) worsening rather than improving symptoms over time while sober, (2) a history of mood or anxiety disorders unrelated to alcohol or substance use, and (3) a strong family history of mood or anxiety disorders (14). While treatment of a mood or anxiety disorder would increase the likelihood of remission from alcohol dependence, this patient does not meet any of the exceptions to start medication treatment for depression. However, the primary care provider can work with James to maintain sobriety from alcohol. At this point, the patient may be managed by continued monitoring to see if his symptoms would improve or worsen. The Patient Health Questionnaire-9 (PHQ-9) may be administered for baseline and then readministered upon follow-up in 2 to 3 weeks. Education should be provided about alcohol withdrawal and related psychiatric symptoms. Sleep hygiene should be reviewed and sedative-hypnotics (which may precipitate alcohol relapse) should be avoided. Liver enzymes and a urine drug screen should be obtained and addressed if abnormal. If on the return visit the patient's depressive and anxiety symptoms continue or worsen, pharmacotherapy and psychotherapy may be initiated and the patient should be asked about suicidal thoughts.*

ICD9	
Alcohol Abuse	*305.00*
Alcohol Dependence	*303.90*
Alcohol-Induced Anxiety Disorder	*291.8*
Alcohol-Induced Mood Disorder	*291.8*

Practical Resources

http://www.niaaa.nih.gov/
http://ncadistore.samhsa.gov/
http://findtreatment.samhsa.gov/
http://www.alcoholics-anonymous.org/
http://www.Al-AnonFamilyGroups.org
http://www.asam.org/

References

1. Fleming MF, Manwell LB, Barry KL, et al. At-risk drinking in an HMO primary care sample: prevalence and health policy implications. *Am J Public Health.* 1998;88(1):90–93.

2. U.S. Department of Health and Human Services. National Institutes of Health. National Institute on Alcohol Abuse and Alcoholism. Updating estimates of the economic costs of alcohol abuse in the United States: estimates, update methods, and data. Rockville, MD: U.S. Department of Health and Human Services; 2000.

3. National Institute on Alcohol Abuse and Alcoholism. *Helping Patients Who Drink Too Much: A Clinician's Guide.* Updated 2005 edition. Bethesda, MD: National Institute on Alcohol Abuse and Alcoholism; 2005.

4. American Psychiatric Association. *Diagnostic and Statistical Manual of Mental Disorders.* 4th ed., text revision. Washington, DC: American Psychiatric Association; 2000.

5. Bayard M, McIntyre J, Hill KR, et al. Alcohol withdrawal syndrome. *Am Fam Physician.* 2004;69(6):1443–1450.

6. Ferguson JA, Suelzer CJ, Eckert GJ, et al. Risk factors for delirium tremens development. *J Gen Intern Med.* 1996;11(7):410–414.

7. U.S. Preventive Services Task Force. Screening and behavioral counseling interventions in primary care to reduce alcohol misuse: recommendation statement. *Ann Intern Med.* 2004;140(7):554–556.

8. Fiellin DA, Reid MC, O'Connor PG. Screening for alcohol problems in primary care: a systematic review. *Arch Intern Med.* 2000;160:1977–1989.

9. Ewing JA. The CAGE questionnaire. *JAMA.* 1984;252:1905–1907.

10. Bush K, Kivlahan DR, McDonell MB, et al. The AUDIT alcohol consumption questions (AUDIT-C): an effective brief screening test for problem drinking. Ambulatory Care Quality Improvement Project (ACQUIP). Alcohol Use Disorders Identification Test. *Arch Intern Med.* 1998;158(16):1789–1795.

11. Bell H, Tallaksen CM, Try K, et al. Carbohydrate-deficient transferring and other markers of high alcohol consumption: a study of 502 patients admitted consecutively to a medical department. *Alcohol Clin Exp Res.* 1994;18(5):1103–1108.

12. Miller PM, Anton RF. Biochemical alcohol screening in primary care. *Addict Behav.* 2004;29:1427–1437.

13. Hasin DS, Stinson FS, Ogburn E, et al. Prevalence, correlates, disability, and comorbidity of DSM-IV alcohol abuse and dependence in the United States: results from the National Epidemiologic Survey on Alcohol and Related Conditions. *Arch Gen Psychiatry.* 2007;64(7):830–842.

14. Brady KT, Malcolm RJ. Substance use disorders and co-occurring axis i psychiatric disorders. In: Galanter M, Kleber H, eds. *Textbook of Substance Abuse Treatment.* Washington, DC: American Psychiatric Publishing, Inc.; 2004:529–538.

15. American Psychiatric Association. *Practice Guideline for the Treatment of Patients with Substance Use Disorders.* 2nd ed. Washington, DC: American Psychiatric Association; 2006.

16. Sullivan JT, Sykora K, Schneiderman J, et al. Assessment of alcohol withdrawal: the revised Clinical Institute Withdrawal Assessment for Alcohol scale (CIWA-Ar). *Br J Addict.* 1989;84(11):1353–1357.

17. Parker AJR, Marshall EJ, Ball DM. Diagnosis and management of alcohol use disorders. *BMJ.* 2008;336:496–501.

18. Kosten TR, O'Connor PG. Management of drug and alcohol withdrawal. *N Engl J Med.* 2003;348(18):1786–1795.

19. Bouza C, Magro A, Munoz A, et al. Efficacy and safety of naltrexone and acamprosate in the treatment of alcohol dependence: a systematic review. *Addiction.* 2004;99:811–828.

20. Anton RF, O'Malley SS, Ciraulo DA, et al. COMBINE Study Research Group. Combined pharmacotherapies and behavioral interventions for alcohol dependence: the COMBINE study: a randomized controlled trial. *JAMA.* 2006;295(17):2003–2017.

21. Morley KC, Teesson M, Reid SC, et al. Naltrexone versus acamprosate in the treatment of alcohol dependence: a multi-centre, randomized, double-blind, placebo-controlled trial. *Addiction.* 2006;101:1451–1462.

22. Johnson BA, Rosenthal N, Capece JA, et al.; for the Topiramate for Alcoholism Advisory Board and the Topiramate for Alcoholism Study Group. Topiramate for treating alcohol dependence: a randomized controlled trial. *JAMA.* 2007;298(14):1641–1651.

23. Bertholet N, Daeppen JB, Wietlisbach V, et al. Reduction of alcohol consumption by brief alcohol intervention in primary care: systematic review and meta-analysis. *Arch Intern Med.* 2005;165:986–995.

24. Fleming M, Manwell LB. Brief intervention in primary care settings. A primary treatment method for at-risk, problem, and dependent drinkers. *Alcohol Res Health.* 1999;23:128–137.

25. Project MATCH Research Group. Project MATCH secondary a priori hypotheses. *Addiction.* 1997;92:1671–1698.

26. Alcoholics Anonymous. *A Brief Guide to Alcoholics Anonymous.* New York: Alcoholics Anonymous World Services, Inc.; 1972.

27. Owen PL, Slaymaker V, Tonigan JS, et al. Participation in alcoholics anonymous: intended and unintended change mechanisms. *Alcohol Clin Exper Res.* 2003;27(3):524–532.

CHAPTER 8

Unexplained Physical Symptoms— Somatoform Disorders

Robert M. McCarron, DO • Glen L. Xiong, MD • Mark C. Henderson, MD, FACP

> A 32-year-old man with no previous medical history presents to an urgent care clinic complaining of "gas in the stomach," shortness of breath, and squeezing back pain that prevents him from working. Other symptoms include a "jumping sensation in the legs" and "poor circulation in the hands and feet." He is unsure about what condition he might have. He is so concerned about his health that he has been sleeping in his car near the hospital for the past few days. He has seen numerous doctors over the past 6 months and, after an extensive medical work-up, has been told there are no obvious medical problems.

Clinical Significance

Patients and primary care practitioners alike often become frustrated with troublesome symptoms that are unexplainable after repeated assessments and unresponsive to multiple treatment regimens. Unexplained physical complaints (UPS) consist of somatic complaints that cannot be satisfactorily explained after a complete general medical work-up. Although UPS may ultimately have general medical and psychiatric etiologies, the focus of this chapter is to help practitioners accurately diagnose and effectively manage patients who have UPS due to psychiatric pathology.

Primary care practitioners encounter unexplained and perplexing complaints in up to 40% of their patients (1, 2). Medical explanations for common physical complaints such as malaise, fatigue, abdominal discomfort, and dizziness are only found 15% to 20% of the time (3). Although it is difficult to reliably determine the prevalence of UPS (loosely termed somatization) due to wide-ranging definitions, most studies estimate a prevalence of 16% to 20% in primary care settings (4).

The common occurrence of UPS, whether from general medical or psychopathologic causes, carries a large financial burden. A retrospective review of over 13,000 psychiatric consultations found that somatization resulted in more disability and unemployment than any other psychiatric illness (5). Moreover, patients with somatization in the primary care setting have more than twice the outpatient utilization and overall medical care costs when compared with patients without somatization. The direct costs related to the management of UPS approach 10% of medical expenditures or over $100 billion annually in the U.S. (6).

CLINICAL HIGHLIGHTS

- Unexplained physical symptoms (UPS) are commonly encountered in the outpatient setting and often require a long-term treatment plan.

- Unlike malingering and factitious disorders, patients who have somatoform disorders do not intentionally feign physical symptoms.

- Psychiatric disorders, such as depression and anxiety, frequently coexist with somatoform disorders. We suggest using the AMPS screening tool

(Continued)

Diagnosis

Although the word *somatization* is often used to describe physical complaints that cannot be completely explained by a physical examination and corresponding diagnostic work-up, a more precise nomenclature should be used. We use the term *UPS* to capture the general *Diagnostic and Statistical Manual of Mental Disorders*, 4th edition, text revision (DSM-IV-TR) diagnostic category of somatoform disorders (7). With a focus on the need to "exclude occult general medical conditions or substance-induced etiologies for the bodily symptoms," the DSM-IV-TR includes seven diagnoses under the category of somatoform disorders: somatization disorder, undifferentiated somatoform disorder, conversion disorder, pain disorder, hypochondriasis, body dysmorphic disorder, and somatoform disorder not otherwise specified.

In order to meet the criteria for any of the somatoform disorders, one must have significant social or occupational dysfunction that is directly related to psychopathology. Also, unlike those with malingering or factitious disorder, patients with somatoform disorders *unconsciously* somatize as a coping mechanism and do not intentionally produce their symptoms (Table 8.1).

Alternatives to the DSM-IV-TR nomenclature have been proposed because of the perceived rigid and imprecise diagnostic criteria, frequent overlap between the somatoform disorders, and resultant impractical and confusing application to clinical practice. For example, in order to establish a DSM-IV-TR diagnosis of somatization disorder, one must manifest four pain symptoms, two gastrointestinal symptoms, one sexual symptom, and one pseudoneurologic symptom during the course of

Table 8.1   Somatoform Disorders: Diagnostic Criteria

DSM-IV-TR	DEFINITION
Somatization disorder	• Many unexplained physical complaints before age 30 • Four pain, two gastrointestinal, one sexual, and one pseudoneurologic symptom
Undifferentiated somatoform disorder	• One or more unexplained physical complaints • Duration of at least 6 months
Conversion disorder	• One or more unexplainable, voluntary motor or sensory neurologic deficits • Directly preceded by psychological stress
Pain disorder	• Pain in one or more sites that is largely due to psychological factors
Hypochondriasis	• Preoccupation with a nonexistent disease despite a thorough medical work-up • Does not meet criteria for a delusion
Body dysmorphic disorder	• Preoccupation with an imagined defect in physical appearance
Somatoform disorder not otherwise specified (NOS)	• Somatoform symptoms that do not meet criteria for any specific somatoform disorder

All the above disorders (1) cause significant social/occupational dysfunction, (2) are not due to other general medical or psychiatric conditions; and (3) are not intentionally produced or related to secondary gain.
From American Psychiatric Publishing, Inc. *Diagnostic and Statistical Manual of Mental Disorders*, 4th ed., text revision. Washington, DC: American Psychiatric Publishing, Inc.; 2000.

the illness. This somewhat arbitrary combination of symptoms is not usually relevant to commonly encountered somatization in the primary care setting. Whether a patient has all of the required symptoms or just a few UPS may not change management strategies. Furthermore, people with a diagnosis of somatization disorder must have had multiple somatic complaints before the age of 30. This information is difficult to obtain as studies have shown that patients beyond the age of 30 often cannot reliably recall their medical history with sufficient detail (8).

The wide clinical spectrum of somatization has prompted some medical specialties to develop their own system to identify unexplained physical symptoms. Some common examples include chronic fatigue syndrome, irritable bowel syndrome, and fibromyalgia. These three disorders all have controversial and elusive etiologies and therefore are challenging to manage. Although several non–DSM-IV-TR somatoform disorder diagnostic alternatives exist, it is both accurate and practical to classify most primary care somatizing patients as having undifferentiated somatoform disorder. Generally speaking, this may be more of a technical point as the long-term treatment plan is similar for most of the somatoform disorders.

PATIENT ASSESSMENT

Other than completing a thorough history and physical examination with indicated laboratory or radiographic tests, there are no specific diagnostic protocols for patients who have a somatoform disorder. Collateral history from other health care providers as well as family members is important to review, because this will help confirm a diagnosis and possibly reduce redundant and unnecessary medical evaluations.

Differential Diagnosis

The differential diagnosis for UPS seen in the primary care setting is extensive. It is important to keep in mind that "unexplainable" physical symptoms may be due to (1) *a medical condition that has not yet been diagnosed* (e.g., hypothyroidism, celiac sprue, multiple sclerosis, or vascular claudication); (2) *a psychiatric condition such as malingering, factitious disorder, or one of the somatoform disorders*; and (3) a *medical condition that is present but not yet known to the medical community at large*. Lyme disease is an example of the latter. Before Lyme disease was discovered, patients were presenting with arthritis, myalgias, cardiac problems, depression, and fatigue, with no known precipitant or cause. It is beyond the scope of this book to explore an all-inclusive differential diagnosis for somatization, but it is noteworthy to stress the importance of doing a complete diagnostic work-up to rule out potential medical causes while considering each somatoform disorder to be "a diagnosis of exclusion" (Figure 8.1).

Before establishing a somatoform spectrum diagnosis, attempt to rule out the intentional production of physical or psychological symptoms. A patient with malingering is focused on feigning illness in an

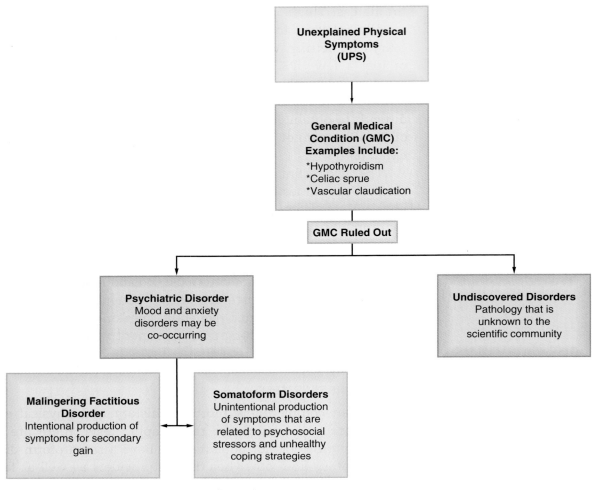

Figure 8.1 Unexplained physical symptoms—differential diagnosis.

attempt to gain external incentives such as financial compensation, shelter, food, or escape from military duty or criminal prosecution. Factitious disorder also involves the purposeful and sometimes elaborate self-report of somatic complaints with the objective of assuming the "sick role." People with factitious disorder have no obvious external secondary gain. When treating either condition, it is important to obtain collateral history (particularly from other area hospitals and providers), conduct a focused physical exam, and, as with any somatoform disorder, consider both as diagnoses of exclusion.

People who are malingering are not usually "antisocial." Instead, they are often emotionally troubled and under so much psychological stress that they engage in maladaptive and deceitful coping strategies, with resultant isolation from family, friends, and medical providers. Once a diagnosis of malingering is established, one should attempt to confront the patient in a supportive and reassuring way while trying to problem solve using a multidisciplinary team approach. Assisting malingerers with urgent stressors can be somewhat effective and a psychiatric referral is not normally indicated. However, if a diagnosis of factitious disorder is made, psychiatric consultation is strongly advised because this disorder is difficult to treat and carries a poor long-term prognosis.

NOT TO BE MISSED

- General medical condition(s)
- Depression
- Anxiety disorders
- Alcohol or substance-induced disorders
- Malingering or factitious disorder

Table 8.2 CARE MD – Treatment Guidelines for Somatoform Disorders

CBT/Consultation	• Follow the CBT treatment plan developed by the therapist and patient
Assess	• Rule out potential general medical causes for the somatic complaints • Treat co-morbid psychiatric disorders
Regular visits	• Short frequent visits with focused exams • Discuss recent stressors and healthy coping strategies • Overtime, the patient should agree to stop over utilization of medical care (e.g. frequent emergency room visits, or excessive calls and pages to the primary care provider)
Empathy	• "Become the patient" for a brief time • During visits, spend more time listening to the patient rather than jumping to a diagnostic test • Acknowledge patient's reported discomfort
Med-psych interface	• Help the patient self-discover the connection between physical complaints and emotional stressors ("the mind-body" connection) • Avoid comments like, "your symptoms are all psychological" or "there is nothing wrong with you medically"
Do no harm	• Avoid unnecessary diagnostic procedures • When possible, minimize unnecessary requests for consultation to medical specialists • Once a reasonable diagnostic work up is negative, feel comfortable with a somatoform disorder diagnosis and initiate treatment

From McCarron R. Somatization in the primary care setting. *Psychiatric Times.* 2006;23(6):32–34.

Biopsychosocial Treatment

The treatment approach to somatoform disorders exemplifies the "art of medicine." Because these disorders occur on a wide-ranging diagnostic continuum, with elusive etiologies, it is difficult to apply a strict, evidence-based approach to treatment (8, 9). We propose a simplified treatment plan that is described by the acronym **CARE MD** (Table 8.2) (10). This approach encourages patients to be active participants in their care and serves as a guide to help primary care practitioners effectively work with people who have somatoform disorders.

COGNITIVE-BEHAVIORAL THERAPY/CONSULTATION

Consultation with mental health professionals and use of CBT has been shown to decrease the severity and frequency of somatic preoccupations (11,12). Kroenke and Swindle, in 2000, reviewed 31 controlled studies and concluded that CBT is an effective treatment for patients with somatization. Group therapy using CBT with an emphasis on education has also been found to be beneficial (13). CBT generally consists of 10 to 20 one-hour psychotherapy sessions with the goal of teaching patients how to take an active role in their treatment and developing skills that last a lifetime. This type of psychotherapy is based on the premise that negative, automatic, or "dysfunctional thoughts" are predominant in patients with somatoform disorders. Examples of such thoughts are "I will always be sick and never get better," "No one understands or believes my pain," and "Everyone thinks it's all in my head." Through a variety of mechanisms, patients learn to recognize and reconstruct dysfunctional thought patterns with resultant decreased somatic complaints.

Patients should be encouraged to use a daily dysfunctional thought record (DTR) to self-monitor depressive or anxious emotions and associated negative thoughts. In collaboration with the therapist, primary care providers can learn to use brief cognitive behavioral techniques and quickly review a DTR during office visits. Additionally, we recommend that patients with somatoform, depressive, or anxiety disorders, as well as treating mental health and primary care practitioners, learn the basics of CBT. One of many practical resources includes the book *Feeling Good: The New Mood Therapy* by Davis Burns, MD (14). The first 80 pages of this book are practical and teach the patient how to recognize dysfunctional thought patterns and complete "homework" that will reverse cognitive distortions, decrease somatization, and improve mood (Figure 8.2).

ASSESS MEDICAL AND PSYCHIATRIC COMORBIDITIES

Assessing patients on each visit for general medical problems that might explain troublesome physical complaints is essential. This is particularly important for patients who have a long history of somatic preoccupation and present with a new complaint or a worsening of existing symptoms. Up to 25% to 50% of patients with conversion disorder eventually have an identifiable, nonpsychiatric disease that explains their symptoms (15). It is also important to screen for other common psychiatric diagnoses. Up to 50% of patients with somatoform disorders have concurrent anxiety or depressive disorders (16, 17). The number of unexplained somatic symptoms is highly predictive of comorbid mood and anxiety disorders as well as functional disability. Primary care clinicians can address frequently co-occurring depression by using the Patient Health Questionnaire (PHQ-9), a patient self-report tool that reliably screens for depression in the primary

Emotions	Automatic Thoughts	Rational Reponse	Outcome
Specify feeling rate 1–10 (10 rated as most intense)	"What is running through your head" (Not an emotion or feeling)	Why is the automatic thought inaccurate (Be specific)?	Re-specify feeling Re-rate feeling using 1–10 scale
"Sad" 8/10	"My pain will *never* go away."	"Not true—I am working hard with my doctor so my pain will get better over time." "Never is a strong word to use."	"Sad" 5/10
"Angry" 9/10	"*Everyone* thinks I'm faking my pain."	"My doctor listens to me and everyone is a lot of people!" "I know my family is trying to understand my pain and depression."	"Angry" 3/10
"Anxious: 9/10	"*Nobody* will ever figure out what is wrong with me and there is no reason to go on living."	"I know I have somatization disorder and doing my CBT homework will only help me." Sometimes I feel like dying but I know I want to live."	"Anxious" 4/10

Figure 8.2 Sample dysfunctional thought record. CBT, Cognitive behavioral therapy. Rating scale: 1 represents least intense specified feeling and 10 is most intense.

care setting (see Chapter 2). All patients with a score greater than 5 should be assessed for a possible major depressive disorder.

REGULAR VISITS

Regular visits with a single clinician are critical to the management of somatoform disorders. Short, frequent appointments or telephone encounters have been shown to decrease outpatient medical costs while maintaining patient satisfaction (18). These encounters should include a brief but focused history and physical exam followed by open-ended questions such as "How are things at home?" "What is your number one, biggest problem?" or, if the patient is exposed to CBT, "Tell me about your most frequent negative thoughts since your last visit." Over time, patients can replace excessive emergency room visits or frequent calls to the clinic with this supportive, caring patient–provider interaction. Longer, less frequent visits can be reserved for assessment and treatment of other general medical disorders and health care maintenance. In sum, spending most of the time during the shorter, frequent visits on worrisome psychosocial stressors will provide an outlet for patients to better cope with somatic preoccupation.

EMPATHY

Empathy or briefly "becoming the patient" is important for developing a strong therapeutic alliance between the patient and the health care provider. The use of empathy can also minimize negative feelings or countertransference from providers. True empathic remarks such as "This must be difficult for you" or "It must be very hard to cope with what you are experiencing" are often therapeutic. This is particularly true when frustrated family or friends are in the exam room when these questions are asked, as it may demonstrate the positive effects associated with the use of empathic remarks. Although there are clear benefits associated with the use of empathy, it can also be emotionally taxing to medical providers. The most important step in dealing with this possible angst is to anticipate and recognize it early on. We recommend the utilization of Balint groups or regularly scheduled, candid, and confidential discussions about challenging patient encounters with colleagues who experience similar clinical situations.

MEDICAL–PSYCHIATRIC INTERFACE

General medicine and psychiatry interface in the treatment of patients with somatoform disorders. Patients with a somatoform disorder should be educated about how emotions and stressors have a direct effect on the body. Understandably, many patients will not accept explanations for their UPS with statements (or indirect communications) such as "It's all in your head," "There is nothing medically wrong with you," or "A psychiatrist will have to take care of your complaints." Instead, primary care practitioners should provide a diagnosis and, if necessary, arrange for a psychiatric consultation while remaining the primary point of contact for all medical issues. During the short but frequent office visits, patients should be asked if the unexplained symptoms worsen as the primary stressor intensifies or if the symptoms improve as the primary stressor lessens. If the answer is affirmative to both questions, allow the patient to slowly make the connection by asking an open-ended question such as "Do you have any thoughts on why this might be?" Essentially, it is best to help the patient self-discover the connection between the unresolved conflict or emotional stress and the UPS.

DO NO HARM

Doing no harm by avoiding unnecessary procedures or consultations is the most important part of treating patients with chronic somatoform disorders. Clinicians should not deviate from normal practice style to appease a patient or minimize provider or frustration. While unnecessary invasive procedures should be avoided, routine health care maintenance studies should be offered and their importance emphasized. The routine studies may be offered over time, rather than completing every test in one visit, in keeping with the principle of utilizing "short and frequent" visits. After taking reasonable steps to rule out a general medical cause for the UPS, make the appropriate somatoform diagnosis and treat accordingly.

PHARMACOTHERAPY

While antidepressants may be considered for the treatment of somatoform disorders, we generally do not recommend starting such medications for UPS, especially on the first encounter. In our clinical experience, offering psychotropic medications for a somatoform disorder too quickly may reinforce the idea that the symptoms are exclusively psychiatric in nature and may impair the development of a trusting therapeutic relationship. On the other hand, antidepressants should be considered when comorbid depressive or anxiety disorders are discovered and treatment accepted by patients. Even in such patients, a significant amount of effort is required to educate patients about the possible psychiatric contribution to the unexplained physical ailment. The provider should only start psychotropic medication after establishing full collaboration with the patient.

Practice pointers

Case 1: Multiple, vague, and unexplained physical symptoms

A 32-year-old man with no previous medical history presents to an urgent care clinic complaining of "gas in the stomach," shortness of breath, and squeezing back pain that prevents him from working. Other symptoms include a "jumping sensation in the legs" and "poor circulation in the hands and feet." He is unsure about what condition he might have. He is so concerned about his health that he has been sleeping in his car near the hospital for the past few days. He has seen numerous doctors over the past 6 months and, after an extensive medical work-up, has been told there are no obvious medical problems.

He does not take any medications. He smokes occasionally and denies illicit drug use. He is currently unemployed. Both parents are healthy with no family history of heart disease or cancer. The physical exam reveals an anxious and somewhat

WHEN TO REFER

- Patients with significant social or occupational dysfunction directly related to a somatoform disorder should be referred to a psychiatrist.

- Patients with comorbid psychopathology such as severe depression or suicidal ideation should receive an urgent psychiatric referral.

- In cases when a psychiatric referral is placed for somatization, the primary care provider should receive input from the psychiatrist but remain the primary care provider.

dramatic man who uses frequent hand gestures. He repeatedly states, "There is something wrong with my heart." The laboratory studies including complete blood count, basic chemistry panel, and thyroid studies are normal.

Two weeks later, the patient returns to inquire about his labs. During this visit, he reports vague physical complaints and recalls that a neurologist had suggested that he might have problems in his spine. He admits to a history of depression more than 3 years ago, which improved on its own. He denies current depressed mood and states, "There is nothing wrong with my head." In fact, he became quite upset when the physician suggested that his symptoms could be related to depression or anxiety. He does concede that things have been stressful for him over the last few months and that he noticed a temporal correlation between the stress and the symptoms. He is motivated to get better and has no desire to collect disability. His physical examination was normal.

Discussion: *This patient exhibits several symptoms that are vague, are seemingly disconnected, and do not suggest any obvious general medical etiology. By enumerating the number of physical symptoms, the patient does not quite meet the criteria for somatization disorder. This patient is not fixated on having a specific disease with related disability and, therefore, does not have hypochondriasis. There is no reason to think he is intentionally feigning the symptoms for either external (e.g., financial) or internal (e.g., assuming the "sick role") gain, and therefore, he does not meet the criteria for either malingering or factitious disorder. Because there is not an apparent general medical cause for the above noted symptoms, coupled with the increased complaints in proportion to life stressors, we favor the working diagnosis of undifferentiated somatoform disorder.*

Patients with undifferentiated somatoform disorder will typically present with one or more unexplained physical complaints that may or may not be specific. Since none of the symptoms leads to a well-defined diagnosis, the provider may become uneasy and frustrated by the lack of diagnostic certainty. Treatment should begin with the establishment of a therapeutic alliance with the patient by creating a supportive, nonjudgmental, and collaborative relationship. It is important that the provider spend sufficient time to understand the patient's symptoms and consequent suffering. The provider may explain to the patient that although the current symptoms may not point to a clear general medical condition, continued monitoring is indicated. It is important to point out the dangers of unnecessary diagnostic tests and procedures as they can lead to false-positive results and increased morbidity. We recommend close attention to health care maintenance and general counseling about diet, exercise, and smoking cessation.

After the establishment of a firm therapeutic alliance, psychoeducation about the nature of unexplained physical symptoms could be gradually introduced. Subsequently, exploration of possible psychosocial precipitants of the distressing physical symptoms should be attempted. Assessment of concurrent psychiatric conditions using the AMPS screening tool should be ongoing. Referral to a mental health professional may also be considered. CBT has been extensively studied and validated as a first-line therapy for somatoform disorders. It is advisable for medical providers to at least become familiar with CBT principles and the use of the DTR, as this is an evidence-based approach that has been studied in primary care settings.

Case 2: "Pseudoseizures"

A 22-year-old female with a history of insomnia, progressive fatigue, and increasingly poor concentration is brought in by her family for the third time in 1 week to the on-call neurologist in the emergency room with complaint of "seizures." The patient was recently laid off from her job and reluctantly reports severe depression without suicidal ideation. When asked to recall what happens during a seizure, she states, "I feel confused and try to talk to people around me but just keep shaking." There is no loss of consciousness, tongue biting, injuries, bowel or bladder incontinence, or postictal disorientation. She is unable to recall any emotional trigger prior to these episodes. When asked about any history of abuse, she denies this after a long pause. There is no other medical history and no report of illicit drug or alcohol abuse. She has recently moved in with her family because of financial constraints. Her mother reports that this is very uncharacteristic of her daughter.

Discussion: Given the self-description of her seizures, it is unlikely she has a true seizure disorder. This young woman has had a recent stressor followed by a nonintentional, voluntary motor abnormality and most likely has pseudoseizures, which would be classified as conversion disorder. Unfortunately, it is often challenging to differentiate pseudoseizures from actual seizures without the use of electroencephalogram monitoring during or immediately after the abnormal behavior. Up to 30% of patients with pseudoseizures have concomitant documented epilepsy. Such a high comorbid prevalence illustrates the importance of completing a thorough examination during each clinical encounter and working closely with a consulting psychiatrist.

The treatment of her depression with an antidepressant and cognitive behavioral therapy should be considered. Providing the patient with healthier coping strategies will also decrease the frequency of pseudoseizures. As a primary care provider or consulting neurologist, it is best to avoid phrases like "There is no medical problem" or "Your problem is strictly psychiatric." One can help the patient slowly self-discover the connection between increased stress and the onset of pseudoseizures by acknowledging that the symptoms experienced by the patient are "real" but associated with maladaptive coping mechanisms (e.g., conversion disorder). There is generally a stressful event that precedes the development of conversion disorders. Identifying and addressing the emotional event may be helpful. In this case, further exploration of physical, sexual, or emotional abuse should be attempted in a private and safe environment and without the presence of family members. The long-term prognosis of conversion disorder is good and the neurologic deficits usually resolve over time.

Case 3: Factitious disorder and malingering

A 44-year-old male with no past medical history is seen in an emergency room with complaint of "I cannot feel my face.... I think I'm having a stroke." He is able to talk on the phone and eat solid and liquid foods without difficulty. He does not give permission to obtain collateral history from his family or friends. A nurse overhears him on the phone say, "It's cold out there and you better let me back in the house." When confronted, he admits his wife separated from him recently and that he is homeless. He also laments, "My face is paralyzed and I need to be hospitalized."

A neurologic examination and brain imaging are both normal. All laboratory values, including blood alcohol and toxicology screens, are also normal. The patient's response to reassurance from the emergency department physician is, "You better admit me...at least for tonight."

Discussion: In this case, a thorough diagnostic work-up was done and it is likely the patient is malingering, with shelter as the external secondary gain. Unlike those who have a somatoform disorder, patients who malinger intentionally report inaccurate information in order to realize a predetermined goal. Although it is often challenging, practitioners should try to empathize with patients who are malingering and focus on a solution to the actual problem. In this case, a discussion about housing options that do not include the hospital should be addressed with the patient in an assertive and nonpunitive manner. Collaboration with social workers and knowledge about local resources is important. The clinician can point out that admitting the patient to the hospital will not solve his housing problem or financial problems.

Lastly, malingering should always be a diagnosis of exclusion and made only after a thorough history and physical examination have been completed.

Factitious disorder should also be considered in this case. This diagnosis would apply if the patient was intentionally feigning symptoms in an attempt to assume the "sick role" and gain medical attention from various health care practitioners. Patients with factious disorder are often resistant to participate in psychiatric evaluations and psychotherapy. The most important part of treatment is to recognize the disorder and do no harm by avoiding unnecessary procedures and consultations. These patients should be fully assessed for general medical, neurologic, and highly comorbid psychiatric disorders. It is important to note that, unlike malingering and factitious disorder, somatoform disorders often originate from unconscious and unhealthy coping mechanism to life stressors.

ICD9	
Body Dysmorphic Disorder	*300.7*
Conversion Disorder	*300.11*
Hypochondriasis	*300.7*
Pain Disorder	
Associated with Medical and Psychological Factors	*307.89*
Associated with Psychological Factors	*307.8*
Somatization Disorder	*300.81*
Somatoform Disorder Not Otherwise Specified (NOS)	*300.82*
Undifferentiated Somatoform Disorder	*300.82*
Factitious Disorder	
With Combined Psychological and Physical Signs and Symptoms	*300.19*
With Predominantly Physical Signs and Symptoms	*300.19*
With Predominantly Psychological Signs and Symptoms	*300.16*
Factitious Disorder NOS	*300.19*
Malingering	*V65.2*

CHAPTER 8 Somatoform Disorders

Practical Resources

Familydoctor.org: http://familydoctor.org/online/famdocen/home/common/pain/disorders/162.html
Merk Manuals on-line: http://www.merck.com/mmhe/sec07/ch099/ch099b.html

References

1. Katon W, Ries RK, Kleinman A. The prevalence of somatization in primary care. *Compr Psychiatry.* 1984;25(2):208–215.

2. Kroenke K. Symptoms in medical patients: an untended field. *Am J Med.* 1992;92:1A.–3S.

3. Kroenke K, Mangelsdorff AD. Common symptoms in ambulatory care: incidence, evaluation, therapy, and outcome. *Am J Med.* 1989;86(3):262–266.

4. de Waal MW, Arnold IA, Eekhof JA, et al. Somatoform disorders in general practice: prevalence, functional impairment and comorbidity with anxiety and depressive disorders. *Br J Psychiatry.* 2004;184:470–476.

5. Thomassen R, van Hemert AM, Huyse FJ, et al. Somatoform disorders in consultation–liason psychiatry: a comparison with other mental disorders. *Gen Hosp Psychiatry.* 2003;25:8–13.

6. Neimark G, Caroff S, Stinnett J. Medically unexplained physical symptoms. *Psychiatry Ann.* 2005; 35(4):298–305.

7. American Psychiatric Association. *Diagnostic and Statistical Manual of Mental Disorders.* 4th ed., text revision. Washington, DC: American Psychiatric Association; 2000.

8. Simon GE, Gureje O. Stability of somatization disorder and somatization symptoms among primary care patients. *Arch Gen Psychiatry.* 1999;56:90–95.

9. Allen LA, Escobar JI, Lehrer PM, et al. Psychosocial treatments for multiple unexplained physical symptoms: a review of the literature. *Psychosom Med.* 2002;64:939–950.

10. McCarron R. Somatization in the primary care setting. *Psychiatric Times.* 2006;23(6):32–34.

11. Speckens AE, van Hemert AM, Spinhoven P, et al. Cognitive behavioural therapy for medically unexplained physical symptoms: a randomised controlled trial. *BMJ.* 1995;311:1328–1332.

12. Warwick HM, Clark DM, Cobb AM, et al. A controlled trial of cognitive behavioural treatment of hypochondriasis. *Br J Psychiatry.* 1996;169:189–195.

13. Kroenke K, Swindle R. Cognitive-behavioral therapy for somatization and symptom syndromes: a critical review of controlled clinical trials. *Psychother Psychosom.* 2000;9:205–215.

14. Burns D. *Feeling Good: The New Mood Therapy.* 2nd ed. New York: Avon Books; 1999.

15. Sadock BJ, Sadock VA. *Synopsis of Psychiatry.* Philadelphia: Lippincott Williams & Wilkins; 2003.

16. Allen L, Gara M, Escobar J. Somatization: a debilitating syndrome in primary care. *Psychosomatics.* 2001;42:1.

17. Kroenke K, Spitzer R, Williams J, et al. Predictors of psychiatric disorders and functional impairment. *Arch Fam Med.* 1994;3:774–779.

18. Smith C, Monson R, Ray D. Psychiatric consultation in somatization disorder. *Engl J Med.* 1986;14:1407–1413.

CHAPTER 8 Somatoform Disorders

CHAPTER 9 Eating Disorders

Margaret W. Leung, MD, MPH • Tracie Harris, MD • Claire Pomeroy, MD, MBA

A 28-year-old female competitive runner presents to a primary care clinic with pain in her right wrist, which developed after she fell at home. She fractured her left ankle 2 months ago. She is anxious to return to training for the next race. Review of symptoms is positive for occasional bloating, abdominal pain, feeling cold, and amenorrhea for the past 4 months.

CLINICAL HIGHLIGHTS

- Eating disorders include anorexia nervosa, bulimia nervosa, and eating disorder not otherwise specified (NOS). Binge eating disorder, currently classified under eating disorder NOS, is a research diagnosis requiring further study. Early detection, especially by the primary care clinician, is critical to successful intervention.

- Psychiatric comorbidities, most commonly depression, anxiety, and substance use disorders, are common in patients with eating disorders.

- In one particularly effective treatment model for eating disorders, the primary care clinician coordinates a multidisciplinary approach, including involvement of a nutritionist and a psychiatrist.

(Continued)

Clinical Significance

Eating disorders are highly prevalent and often associated with serious physical and psychiatric complications. Of all psychiatric diagnoses, eating disorders have the highest lethality, with anorexia nervosa carrying the highest death rates among eating disorders (1). Moreover, female patients with anorexia nervosa have more than 12 times the mortality rate when compared with women in the general population (2).

The U.S. lifetime prevalence of anorexia nervosa, bulimia nervosa, and binge eating disorder is 0.9%, 1.5%, and 3.5% in women, and 0.3%, 0.5%, and 2% in men, respectively, with the median age of onset ranging from 18 to 21 years old (2). In outpatient settings, eating disorders NOS (which include binge eating disorder) account for 60% of cases, compared with 14% for anorexia nervosa and 25% for bulimia nervosa, suggesting that "classic" presentations of anorexia nervosa and bulimia nervosa may be in the minority (3). The degree to which binge eating disorder contributes to the obesity epidemic in Western cultures is largely unknown. Recognizing eating disorders can be challenging for the primary care clinician because signs and symptoms are often not apparent in the early stages of these diseases.

A compassionate, nonjudgmental therapeutic relationship between the clinician and the patient is essential to maintain regular general medical and psychiatric follow-up. Eating disorders—much like other chronic diseases—vary in severity, relapse, and chronicity over the course of illness. While identification and medical management of eating disorders are core clinical tasks, the primary care clinician's role also includes encouraging healthy eating to help prevent these disorders. The clinician should emphasize basic nutritional and health education to patients, families, and schools, focusing on healthy eating habits and healthy weight maintenance. Within clinical practice, the primary care clinician can prevent further medical complications in the high-risk patient by refusing requests for prescriptions for diuretics, laxatives, and appetite-suppressant pills.

Diagnosis

An abbreviated summary of the *Diagnostic and Statistical Manual of Mental Disorders*, 4th edition, text revision (DSM-IV-TR) criteria for anorexia nervosa, bulimia nervosa, binge eating disorder, and eating disorder not otherwise specified is provided in Table 9.1 (4). Binge eating disorder, currently classified under eating disorder NOS, is discussed in the DSM-IV-TR with

Table 9.1 DSM-IV-TR Criteria

EATING DISORDER (SUBTYPES)	CRITERIA
Anorexia nervosa • Restricting • Binge eating/ purging	All four criteria need to be met for diagnosis • Refusal to maintain body weight at or above normal weight for age and height (<85% expected body weight) • Intense fear of gaining weight even though underweight • Disturbed thoughts about body weight or shape and denial of symptom severity • Amenorrhea
Bulimia nervosa • Purging • Nonpurging type	• Binge eating characterized by ○ Eating an amount of food larger than most people would consume in a similar period of time and circumstance ○ Loss of control during the binge • Recurrent inappropriate compensatory behaviors (i.e., exercise, diuretics, laxatives, purging) to prevent weight gain • Binge eating and behaviors occur at least twice a week for 3 months • Self-evaluation unduly influenced by body shape and weight
Binge eating disorder	• Recurrent episodes of binge eating characterized by ○ Eating larger amount of food than normal during short period of time ○ Lack of control over eating during binge period • Binge eating episodes are associated with ○ Eating until uncomfortably full ○ Eating large amounts of food when not physically hungry ○ Eating more rapidly than normal ○ Eating alone because of embarrassment by how much food is consumed ○ Feeling disgusted, depressed, or guilty after overeating • Binge eating occurs at least 2 days a week for 6 months • Binge eating not associated with regular inappropriate compensatory behavior
Eating disorder NOS	• Disordered eating that does not meet full criteria for anorexia nervosa or bulimia nervosa

Modified from American Psychiatric Association. *Diagnostic and Statistical Manual of Mental Disorders.* 4th ed., text revision. Washington, DC: American Psychiatric Publishing, Inc.; 2000.

Table 9.2 Symptoms Reported in Patients with Anorexia Nervosa, Bulimia Nervosa, and Binge Eating Disorder

ANOREXIA NERVOSA	BULIMIA NERVOSA	BINGE EATING DISORDER
Generalized weakness and lassitude	Abdominal bloating	Anxiety
Difficulty concentrating	Constipation	Depression
Palpitations	Sore throat	Dyspepsia and bloating
Abdominal pain and bloating	Dyspepsia	
Cold sensitivity	Menstrual irregularities	
Amenorrhea or menstrual irregularities	Anxiety	
Loss of libido	Depression	
Anxiety		
Depression		

descriptive research criteria requiring further study. Nonetheless, as it has relevance as a clinical phenomenon, it is discussed here.

ANOREXIA NERVOSA AND BULIMIA NERVOSA

Disordered eating ranges along a spectrum from early preoccupation with food and/or body image to late-stage medical complications. Eating disorders often present with nonspecific generalized symptoms (Table 9.2). A patient with anorexia nervosa does not complain of weight loss per se, though may report fatigue, constipation, abdominal pain, irregular menses, hair and skin changes, and cold intolerance. Persons with bulimia nervosa may report lethargy, abdominal bloating, and constipation but are often secretive about their binge and purging behavior.

The DSM-IV-TR classifies anorexia nervosa into two categories, restricting and binge eating/purging. Anorexia nervosa includes (1) a psychological component of fear of gaining weight despite being underweight, (2) disturbed thoughts about body weight, (3) amenorrhea, and (4) less than 85% expected body weight. The body image distortion in anorexia nervosa is significant in its context and severity with patients overestimating their bodies on a body fat dimension, whereas patients with bulimia nervosa wish to have a body with less fat (5).

Bulimia nervosa is divided into two subtypes, purging and nonpurging. It is characterized by disordered self-perception unduly influenced by body shape and weight concerns, multiple episodes of binge eating over a specific time, and compensatory behaviors that may or may not include purging, such as excessive exercise. In general, anorexia nervosa is an easier diagnosis to make than bulimia nervosa because the former presents with severe weight loss and the desire to lose more weight. Bulimia nervosa is harder to diagnose based on physical appearance because a patient may be either average weight or slightly overweight.

BINGE EATING DISORDER

Binge eating disorder has emerged as a specific DSM-IV-TR research disorder that often presents with symptoms associated with obesity such as orthopnea from obstructive sleep apnea or polyuria from untreated diabetes mellitus induced by obesity. What distinguishes the obese individual without binge eating disorder from the obese individual with binge eating disorder is the severity of binge eating, not the degree of obesity (6). Binge eating disorder shares many clinical characteristics with bulimia nervosa but lacks the compensatory behavior seen in bulimia nervosa (no purging, etc.).

The patient with disordered eating who does not meet full criteria for anorexia nervosa and bulimia nervosa is diagnosed with eating disorder NOS. A common example is a patient who meets many of the clinical criteria for anorexia nervosa but who has of yet not developed secondary amenorrhea.

GENERAL MEDICAL ASSESSMENT

Monitoring for signs and symptoms of eating disorders should be routine and especially kept in mind when evaluating high-risk populations such as participants in gymnastics, wrestling, and ballet. These individuals often place a high value on a thin body habitus or have rigid weight maxima for competition (7). When there are clinical concerns for an eating disorder, particular components of the history can identify physical complications (8). A complete weight history includes a timeline of maximum and minimum weights, and how much the patient feels he or she "ought to" weigh compared with "standardized" height and weight values. A diet history documents the number and types of past weight loss diets, use of weight loss medications, preoccupations with food, excessive calorie counting, avoidance of "taboo" foods, and types of food consumed, especially in binge eating episodes. An exercise history provides information about the frequency and intensity of exercise. A medication history can elucidate methods of purging with diuretics, ipecac, and laxatives. A specific question about over-the-counter or "borrowed" medication usage may be needed. For women, a menstrual and fertility history is important to determine the impact of the eating disorder on metabolic and endocrinologic homeostasis, such as amenorrhea. Given the high frequency of psychiatric comorbidities in eating disorders, it is important to obtain a psychiatric history and document the presence of depression, anxiety, psychosis, or substance use. Information from the social history can highlight potential risk factors such as a history of trauma or childhood or sexual abuse, which may affect personality functioning and be partially implicated in the genesis of eating disorder in some patients. The family history includes an inquiry particularly about first-degree relatives with eating disorders. The relative risk for full or partial syndromes of anorexia nervosa and bulimia nervosa in patients with a first-degree relative with an eating disorder was 11- and 4-fold, respectively (9).

Pregnancy and diabetes present unique challenges to the primary care clinician providing care to the patient with or at risk for an eating disorder. In pregnancy, hyperemesis gravidarum, a history of eating disorder, or a lack of weight gain in two consecutive visits in the second trimester should prompt a full assessment for an eating disorder (10).

Table 9.3 SCOFF: Validated Screening Questions for Eating Disorders in Primary Care Settings

- Do you make yourself **s**ick because you feel uncomfortably full?
- Do you worry that you have lost **c**ontrol over how much you eat?
- Have you recently lost more than **o**ne stone (14 pounds or 6.3 kg) in a 3-month period?
- Do you belief yourself to be **f**at when others say you are too thin?
- Would you say that **f**ood dominates your life?

Two positive answers are highly predictive of either anorexia nervosa or bulimia nervosa.

From Morgan JF, Reid F, Lacey H. The SCOFF questionnaire: assessment of a new screening tool for eating disorders. *BMJ*. 1999;319:1467–1468.

Eating disorder risk increases dramatically in the postpartum period and plateaus 6 months after delivery. An insulin-dependent diabetic may control his or her weight by withholding insulin, thereby increasing the risk for severe hyperglycemia, diabetic ketoacidosis, and long-term complications of diabetes mellitus.

Once a thorough history has been obtained, various screening tools can be applied. The SCOFF is a validated screening questionnaire for eating disorders in the primary care setting (11). Five questions screen for weight loss, attitude about food, sense of control over food, and self-evaluation of body image (Table 9.3). In one study, positive answers to two of the questions yielded a 100% sensitivity and 87% specificity for detecting anorexia nervosa or bulimia nervosa (11).

A thorough physical exam of someone with an eating disorder should be completed, beginning with height and weight. Aberrant vital signs may include bradycardia or orthostatic hypotension. An oral exam may reveal dry mucous membranes, enlarged parotid glands, dental caries, or enamel erosion (Table 9.4). Auscultation of the cardiovascular system may reveal arrhythmias. Mitral valve prolapse may occur secondary to loss of left ventricle muscle mass in anorexia nervosa. The abdominal exam can aid in the detection of pancreatitis and cholecystitis. The genital and gynecologic exam may reveal hypogonadism and related estrogen deficiency. The dermatologic exam may reveal dry, cool skin with lanugo hair. A mental status exam and psychiatric review of systems should be performed to detect the presence of depression, mania, anxiety, psychosis, or other psychiatric comorbidities.

The history and physical exam aid the clinician to choose appropriate laboratory studies. Basic laboratory tests can gauge the extent of the medical complications of eating disorders (Table 9.4). There are no specific consensus guidelines for a basic laboratory work-up; the extent of the work-up will be based on clinical judgment. A complete blood cell count is helpful for the assessment of anemia due to malnutrition and/or gastrointestinal blood loss secondary to repeated emesis. Abnormal serum electrolytes, especially potassium, phosphorous, magnesium, and bicarbonate, may reflect compensatory bulimic behaviors of vomiting and laxative and diuretic abuse. Serum amylase level may be elevated

Table 9.4 Signs, Medical Complications, and Common Lab Findings in Eating Disorders

	ANOREXIA NERVOSA	BULIMIA NERVOSA	BINGE EATING DISORDER
Signs	• Low BMI and body weight[a] • Orthostatic hypotension • Skin cool to touch • Lanugo • Jaundice-like skin color • Arrested development of secondary sex characteristics	• Loss of tooth enamel • Tender or swollen parotid and submandibular glands • Knuckle calluses and hypertrophy	• High BMI
ECG	• Low voltage • Bradycardia • Prolonged QT interval • Prolonged PR interval • ST-T–wave abnormalities	• Low voltage • Bradycardia • Prolonged QT interval • U waves	• ST-T–waves changes suggestive of atherosclerotic changes
Labs	• Hyponatremia (excessive water intake) • Hypophosphatemia (distinguished from the refeeding syndrome) • Hypoglycemia • Sick euthyroid syndrome	• Hypochloremia • Hypokalemia • Metabolic alkalosis • Elevated serum amylase	• Hypercholesterolemia • Transaminitis
Major manifestations of eating disorders	• Electrolyte abnormalities • Arrhythmias • Dehydration • Superior mesenteric artery syndrome • Refeeding hypophosphatemia • Osteoporosis and fractures • Infections	• Electrolyte abnormalities • Dehydration • Esophageal rupture • Postbinge pancreatitis • Aspiration pneumonitis • Pneumothorax or rib fracture	• Coronary heart disease • Cholecystitis, cholelithiasis • Gastric dilation/rupture • Degenerative joint disease • Dyslipidemia • Diabetes mellitus • Sleep apnea • Nonalcoholic steatohepatitis

BMI, body mass index; ECG, electrocardiogram.
[a] BMI = kg/m^2 (underweight BMI <18.5, normal weight 18.5–24.9 kg/m^2, overweight 25.0–29.9 kg/m^2, class I obesity 30–34.9 kg/m^2, class II obesity 35.0–39.9 kg/m^2, class III obesity [severe or morbid obesity] ≥40 kg/m^2).
Ideal body weight for men = 106 pounds (per 5 feet) + 6 pounds/inch (per inch over 5 feet) ± 10%.
Ideal body weight for women = 100 pounds (per 5 feet) + 5 pounds/inch (per inch over 5 feet) ± 10%.
Adapted from Pomeroy C. Medical evaluation and medical management. In: Mitchell J, ed. *The Outpatient Treatment of Eating Disorders: A Guide for Therapists, Dietitians, and Physicians*. Minneapolis: University of Minnesota Press; 2001:306–348.

in self-induced vomiting or pancreatitis. Elevated liver function tests may point to gallbladder disease or nonalcoholic steatohepatitis in binge-eating patients. Poor nutritional status is reflected in low albumin and transferrin. Levels of thyroid-stimulating hormone and thyroxine (i.e., free T_4) help exclude thyroid dysfunction. Urinalysis and stool tests are useful in bulimia nervosa to detect diuretic or laxative abuse. Urine toxicology can detect the presence of stimulants, which are often used to suppress appetite. A baseline electrocardiogram should be checked with all patients who have an eating disorder. Depending on the clinical situation, a bone density scan can be obtained for patients with anorexia nervosa, as they often are at increased risk for osteoporosis (12).

PSYCHIATRIC ASSESSMENT

Psychiatric comorbidities frequently complicate eating disorders. Starvation can mimic symptoms of a mood disorder. Since a starving patient can become depressed, irritable or have decreased cognitive capacity, a definitive psychiatric diagnosis cannot always be determined on a single visit. Nevertheless, early screening for psychiatric disorders and re-evaluations during treatment are recommended to optimize management. Depression may occur prior to or after the onset of an eating disorder, with the prevalence ranging from 20% to 83% (13). Among anxiety disorders, obsessive compulsive disorder and social phobia are the most common in eating disorder patients (14). A patient may become anxious when he or she is forced to eat a normal-calorie meal or eat in front of others, or is unable to purge. Substance use disorders, particularly amphetamine and cocaine abuse, are more prevalent among patients with eating disorders than the general population (15). Although obsessive compulsive personality disorders are common in patients with eating disorders, a subset including patients with anorexia nervosa (purging subtype) and bulimia nervosa exhibit Cluster B personality traits, such as borderline personality disorder (16).

Differential Diagnosis

Eating disorders affect numerous organ systems, resulting in a large differential diagnosis (Table 9.5). The main feature distinguishing general

Table 9.5 Differential Diagnosis of Eating Disorders

SYMPTOM	DIFFERENTIAL
Amenorrhea	Pregnancy Polycystic ovarian syndrome Hypothalamic dysfunction Prolactinoma Outflow tract abnormalities Congenital adrenal deficiency
Diarrhea	Laxative abuse Inflammatory bowel disease Malabsorption (e.g., celiac disease) Inflammatory bowel disease Superior mesenteric artery disorder
Intractable nausea and vomiting	Brain tumors Diabetes mellitus Disordered gastrointestinal dysmotility Hyperemesis gravidum Pancreatitis
Endocrinologic abnormalities	Hyperthyroidism/hypothyroidism Adrenal insufficiency Hypopituitarism Diabetes mellitus
Severe wasting	Malignancy Tuberculosis Human immunodeficiency virus
Psychiatric	Depression Anxiety Schizophrenia
Excessive eating	Temporal lobe or limbic seizures Lesions of the hypothalamus or frontal lobe Prader-Willi syndrome Kleine-Levin syndrome

medical disorders from eating disorders is the psychological presence of an altered body image or evaluation of oneself based on body habitus. A distorted body image is a feature of anorexia nervosa distinct from bulimia nervosa in which self-evaluation is affected by body shape. The general medical differential diagnosis of eating disorders is broad but can be organized according to symptoms. For example, diarrhea may be secondary to laxative abuse in eating disorders but may also be associated with inflammatory bowel disease and malabsorption. Amenorrhea occurs in pregnancy, hypothalamic dysfunction, and polycystic ovarian syndrome. Metabolic abnormalities such as hypothyroidism and adrenal insufficiency should be considered in the differential diagnosis of eating disorders.

Psychiatric disorders are also included in the differential diagnosis of eating disorders. Body dysmorphic disorder differs from eating disorders by the preoccupation with a perceived distortion of a specific body part rather than overall body shape. A patient with body dysmorphic disorder may seek and/or undergo unnecessary surgical alterations instead of binging, purging, restricting food, or excessively exercising. Depression manifests in changes in appetite, leading to either weight gain or loss. Schizophrenia may produce delusions about food or odd eating behaviors. Finally, obsessions and compulsions related to food or social fears of eating with others or in public may be associated with anxiety disorders.

Biopsychosocial Treatment

Because treatment of eating disorders encompasses medical, nutritional, psychological, and behavioral aspects of care, a multidisciplinary approach to care is ideally provided by a team consisting of the primary care clinician, a nutritionist, and a mental health professional. Ideally, the latter two individuals have experience working with eating disorders. The primary care clinician should have a low threshold to consult and refer to specialists since eating disorders are chronic medical and psychiatric illnesses that require ongoing monitoring for medical complications. As in any other medical condition, early detection facilitates early treatment. A nonconfrontational approach to patient care can be a means to educate the patient about medical complications of anorexia nervosa, bulimia nervosa, and binge eating disorder. The appendix provides online resources of local and national referrals for self-help support groups, private treatment centers, and mental health professionals with expertise in eating disorders.

A patient with an eating disorder will often try to assert his or her own independence and subvert the treatment plan. As such, the team needs to work with the patient to establish explicit goals and limitations and a contract for monitoring recovery. Contracts for eating disorder treatment outline indications for more advanced care beyond the outpatient setting (e.g., medical complications and severe low weight despite aggressive treatment) and frequency and duration of patient follow-up with each member of the team. Relapses and chronic persistence of symptoms are common in eating disorders.

ANOREXIA NERVOSA

In anorexia nervosa, a common goal is to restore weight to within 10% of ideal body weight. To put it simply, food is medicine. During refeeding, the patient consumes calorie-rich, nutritious food (e.g., avoid diet sodas) and is encouraged to eat in social settings. A patient with an ideal body weight greater than 75% and who is medically stable can receive outpatient management (Figure 9.1).

In the outpatient setting, physical health and body weight are regularly assessed and monitored. The patient is weighed in a gown at each visit after voiding to avoid artificial inflation of weight including excessive water intake prior to weigh-ins and extra weight from clothes and shoes. Indications for hospitalization in anorexia nervosa are listed in Table 9.6. In general, a patient who presents with persistent weight loss despite aggressive treatment, unstable vital signs, dehydration, electrolyte abnormalities, or medical complications such as cardiac arrhythmias, pancreatitis, and seizures requires hospitalization.

The role of the nutritionist is to plan a diet designed to help the patient gain weight slowly and safely. Diets initially begin with 800 to

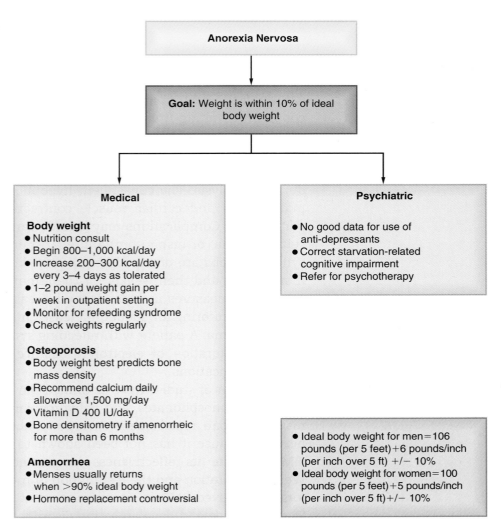

Figure 9.1. Outpatient treatment of anorexia nervosa.

Table 9.6   Indications for Hospitalization in Anorexia Nervosa

- <75% ideal body weight, or ongoing weight loss despite aggressive treatment
- Autonomic instability: bradycardia, <50 beats per minute; hypotension, systolic blood pressure <90; hypothermia, temperature <96°F; orthostatic changes
- Refusal to eat
- Dehydration
- Electrolyte abnormalities
- Cardiac arrhythmia
- Failure of outpatient management
- Acute psychiatric emergencies such as suicidal ideation or psychosis
- Intractable vomiting
- Medical complications from malnutrition such as cardiac failure, pancreatitis, seizures, and syncope

From *Practice Guidelines for the Treatment of Patients with Eating Disorders.* 3rd ed. Washington, DC: American Psychiatric Publishing, Inc.; 2006.

1,000 kcal/day, and gradually increase by 200 to 300 kcal every 3 to 4 days as tolerated with the goal of gaining at least 1 to 2 pounds per week in the outpatient setting and 2 to 3 pounds per week while hospitalized (20). In early refeeding, the initial weight gain is fluid retention. Refeeding may also cause bloating and constipation, which can be minimized or avoided with stool softeners, bulk-forming laxatives, and decreased use of gastric motility agents.

A feared complication in the medical treatment of anorexia nervosa is the refeeding syndrome. The refeeding syndrome is a potentially fatal condition resulting from severe electrolyte and fluid shifts in malnourished patients undergoing refeeding. In starvation, phosphorous stores are depleted. As carbohydrate intake increases, primary metabolism switches from fat to glucose and the demand for phosphate increases during glycolysis. The consequent hypophosphatemia can cause abnormal skeletal and cardiac muscle contraction, neurologic deficits, and pancreatitis. Complications may include cardiac failure, rhabdomyolysis, seizure, coma, or respiratory failure. To minimize risks of the refeeding syndrome, labs are obtained before refeeding, every 2 or 3 days for the first 10 days and then weekly for the remainder of refeeding (18). Other preventive measures include slowly increasing the calorie content each day and monitoring for sudden increases in pulse or the presence of significant edema. A patient with refeeding syndrome needs to be hospitalized for restoration of electrolyte balance and to prevent potentially lethal complications.

A number of studies have examined the use of hormone replacement therapy, bisphosphonates, and dehydroepiandrosterone to treat osteoporosis. Hormone replacement therapy is not recommended in anorexia nervosa because it has not been shown to increase bone mass density (BMD) despite its effectiveness in postmenopausal osteoporosis (12). Weight restoration and the resumption of menses are the greatest predictors of improved BMD in anorexia nervosa. Females who are 11 through 24 years of age and have an eating disorder should consume a daily dose of 1,500 mg of calcium and 400 international units of vitamin D (12).

Menses will usually resume as the patient approaches 90% of ideal body weight.

Attempts to identify psychopharmacologic treatments for anorexia nervosa have been disappointing. Fluoxetine did not differ from placebo in the time to relapse even with the addition of CBT for anorexia nervosa (19). Other medications such as cyproheptadine, zinc, tetrahydrocannabinol, and cisapride showed mixed outcomes and are not routinely used for anorexia nervosa in the primary care setting.

While medication management has little success in anorexia nervosa, psychosocial support has been a central aspect of care. Although the treatment team may concurrently address both the general medical and psychiatric aspects of an eating disorder, the primary care practitioner may consider treating urgent medical issues before beginning psychotherapy. In the latter case, deferral of psychotherapy may be appropriate until the cognitive deficits associated with starvation are corrected. A Cochrane review did not find one specific psychotherapy modality to be superior over another in the treatment of anorexia nervosa when comparing among time-limited individual psychotherapy, CBT, and interpersonal therapy (20).

BULIMIA NERVOSA

The treatment goals for bulimia nervosa are to eliminate binges and purges and normalize eating patterns (Figure 9.2). Behavioral contracts with the patient are established to eliminate purging (e.g., patient agrees not to buy laxatives) and decrease excessive weight loss (e.g., exercise is

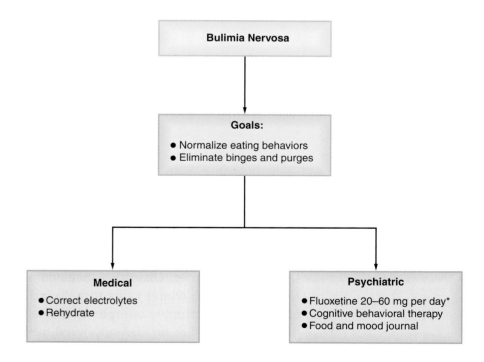

*Alternative serotonin reuptake inhibitors (SSRI) have been used although fluoxetine is the only FDA-approved SSRI approved for the treatment of bulimia nervosa.

Figure 9.2. Outpatient treatment of Bulimia Nervosa.

limited to no more than 1 hour per day). The intensity of medical treatment and the preferred setting will depend on the severity of the illness. Medical treatment of bulimia nervosa usually includes electrolyte and fluid repletion. An insulin-dependent diabetic patient should be educated about the necessity of a balanced diet and the continued usage of insulin.

There are no differences in efficacy and tolerability among antidepressants studied, although fluoxetine is the only Food and Drug Administration (FDA)-approved medication for the treatment of bulimia nervosa. After gradual titration to 60 mg/day, fluoxetine has been shown to reduce binge eating and purging episodes, prolong time to relapse, and decrease relapse rates (21). Bupropion use in a patient with depression and an eating disorder is contraindicated because of the increased risk of seizures.

Behavioral management is useful for maintaining recovery from bulimia nervosa. While the primary care clinician is not expected to engage patients in long-term psychotherapy, the primary care provider can help the patient understand how emotions and thoughts influence behavior. Table 9.7 shows how a food and mood response journal can help a patient with bulimia nervosa to identify reproducible patterns of behavior in response to triggers and mood (22). The emotions recorded before, during, and after eating become a source of discussion for how emotions affect binges and purges. Evidence-based research supports CBT as the first-line psychotherapy treatment for bulimia nervosa. CBT helps patients identify disturbed eating patterns, change dysfunctional thoughts, and build better coping skills.

BINGE EATING DISORDER

The treatment goals of binge eating disorder are to reduce binge eating episodes, lose weight or prevent weight gain, and manage medical complications and psychiatric comorbidities. Conventional behavioral weight loss treatments such as commercial weight loss programs are as effective as psychotherapy. Behavioral weight loss treatment modifies eating behaviors through increased organization of regular eating patterns involving moderate caloric restriction. Different modalities of psychotherapy including CBT, interpersonal therapy, and dialectical behavioral therapy have effectively reduced binge eating. Compared with CBT, which focuses on correcting an individual's negative beliefs and behaviors and replaces them with healthy, positive ones, interpersonal therapy focuses on improving interpersonal relationships and the interpersonal context of the eating disorder. Dialectical behavioral therapy is a variation of CBT that teaches behavioral skills to help individuals tolerate stress, regulate emotions, and improve interpersonal relationships.

While there are no FDA-approved medications for binge eating disorder, clinical trials show topiramate, orlistat, sibutramine, and zonisamide to be more effective in treating binge eating disorder and reducing obesity. In general, CBT is considered first-line treatment and the use of medications is not routinely employed for initial management.

Table 9.7 Food and Mood Response Journal

FEELINGS ABOUT FOOD (WERE YOU HUNGRY OR WAS IT CONVENIENT TO EAT?)

TIME	FOOD/EXERCISE	WHERE DID I EAT AND WITH WHOM?	BEFORE	DURING	AFTER
8:00 a.m.	1 cup milk 1 cup corn flakes 2 scrambled eggs	Dorm cafeteria with my roommates	Hungry	Chewed slowly	Satisfied with eating small breakfast
10:15 a.m.	3 glazed donuts	Dorm room, by myself	Couldn't focus on lecture because I was starving and other people around me were eating	Wanted to satisfy my craving for something sweet	Glutinous, angry for upsetting my diet; I think I gained 5 pounds from those donuts
11:15 a.m.	Gym: ran on the treadmill for 45 minutes to burn off the donuts		Angry for lack of control in eating donuts	Relieved to be exercising	Wanted to go on treadmill for another 30 minutes but I had to meet my study group
4:00 p.m.	1 small bag baby carrots	On campus by myself	Couldn't concentrate with my study group because I was still hungry	Wanted to eat something other than carrots but I knew that it would mean extra unnecessary calories	Still hungry
8:00 p.m.	1 small salad without dressing 1 cup vegetable soup	Dorm cafeteria with my roommates	Hungry	Relieved to eat something to stop the stomach pangs	Happy to eat something healthy
10:00 p.m.	½ pint chocolate ice cream, finished half box Oreo cookies, 1 slice pie	Dorm room, by myself	I didn't care what I ate because I was so hungry; I was upset my boyfriend didn't call me	I didn't care what I ate because I knew I was going to purge	Disgusted with self for binging, self-induced vomiting, happy to get the food out of my body, determined to work out at gym tomorrow for 2 hours

This is a food diary of a college-aged student with bulimia nervosa–type symptoms. Note that the patient compensated for her binge on donuts by exercising and skipping lunch.
Adapted from Becker AE. Outpatient management of eating disorders in adults. *Curr Womens Health Rep.* 2003;3:221–229.

WHEN TO REFER   ?

- Early in the course of the illness
- Signs of cardiovascular, renal, or hepatic compromise
- Electrolyte abnormalities
- Rapid or persistent decline of weight despite intensive intervention
- Lack of a strong social support system
- Comorbid substance use disorder, suicidality, or comorbid psychiatric diagnoses

MULTIDISCIPLINARY MANAGEMENT

The treatment of medical and psychiatric complications related to eating disorders is challenging. Managing medical complications of eating disorders including electrolyte imbalances and dehydration while ignoring the underlying causes does not serve the patient well. Support from other professionals including nutritionists, therapists, and psychiatrists who are familiar with this type of illness is necessary to address the complex issues related to eating disorders. Moreover, a multidisciplinary approach can allow the primary care provider to focus on coordination of care and maintain an overall picture of the patient's treatment goals. Transitioning care from the outpatient to inpatient setting is indicated if the patient presents with unstable vital signs; signs of cardiovascular, renal, or hepatic compromise; electrolyte abnormalities; severe dehydration; rapid or persistent decline of weight despite intensive intervention; lack of a strong social support system; and need for meal supervision or the patient will otherwise restrict, binge, or purge. When the patient presents with comorbid substance use disorder, suicidality, or comorbid psychiatric diagnoses, a referral to a psychiatrist is most likely indicated.

ADVOCACY

The primary care clinician plays a critical role in advocating for comprehensive, coordinated care that addresses the medical, psychiatric, and social needs of a patient with an eating disorder. Eating disorders are at the interface of traditionally disparate disciplines of general medicine and psychiatry, and as such, access to treatment may be limited and insurance coverage may be variable. As with other psychiatric disorders, lack of mental health parity may limit the availability of treatment options, especially for a patient with limited economic resources. The patient may also likely encounter limits on length of hospitalizations, lack of eating disorder facilities, and insufficient availability of mental health services. The primary care clinician can work with insurance companies and policy makers to extend benefits while challenging the myth that eating disorders can be cured simply by refeeding or ordering the patient to stop purging. At the community level, primary care providers can work alongside schools and athletic departments to prevent eating disorders by emphasizing nutrition and physical activity and raising awareness of eating disorders.

Practice Pointers

Case 1: A competitive runner with Colles fracture and osteoporosis

A 28-year-old competitive runner presents to a primary care clinic with pain in her right wrist, which developed after she fell at home. She fractured her left ankle 2 months ago. She is anxious to return to training for the next race. A review of symptoms is positive for occasional bloating, abdominal pain, feeling cold, and amenorrhea for the past 4 months. On physical exam, her height is 66 inches (167 cm) and she weighs 110 pounds (50 kg). Her vitals are 98°F, blood pressure 92/60 mmHg, heart rate 55 beats per minute, and respirations 16. Her skin is cool to touch and lanugo hair is present on her face, abdomen, and back. A wrist radiograph shows a Colles fracture and osteoporosis.

Discussion: Competitive female athletes are at increased risk for eating disorders. This patient the meets criteria for anorexia nervosa, restrictive subtype, as her body mass index (BMI) is 17.8 and her weight is less than 85% ideal body weight. This patient has features of the athletic triad: disordered eating, amenorrhea, and osteoporosis. For athletes, evaluation includes asking about exercise history with information on frequency, duration, and intensity of training. In cases like this, it is also important to inquire about previous fractures and/or overuse injuries. The patient's previous fracture was a missed opportunity for an eating disorder evaluation. Her medical work-up should now include electrolytes and liver function tests, as well as a baseline electrocardiogram (ECG). Since the patient's blood pressure and heart rate are low, orthostatic blood pressure changes may suggest dehydration. The patient should also be encouraged to consult with a nutritionist to plan a diet that increases calories safely. She will need close medical follow-up with careful laboratory monitoring and regular weigh-ins. The primary care provider could consider referral to a multidisciplinary team that specializes in eating disorders, especially if the patient fails to gain weight in subsequent follow-up visits. In resource-limited areas, the primary care provider may need to assemble a team of practitioners to build local expertise. A psychiatric evaluation should assess for mood disorders and substance abuse, particularly use of performance-enhancing drugs.

Case 2: A depressed woman with a normal BMI

A 22-year-old college student with a history of depression presents to the student health center requesting diuretics. She successfully lost 3 pounds over the past week by exercising. She reports that she eats mostly vegetable soup and a few crackers most days of the week. She is fastidious in tracking the number of calories she consumes. However, she finds that she is so hungry at the end of the day that she occasionally loses control and "gorges" on mostly "junk food" estimated at 4,000 calories in one sitting. She attempts to lose the extra calories by exercising 3 hours the following day. On her physical exam, her height is 65 inches (165 cm) and she weighs 140 pounds (63.5 kg). Oral exam reveals erosion of the teeth enamel and halitosis.

Discussion: In an otherwise healthy woman, there is no indication for diuretics. This patient's request raises concerns that she is seeking diuretics to lose weight. This patient has a normal BMI of 23.3, as do many patients with bulimia nervosa. Her eating behaviors, including her detailed documentation of caloric intake and cycles of binging and purging, are indicative of an eating disorder. The patient reports an excessive amount of exercise but neglects to mention self-induced vomiting, as suggested by the physical exam findings of enamel erosion. In addition to her bulimia nervosa, this patient also presents with a history of depression. Comorbid psychiatric disorders are frequent in eating disorders and need to be evaluated. This patient could benefit from starting on a low dose (10 to 20 mg/day) of fluoxetine and gradually titrating to the maximum dose of 60 mg/day, as tolerated. A referral to a therapist familiar with CBT for eating disorders will help the patient normalize her eating behaviors and correct distorted thoughts about her body image.

Case 3: An overweight man who copes by eating

A 34-year-old man who has not seen a doctor in many years presents to his primary care office to establish care after learning his uncle had recently died from a heart attack. On physical exam, he weighs 235 pounds (106 kg) and is 77 inches (196 cm) tall. Fasting laboratory values are significant for triglycerides 230 mg/dL, low-density lipoprotein 218 mg/dL, high-density lipoprotein 30 mg/dL, and glucose 198. Despite your attempts to counsel him on lifestyle modifications and treat the hyperlipidemia and diabetes, he continues to gain weight each time he visits you. When you ask about his continued weight gain, the patient replies that he has struggled with his uncle's death. He reluctantly reveals that his now deceased uncle had sexually abused him as a child. As a result of his early childhood trauma, he soothed his pain by excessively eating. He binges nearly every day with a typical episode consisting of half a pie, a large bag of potato chips, two hamburgers, two frozen pizzas, and four sodas. All this food is consumed in a 2-hour period. The patient is extremely frustrated with his weight and requests bariatric surgery.

Discussion: *This patient probably has binge eating disorder that has been ongoing since childhood. A history of childhood abuse is a risk factor for eating disorders. This patient recognizes his binging behaviors but reports no compensatory behavior, thus distinguishing the diagnosis from bulimia nervosa. In this case, the patient's binge eating has led to obesity and significant metabolic derangements. While bariatric surgery is an option for morbidly obese patients, this patient is not an optimal candidate at this time, as he is at high risk of returning to his binge eating despite surgery. Surgery alone cannot solve the psychological and behavioral problems from which this patient suffers. This patient would benefit from an intensive weight loss program and psychotherapy to address his past history of being abused. Further assessment of his mood disorder and substance use disorder should be performed. Pharmacologic and psychotherapeutic treatments, especially for his depression, should be considered.*

ICD9	
Anorexia Nervosa	307.1
Bulimia Nervosa	307.51
Eating Disorder NOS	307.50

Practical Resources

Anorexia Nervosa and Related Eating Disorders: http://www.anred.com
National Eating Disorders Association: http://www.nationaleatingdisorders.org
Academy for Eating Disorders: http://www.aedweb.org
Eating Disorder Referral and Information Center: http://www.edreferral.com
Eating Disorders Coalition: http://www.eatingdisorderscoalition.org
National Association of Anorexia Nervosa and Associated Disorders: http://www.anad.org
Something Fishy: http://www.something-fishy.org
Overeaters Anonymous: http://www.oa.org
Food Addicts Anonymous: http://www.foodaddictsanonymous.org

References

1. Sullivan PF. Mortality in anorexia nervosa. *Am J Psychiatry.* 1995;152:1073–1074.

2. Hudson JL, Hiripi E, Pope HG, et al. The prevalence and correlates of eating disorders in the National Comorbidity Survey Replication. *Biol Psychiatry.* 2007;61:348–358.

3. Fairburn CG, Bohn K. Eating disorder NOS (EDNOS): an example of the troublesome "not otherwise specified" (NOS) category in DSM-IV. *Behav Res Ther.* 2005;43:691–701.

4. American Psychiatric Association. *Diagnostic and Statistical Manual of Mental Disorders.* 4th ed., text revision. Washington, DC: American Psychiatric Association; 2000.

5. Benninghoven D, Tetsch N, Kunzendorf S, et al. Perceptual body image of patients with anorexia or bulimia nervosa and their fathers. *Eat Weight Disord.* 2007;12:12–19.

6. Telch CF, Agras WS. Obesity, binge eating and psychopathology: are they related? *Int J Eat Disord.* 1994;15:53–61.

7. Herpertz S, Albus C, Kielmann R, et al. Comorbidity of diabetes mellitus and eating disorders: a follow-up study. *J Psychosom Res.* 2001;51:673–678.

8. Pomeroy C. Medical evaluation and medical management. In: Mitchell J, ed. *The Outpatient Treatment of Eating Disorders: A Guide for Therapists, Dietitians, and Physicians.* Minneapolis: University of Minnesota Press; 2001:306–348.

9. Strober M, Freeman R, Lampert C, et al. Controlled family study of anorexia nervosa and bulimia nervosa: evidence of shared liability and transmission of partial syndromes. *Am J Psychiatry.* 2000;157:393–401.

10. Franko DL, Spurrell EB. Detection and management of eating disorders during pregnancy. *Obstet Gynecol.* 2000;95:942–946.

11. Morgan JF, Reid F, Lacey H. The SCOFF questionnaire: assessment of a new screening tool for eating disorders. *BMJ.* 1999;319:1467–1468.

12. Mehler PS. Osteoporosis in anorexia nervosa: prevention and treatment. *Int J Eat Disord.* 2003;33:113–126.

13. Fernandez-Aranda F, Pinheiro AP, Tozzi F, et al. Symptom profile of major depressive disorder in women with eating disorders. *Aust N Z J Psychiatry.* 2007;41:24–31.

14. Kaye WH, Bulik CM, Thornton L. Comorbidity of anxiety disorders with anorexia and bulimia nervosa. *Am J Psychiatry.* 2006;163:2215–2221.

15. Herzog DB, Franko DL, Dorer DJ, et al. Drug abuse in women with eating disorders. *Int J Eat Disord.* 2006;39:364–368.

16. Jordan J, Joyce PR, Carter FA, et al. Specific and nonspecific comorbidity in anorexia nervosa. *Int J Eat Disord.* 2008;41:47–56.

17. *Practice Guidelines for the Treatment of Patients with Eating Disorders.* 3rd ed. Washington, DC: American Psychiatric Association; 2006.

18. Mehler PS, Crews CK. Refeeding the anorexia patient. *Eat Dis J Treat Prevent.* 2001;9:167–171.

19. Walsh BT, Kaplan AS, Attia E, et al. Fluoxetine after weight restoration in anorexia nervosa: a randomized controlled trial. *JAMA.* 2006;295:2605–2612.

20. Hay P, Bacaltchuk J, Claudina A, et al. Individual psychotherapy in the outpatient treatment of adults with anorexia nervosa. *Cochrane Database System Rev.* 2003;4:CD003909.

21. Fluoxetine Bulimia Nervosa Collaborative Study Group. Fluoxetine in the treatment of bulimia nervosa. *Am J Psychiatry.* 1992;49:139–147.

22. Becker AE. Outpatient management of eating disorders in adults. *Curr Womens Health Rep.* 2003;3:221–229.

CHAPTER 10 Personality Disorders

Shannon Suo, MD • Maga Jackson-Triche, MD, MSHS
• Mark Servis, MD

> A 21-year-old female college student presents to your continuity clinic. She has been the patient of one of your partners for 2 years and states, "He was horrible and didn't understand me." She complains of anxiety due to recent fights with her boyfriend and also describes feeling as though she's "not good enough" for her boyfriend. Toward the end of the interview, she says, "My boyfriend will regret it if anything happens to me." She denies any history of manic or psychotic symptoms and denies drug or alcohol use.

CLINICAL HIGHLIGHTS

- Personality disorders are commonly encountered in primary care settings and may disrupt the patient–provider relationship and compromise the quality of care.

- Primary care clinicians should be aware of their own feelings toward patients with personality disorders and ensure that treatment is not adversely influenced by emotionally charged and negative feelings.

- The presence of a personality disorder can significantly increase the risk of comorbid psychiatric conditions. As such, it is

Clinical Significance

Personality disorders develop early in life, result in ongoing emotional angst, and tend to be challenging to manage and virtually impossible to "cure." Table 10.1 describes the *Diagnostic and Statistical Manual of Mental Disorders*, 4th edition, text revision (DSM-IV-TR) criteria for personality disorders (1). The specific types of personality disorders will be discussed individually and as "clusters."

Collectively, personality disorders are estimated to occur in the general population at rates from 10% to 15% (2). They are more frequently encountered in primary care settings with an average prevalence of 20% to 30% (3, 4). Patients with personality disorders are more likely to have had increased outpatient, emergency, and inpatient visits (5). Other studies have found higher levels of dissatisfaction with care, lower scores on functioning scales, and increased antidepressant prescriptions in patients who have a personality disorder (5, 6).

Primary care providers rarely receive sufficient training in psychiatry, and most clinical rotations do not cover Axis II pathology but instead focus almost exclusively on Axis I disorders. The medical literature has historically labeled personality disordered patients as "difficult" or even "hateful" rather than identifying the specific disorders or traits that lead to the difficult patient–provider interactions (7). Nonetheless, it remains important for primary care clinicians to identify those patients with personality disorders or personality disorder traits, because these patients are at increased risk for a multitude of other conditions, including alcohol and SUD disorders, depression, bipolar disorder, and somatization disorder (8–10).

(Continued)

Patients with Cluster A personality disorders (i.e., paranoid, schizoid, and schizotypal personality disorders) are more prone to substance use and social isolation. Individuals with Cluster B disorders (i.e., antisocial, borderline, histrionic, or narcissistic personality disorders) may engage in deliberate self-injury and high-risk physical and sexual behaviors, with consequent increased risk of injury, disease, and infection. The lifetime prevalence of suicidal ideation in patients with borderline personality disorder (BPD) is approximately 75%, and up to 10% of BPD patients complete suicide (11). These patients are also more sensitive to perceived "abandonment," and may act in inappropriate ways to retain contact with their providers. Patients with Cluster C pathology (i.e., avoidant, dependant, or obsessive compulsive personality disorders) may be more avoidant, less compliant with treatment, and more anxious on an everyday basis.

Diagnosis

Personality disorders are categorized in Axis II of the five-axis DSM-IV-TR diagnostic classification. While there is no specific nomenclature for such, mental health professionals often note "traits" of personality disorders on Axis II if they are unable to make a diagnosis of the full personality disorder. Features that distinguish "normal" personality traits from pathologic ones include inflexibility and maladaptive behavior. Common characteristics of personality disorders and the clusters to which they belong are listed in Table 10.2. Although personality disorder diagnoses are intended to be made based on enduring patterns of behavior, patients may not meet criteria for the full disorder at a later (or earlier) time period based on mitigating circumstances or severity of comorbid Axis I conditions. For example, the National Institute of Mental Health (NIMH) Collaborative Longitudinal Personality Disorders Study found that only 44% of patients diagnosed with BPD retained the

---

Table 10.1 DSM-IV-TR General Diagnostic Criteria for a Personality Disorder

A. An enduring pattern of inner experience and behavior that deviates markedly from the expectations of the individual's culture. This pattern is manifested in two (or more) of the following areas:

1. Cognition (i.e., ways of perceiving and interpreting self, other people, and events)
2. Affectivity (i.e., the range, intensity, lability, and appropriateness of emotional response)
3. Interpersonal functioning
4. Impulse control

B. The enduring pattern is inflexible and pervasive across a broad range of personal and social situations.
C. The enduring pattern leads to clinically significant distress or impairment in social, occupational, or other important areas of functioning.
D. The pattern is stable and of long duration, and its onset can be traced back to adolescence or early adulthood.
E. The enduring pattern is not better accounted for as a manifestation or consequence of another mental disorder.
F. The enduring pattern is not due to the direct physiologic effects of a substance (e.g., a drug of abuse, a medication) or a general medical condition (e.g., head trauma).

From American Psychiatric Association. Personality disorders. In: *Diagnostic and Statistical Manual of Mental Disorders*. 4th ed., text revision. Washington, DC: American Psychiatric Publishing, Inc.; 2000:685.

Table 10.2 DMS-IV-TR Personality Clusters, Specific Types, and Their Defining Clinical Features

CLUSTER	TYPE	CHARACTERISTIC FEATURES
A		**Odd or eccentric behavior**
	Paranoid	• Pervasive distrust and suspiciousness (not "delusional") of others such that their motives are interpreted as malevolent
	Schizoid	• Pervasive pattern of detachment from social relationships and restricted range of expression of emotions in interpersonal settings
	Schizotypal	• Pervasive pattern of social and interpersonal deficits marked by acute discomfort with, and reduced capacity for, close relationships as well as by cognitive or perceptual distortions and eccentricities of behavior
B		**Dramatic, emotional, or erratic behavior**
	Antisocial	• History of conduct disorder before age 15; pervasive pattern of disregard for and violation of the rights of others; current age at least 18
	Borderline	• Pervasive pattern of instability of interpersonal relationships, self-image, and affects, and marked impulsivity
	Histrionic	• Pervasive pattern of excessive emotionality and attention seeking
	Narcissistic	• Pervasive pattern of grandiosity (in fantasy or behavior), need for admiration, and lack of empathy
C		**Anxious or fearful**
	Avoidant	• Pervasive pattern of social inhibition, feelings of inadequacy, and hypersensitivity to negative evaluation
	Dependent	• Pervasive and excessive need to be taken care of that leads to submissive and clinging behavior and fears of separation
	Obsessive compulsive	• Pervasive pattern of preoccupation with orderliness, perfectionism, and mental and interpersonal control at the expense of flexibility, openness, and efficiency

Adapted from American Psychiatric Publishing, Inc. Personality disorders. In: *Diagnostic and Statistical Manual of Mental Disorders.* 4th ed., text revision. Washington, DC: American Psychiatric Association; 2000:685.

diagnosis 2 years later (12). Therefore, the patient who exemplified BPD one year may seem vastly different and no longer meet the diagnostic criteria a few years later. Moreover, it may take several encounters with a patient to accurately recognize long-standing and pervasive character pathology (e.g., an individual may appear "borderline" while on an isolated "bad day" but is usually capable of coping with stressors in a healthy and adaptive manner). As such, health care providers are encouraged to obtain collateral history and see patients several times before definitively giving a personality disorder diagnosis.

Our visceral response or feelings about a patient encounter can often be helpful when considering an Axis II diagnosis. It is helpful to consider underrecognized feelings and emotions that may subtly influence the patient–provider relationship. *Transference* is loosely defined as the unconscious reenactment of feelings or behaviors toward the provider based on previous experiences of the patient with significant others or caretakers. In challenging therapeutic encounters, it is often useful to discuss the provider's thoughts and feelings about patients (*countertransference*) as they may relate to identification of personality pathology and treatment of the patient. Table 10.3 identifies feelings that may arise in health care providers and the disorders that are typically associated with such feelings. Particularly problematic may be feelings of anger, leading to retaliation against or punishment of the patient that is not appropriate to the circumstance. This contrasts with clearly defined

Table 10.3 Feelings of Countertransference and Reactions to Avoid

PROVIDER'S FEELING	PERSONALITY DISORDER	POTENTIAL PROVIDER PITFALLS	SUGGESTED ACTION
Anger (patient is viewed as manipulative)	• Borderline • Antisocial • Narcissistic	• Overreaction to provocation, retaliation (e.g., verbal/physical abuse of patient, substandard care, inappropriate comments in charting)	• Be aware of feelings • Process in Balint groups • Strictly adhere to evidence-based standard of care
Fear of patient (physical or legal threat)	• Antisocial • Paranoid	• Immediate emotional or physical overresponse (out of proportion to threat)	• Maintain personal safety • Document thoroughly
Sympathy	• Borderline (sympathy by some providers associated with negative views by other providers may represent *splitting* by the patient) • Dependent	• Overindulgence or tendency to rescue the patient	• Provide regular, structured, and scheduled visits with the same provider that do not run over scheduled time • Manage splitting in interdisciplinary meetings to make sure all members of team are acting in accordance with treatment plan and not providing "special" treatment
Self-doubt	• Narcissistic	• Putting down the patient instead; questioning your own abilities in a nonrealistic way	• Be aware of your behavior • Examine your abilities in a realistic way • Process in Balint groups
Frustration	• Borderline • Avoidant • Dependent	• Patients may not follow through with treatment recommendations or rely overly on provider	• Set clear expectations • Ally yourself with patient's family/friends to assist (as permitted by privacy restrictions)
Attraction	• Histrionic • Borderline	• Inappropriate relationship with patient	• Consider using a chaperone for exams requiring examination of genitalia • Do not see patient after hours or in social settings

consequences that *should* follow inappropriate behavior by the patient, including termination of care following repeated breaches of clinic rules despite explanations of limits and responses to violations of those limits. Equally dangerous are feelings of attraction to patients that lead to indiscretions of a sexual or romantic nature. Balint groups provide a forum for health care professionals to discuss the emotional content of the patient–provider relationship and can be helpful in processing the strong feelings evoked by patients with a personality disorder. These groups are led by health care professionals with psychological training and provide guidance to the members about countertransferential feelings to ensure the preservation of healthy clinical relationships.

A routine physical examination should be completed on all patients thought to have a personality disorder. Providers should check for self-inflicted injuries in patients with borderline pathology, including cuts, burns, or other forms of self-mutilation. Patients who self-inflict injuries often hide their wounds by wearing long sleeves or pants. Patients with borderline or dependent personality disorders are at increased risk for domestic violence and should be carefully assessed for signs of physical abuse. All patients with a suspected personality disorder should be asked about alcohol and illicit substance use. Obtaining collateral information from other care providers as well as family members and friends can help establish a diagnosis or confirm the presence of traits.

BORDERLINE PERSONALITY DISORDER: SPECIAL DIAGNOSTIC CONSIDERATIONS

Of the personality disorders, BPD has received the most attention in terms of epidemiologic research and evidence-based treatment approaches. In our experience, an open discussion with patients about a possible diagnosis of BPD can be both therapeutic and rewarding. While many providers fear informing patients of a diagnosis of BPD, this fear proves largely unfounded. The stigma that providers associate with BPD fuels this concern, while patients are often relieved when someone can explain why they behave the way they do, especially when informed that effective treatment options are available. However, every patient with BPD or borderline traits does not require an in-depth discussion of BPD, so such discussions should be limited to when they are clinically indicated, such as when referring to mental health or when reflecting on maladaptive patterns of behavior.

When considering a diagnosis of BPD, we recommend a stepwise approach. First, summarize the emotional, behavioral, and interpersonal difficulties the patient seems to be having. Second, inquire about the patient's understanding of his or her difficulties and what role they play in the problems. Third, introduce BPD as a possible but not definitive explanation. Lastly, recommend that the patient learn about BPD either through reading or consultation with a mental health professional. Upon follow-up, the provider can reassess the patient's understanding of BPD. If significant conflicts arise or a definitive diagnosis is required, primary care providers should refer to a mental health professional for ongoing assessment and treatment.

Differential Diagnosis

There can be considerable overlap between symptoms of personality disorders and other psychiatric diagnoses, and it is important to assess and appropriately rule out conditions that may lead to an entirely different treatment plan. Also, patients with personality disorders often have both Axis I and Axis II conditions, therefore requiring treatments that address the comorbid diagnoses. The AMPS screening tool may be used to systematically screen for comorbid psychiatric conditions (see Chapter 1). Anxiety disorders, mood disorders (e.g. bipolar and depressive disorders), psychotic disorders and substance abuse disorders, as well as changes induced by general medical conditions are important to consider as either alternate or co-occurring conditions. BPD and bipolar disorder, in particular, can be difficult to differentiate due to the overlap of symptoms in impulsivity and affective lability. Some distinguishing features between bipolar disorder and BPD include decreased *need* for sleep with mania and *episodic* mood swings lasting days to weeks, both found in the former. Keep in mind that borderline personality and bipolar disorder can coexist and bipolar disorder has been found to be more prevalent in people with BPD than in people with other personality disorders (13). Table 10.4 highlights common primary care complaints and comorbid conditions frequently encountered in patients with personality disorders.

Information about long-standing patterns of behavior, affect, thought disorder, and behavioral lability can help distinguish between personality and Axis I disorders. Personality symptoms that only occur during the course of a diagnosed comorbid psychiatric disorder should not be diagnosed as a personality disorder. Personality changes caused by medical conditions (e.g., endocrine disorders, traumatic brain injury, and seizure disorders) can usually be distinguished by the development of symptoms with the onset of the medical condition.

Biopsychosocial Treatment

The following discussion on the treatment for personality disorders will focus primarily on paranoid, borderline, antisocial, and dependent personality disorders, as they are more commonly encountered in the primary care setting.

PHARMACOTHERAPY: OVERVIEW

While psychotherapy remains the mainstay treatment for personality disorders, medications may facilitate psychotherapy and stabilize a patient to tolerate the process of psychotherapy (1). No medications have been approved by the Food and Drug Administration (FDA) for the treatment of personality disorders, and therefore, all recommendations for medication management are for off-label use only. As a general rule, medication should be selected to first target the comorbid Axis I psychiatric disorder. For *paranoid personality disorder*, low-dose antipsychotics may reduce anxiety and paranoid tendencies but patients are often reluctant to take medications, especially if they believe medications impair their ability to remain hypervigilant. For *dependent personality disorder,* antidepressants used for comorbid anxiety or depression may need to be used at higher than usual doses and with a longer treatment duration to evaluate clinical response. Antidepressants have the potential to improve assertiveness and outgoing behavior in those who have dependent personality disorder (1). Antisocial personality disorder is usually managed by firm limit setting and not with the use of psychiatric medications.

PHARMACOTHERAPY OF BORDERLINE PERSONALITY DISORDER

Pharmacotherapeutic options for BPD have been studied more than any other personality disorder. Although the collective findings are not robust, it is generally accepted that selective serotonin reuptake inhibitors (SSRIs), mood stabilizers, and antipsychotics provide the greatest

NOT TO BE MISSED

- Depression
- Anxiety disorders
- Bipolar disorder
- Substance use disorder
- Psychotic disorders (e.g., schizophrenia)
- General medical condition(s)
- Suicidal intent and plan

Table 10.4 Differential Diagnosis of Personality Disorders

PERSONALITY DISORDER	COMMON PRIMARY CARE PRESENTATIONS AND CONCERNS	DIFFERENTIATION FROM OTHER PSYCHIATRIC DISORDERS	COMMON AXIS I COMORBIDITY
Paranoid	• Guarded, hypervigilant, anxious, irritable/hostile, business-like, suspect of harm from clinicians • Preoccupied with justice and rules	Psychotic disorder, which has overt delusional or psychotic content	• Depression • Substance use • Obsessive compulsive disorder (OCD) • Agoraphobia
Schizoid	• Eager for visits to end • Offers little comment or elaboration • May delay seeking care until conditions are advanced	Avoidant personality disorder, in which patients crave intimate relationships	
Schizotypal	• Odd, peculiar behavior, idiosyncratic speech/dress • Difficulty with face-to-face communication • Eccentric beliefs, paranoid tendencies, may appear guarded • Uncomfortable with physical exam, especially gynecologic/rectal exams	Psychotic disorder, in which a fixed and false belief is generally bizarre or paranoid in nature	• Depression
Antisocial	• Superficially cooperative and charming • Impulsive and manipulative • Lacking guilt or remorse for behavior • Little or no regard for the rights of others • Usually deceitful	Adult antisocial behavior, which consists of purely criminal behavior	• Impulse control disorders • Depression • Substance use • Pathologic gambling • Anxiety • Malingering
Borderline	• Interpersonally intense with superficial sociability and periods of intense anger • Idealization/devaluation • Impulsive self-destructive behavior • Identity disturbance (unstable choices in career, sexual orientation, appearance)	Bipolar disorder, in which lability of mood and affect is episodic and occurs for days to weeks (not a fixed personality trait)	• Substance use • Mood disorders (higher risk of suicide) • Eating disorder • Posttraumatic stress disorder
Histrionic	• Dramatic, exhibitionistic, attention seeking • Avoids/forgets unpleasant feelings or ideas (such as appointments, seriousness of medical conditions) • Exaggerated displays of emotion to manipulate/seduce	Borderline personality disorder, which includes an unstable self-image and feelings of emptiness	• Depression • Somatization disorder
Narcissistic	• Egocentric, entitled, hypersensitive to criticism and preoccupation with being envied • Seek the "best" clinician and demand special attention • Difficulty accepting diagnoses that are incompatible with their self-image	Antisocial personality disorder The narcissist knows the rules and thinks he or she is above them; the antisocial does not wish to know the rules	• Depression (especially with "failure") • Substance use
Avoidant	• Extreme sensitivity and fear of rejection, shy, anxious about what others think of them	Schizoid personality and social phobia	• Mood disorders • Social phobia

(Continued)

Table 10.4 Differential Diagnosis of Personality Disorders (*Continued*)

PERSONALITY DISORDER	COMMON PRIMARY CARE PRESENTATIONS AND CONCERNS	DIFFERENTIATION FROM OTHER PSYCHIATRIC DISORDERS	COMMON AXIS I COMORBIDITY
	• Reluctant to disagree or ask questions • May delay seeking medical care for fear of appearing foolish	Avoidant personality disorder shows general feelings of inadequacy/inferiority/ineptness and general reluctance to take risks and engage in new activities	
Dependent	• Excessive reliance on others, trying to get others to be responsible for health care (e.g., a diabetic seeks others to give insulin injections) • Asks many questions to avoid terminating the interview • Brings family or friends to appointments and inappropriately asks them to provide answers or decisions	<u>Histrionic personality disorder</u> Patients with dependent traits want attention, but are not flamboyant or seductive	• Mood disorders • Anxiety disorders • Adjustment disorder
Obsessive compulsive	• Perfectionistic, obsessed with the "right" way • Facts preferable to emotions • Responds negatively to clinician being late • Keeps detailed notes to track illness • May seek opinions from multiple clinician sources	<u>Obsessive compulsive disorder</u>, which, as an Axis I disorder, has specific obsessions and compulsions and tends to be more severe	• Depression • Anxiety disorders • Obsessive compulsive disorder

effect in treatment of the disorder (17). Antidepressants may be used to target depression, rejection sensitivity, anger, and self-harm behavior. Mood stabilizers and second-generation antipsychotics may be selected to target affective instability and impulsivity. For paranoia, dissociation, and other psychotic features, a second-generation antipsychotic may be prescribed (17, 18). Standard doses for mood stabilizers, antipsychotics, and antidepressants are recommended (see corresponding chapters on bipolar, psychotic, and depressive disorders for dosing protocols). Before prescribing antidepressants, all patients should be thoroughly screened for a history of mania to avoid iatrogenic induction of a manic or mixed episode in a patient with an undiagnosed bipolar spectrum disorder. Patients should also be closely monitored for the presence of suicidal ideation, intent, and plan upon the initiation of an antidepressant.

THERAPEUTIC RELATIONSHIP AND LIMIT SETTING

The management of patients with personality disorders is challenging to even the most experienced clinicians. BPD is usually associated with intense dependency, maladaptive use of self-destructiveness, and alternating idealization and devaluation of interpersonal relationships, which often generate intense feelings of anger and sometimes inappropriate attraction in health care providers. Impulsively acting on these feelings is counterproductive and can be dangerous as these actions not

Table 10.5 Using $E = MC^2$ as Part of the Treatment for Borderline Personality Disorder

Empathy – Try to fully understand the details of one's turbulent and chaotic life.

"Manage," not "cure" – Personalities are formed early and can be difficult to modify. Improvement may be gradual and temporary with frequent "relapses" of behavior.

Countertransference – Consider why you are feeling a certain way before you respond to a patient.

Comorbidity – Screen for other psychopathology (e.g., mood, anxiety, and substance use disorders).

only jeopardize the therapeutic relationship, but also leave the provider vulnerable to possible legal or disciplinary action. The clinician should try to recognize and acknowledge these intense feelings (countertransference), consult with colleagues, actively set limits, and avoid the seduction of idealization.

All patients with personality disorders who make "special" demands should be managed with an explicit explanation of clinic rules (e.g., number and frequency of phone calls, length and frequency of appointments, only seeing the patient in the office) and reasonable expectations for what the clinician can provide (8). The clinician who tries to meet unreasonable requests will quickly be dealing with escalating demands. Limit setting may be challenged and the clinician should remain calm while repeatedly reinforcing clear boundaries. The $E = MC^2$ mnemonic for treatment of BPD can be used to minimize frustration and facilitate the delivery of compassionate and effective care for patients with personality disorders (Table 10.5).

Shaping of patient behavior through positive reinforcement is possible and rewards for desirable behavior should be clear and consistent. Similarly, negative consequences for harmful behaviors should be explicit and enforceable. In order to prevent impulsive and self-destructive behaviors, the provider should encourage the patient to put feelings into words rather than counterproductive actions. Rage and aggression are common problems in patients with cluster B personality disorders, and the clinician should identify underlying anger in the behavior of patients, tolerate patient tirades when they are not abusive, and redirect aggression to healthy and adaptive outlets such as hobbies or leisure activities.

PSYCHOTHERAPY

The best long-term treatment for personality disordered patients is psychotherapy, and several evidence-based studies demonstrate the efficacy of specific psychotherapies for borderline, narcissistic, and dependent personality disordered patients (14, 15). BPD patients benefit from both dialectical behavior therapy (DBT), a form of cognitive behavioral therapy that also utilizes mindfulness meditation techniques, and from transference-based psychodynamic psychotherapy.

DBT involves once-weekly group and once-weekly individual therapy focused on optimizing coping skills and modifying maladaptive behaviors. The initial goal of DBT is to reduce "para-suicidal" behaviors, such as cutting and self-mutilation, while progressing to the development of behaviors that further improve the quality of life. A firm, detailed, and explicit treatment contract is established with the patient that addresses attendance, vacations, homework, and boundary issues such as limits on extra sessions and telephone and e-mail contact. DBT is highly structured and compels the patient to identify deficits, learn skills, and apply these skills to replace dysfunctional behaviors that the patient has developed in response to intense emotional dysregulation and conflicts in relationships.

Transference-based psychodynamic psychotherapy is also an effective treatment for BPD. This type of psychotherapy involves once- or twice-weekly individual therapy that is mainly focused on the patient's internal experiences and relationships. Both psychotherapeutic approaches usually take place outside of the primary care setting and require a mental health referral with long-term treatment. Patients with dependent personality disorder benefit from individual and group psychotherapy using supportive psychotherapy techniques that teach, model, and reinforce adaptive coping skills and discourage maladaptive behaviors. Paranoid and antisocial personality disorders are difficult to treat and do not typically respond to psychotherapy. In most primary care settings, psychotherapy requires a referral to mental health professionals, although certain techniques of cognitive behavioral therapy (CBT) may be useful in clinical encounters.

PSYCHOSOCIAL INTERVENTIONS

Whenever possible, it is important to include the patient's family and support network as part of the treatment plan. With due diligence to patient privacy, educating the patient and his or her caregivers about the nature of behavioral patterns related to a personality disorder may assist the patient in anticipating and avoiding some of the more harmful consequences. As mentioned previously, it is often an enormous relief to patients when they are informed about their diagnosis of BPD. Caregivers and friends may have greater patience and sympathy for the patient's frustrating behaviors if the nature of the illness is explained to them. Involved family and friends may also need to learn about boundaries and how not to overreact when the patient seems out of control.

Community organizations, such as the National Alliance on Mental Illness (NAMI), offer additional support and education for patients and their families. Support groups, where a patient can meet others who share similar difficulties, provide the additive advantage of peer-to-peer feedback. For BPD, dialectical behavioral therapy groups are becoming more popular in both public mental health systems and in the private sector.

Practice Pointers

Case 1: Borderline personality disorder diagnosis
A 21-year-old female college student presents to your continuity clinic. She has been the patient of one of your partners for 2 years and states, "He was horrible and didn't understand me." She complains of anxiety due to recent fights with

WHEN TO REFER

- Persistently negative thoughts and feelings (countertransference) can cause significant angst among providers who care for patients with severe personality disorders and, in cases like these, referrals for psychiatric consultation and treatment are usually indicated

- Psychiatric referrals should be made when a personality disorder co-occurs with one or more comorbid Axis I disorders

- High risk for suicide or self-harm

- Need for ongoing individual or group CBT, DBT, and other psychotherapies her boyfriend and also describes feeling as though she's "not good enough" for her boyfriend. Toward the end of the interview, she says, "My boyfriend will regret it if anything happens to me." She denies any history of manic or psychotic symptoms and denies drug or alcohol use.

The physical examination shows an attractive, well-developed, well-nourished woman with superficial, healing, linear scratches and scars on her left forearm. Upon questioning, she admits that she has inflicted these wounds herself when she got upset. She denies any suicidal ideation, but admits to having overdosed on medications in the past. She says she slept for a day and a half and did not seek medical attention.

After completing the exam, you advise the patient that you feel she needs a referral for mental health care. She responds positively, but asks for your direct phone number and pager in case she "has any emergency meltdowns." The following Friday you are paged by the triage nurse because the patient is agitated in the lobby and demanding to see you. After ushering her into an exam room, the patient bursts into tears and says that her boyfriend broke up with her and that she wants to kill herself. She knows you can help her because "you're the best doctor I've ever had!"

Discussion: *This patient presents with a history and several symptoms that are consistent with BPD: female gender, unstable relationships and self-image, affective lability, suicidal and para-suicidal gestures, and idealization intermixed with devaluation of her physicians. She does not admit to comorbid substance use and denies any episodic symptoms of mania that would suggest bipolar disorder. She denies a history of domestic violence but remains at risk for such due to her refusal to be "abandoned." She could be further evaluated for posttraumatic stress disorder.*

Her presentation of suicidal ideation following a break-up demonstrates a frantic attempt to avoid abandonment. This represents her intolerance and inability to cope with being "left alone." She has responded the only way she knows how—with thoughts of ending her life. If truly suicidal, the patient may need an emergency psychiatric evaluation and consideration for an involuntary psychiatric hospitalization. If she is able to articulate a plan for safety as an alternative to suicide (such as staying with family and calling a crisis line with worsening symptoms) and is able to calmly discuss her alternatives rationally, an involuntary hold may be averted.

Your availability to this patient should be limited to what is the standard within your practice. The patient should be given clear instructions about how to contact you and not be given special treatment, as this will only increase her maladaptive dependency. Patients with BPD can present with multiple challenges that may intermittently "test" provider responses and limits. Be careful not to impulsively retaliate to such "tests," as many BPD patients are highly sensitive to perceived abandonment. However, if the patient is in clear violation of prespecified expectations, this needs to be explained and boundaries firmly reinforced. Once referred, you should remain in contact with her mental health professional to discuss risky behaviors or warning signs. Successful long-term management may be achieved with concurrent treatment of comorbid Axis I disorders and participation in a psychotherapy program.

Case 2: An unreasonable request for pain killers

A 32-year-old man presents to an urgent care clinic with new-onset back pain. He states that he was lifting boxes at work yesterday and experienced sudden pain in his lower back. He denies any neurologic symptoms and jokes about how he got his injury, though grimaces when describing the pain. Physical exam is significant for normal vital signs and mild tenderness in the right L4–L5 paraspinous muscles, but strength, reflexes, and sensation are intact. The straight leg raise test is negative.

You explain that he has an acute back strain and recommend conservative management (e.g., rest, no heavy lifting for 3 weeks, and nonnarcotic analgesic medications). He thanks you for your advice, but asks if he can have "something stronger" for the pain and hands you some disability forms. You give him a prescription for 10 hydrocodone/acetaminophen tablets and complete the disability forms. Two days later you receive a message from the patient that he lost the prescription before he could get it filled, but thinks he might need more than 10 pills since he has not been able to sleep. You advise him to return to the urgent care clinic for re-evaluation.

On exam, he is still limping and his physical examination is unchanged. He says he has a "high tolerance" to pain medications. You see a previous note that shows the patient reported a bottle of opioid analgesics stolen by a friend. You explain that you cannot write for more hydrocodone and again recommend conservative management. He responds by snarling, "I told you, that's not enough and I will do what I need to do to get it!"

Discussion: *Acute low back strain is one of the most common presenting problems in primary care. Certainly not all patients with this presentation will be behaviorally problematic. However, this patient displays a superficial charm and pleasantness that quickly fades when he does not achieve his own goals. He implies a superiority or "specialness" when speaking of his high tolerance to pain medications. Upon being challenged, he escalates to threatening behavior and the provider should make safety the number one priority. Every clinic should have policies about the management of potentially violent patients. Being sympathetic to reasonable complaints or expressing regret about the inability to fulfill unreasonable requests may diffuse some anger. However, if a patient is unable or unwilling to calm down so that his complaints can be addressed, the clinician should have a low threshold to leave the exam room and seek assistance. If a patient becomes threatening, the office staff should contact a peace officer.*

Patients with antisocial personality disorder are at high risk for substance abuse and dependence. If an opioid analgesic is warranted, providers should require a narcotic contract. Giving into the unreasonable demands of patients who have antisocial personality disorder will only feed into their feeling of superiority and increase their incentive to threaten or manipulate other providers (and the health care system) in the future. Providers should realize that they cannot meet all the demands of patients with antisocial personality disorder, nor would it be appropriate to do so.

Case 3: "I'm just too weak"

A 57-year-old woman, well known to you as a long-standing patient with hypertension and osteoporosis, comes into clinic for follow-up. At her last visit 3 weeks ago, she reported abdominal pain and dizziness. Today she says the abdominal pain has improved, but she still has dizziness and now complains of feeling weak. Review of systems is otherwise unremarkable; she denies feeling depressed, but admits she is feeling anxious about her physical problems. For the very first time, she presents with a walker and is unable to explain why she is using it. Her vital signs are normal and virtually unchanged from her previous visit. Although her leg strength is 5/5, she still ambulates with difficulty, stating, "I'm just too weak."

You explain that her examination is normal and that you cannot provide an explanation for her dizziness and weakness. However, she refuses to walk without the walker, and insists there must be something wrong. Her daughter has accompanied her to today's appointment and asks you to do something because the patient has been calling her several times a day to complain about the dizziness, but adds that she has consistently called her about trivial issues nearly every day for over 30 years.

Discussion: *Patients with dependent personality disorder can be challenging for caregivers and providers alike due to their constant need for reassurance. This patient has become hypervigilant about symptoms that remain unexplained. Her refusal to walk unfortunately compounds the problem because she may develop deconditioning. It may be helpful to establish regularly scheduled brief visits for patients with dependent personality disorder to provide a predetermined time to discuss problems rather than them coming in urgently (and frequently) for every worry.*

Since psychiatric comorbidity is high with people who have dependent personality disorder, the AMPS screening tool should be used to assess for anxiety, mood, psychotic, or substance use disorders. In this case, the patient may additionally have a depressive or an anxiety disorder and should be treated accordingly.

ICD9

Paranoid Personality Disorder	301.0
Schizoid Personality Disorder	301.20
Schizotypal Personality Disorder	301.22
Antisocial Personality Disorder	301.7
Borderline Personality Disorder	301.83
Histrionic Personality Disorder	301.50
Avoidant Personality Disorder	301.82
Dependent Personality Disorder	301.6
Obsessive Compulsive Personality Disorder	301.4
Personality Disorder NOS	301.9
Narcissistic Personality Disorder	301.81

Practical Resources

National Institute of Mental Health: http://www.nimh.nih.gov/health/publications/borderline-personality-disorder.shtml
Mentalhelp.net: http://www.mentalhelp.net/poc/view_doc.php?type=doc&id=450&cn=8
Psychiatryonline.com: http://www.psychiatryonline.com/pracGuide/pracGuideTopic_13.aspx

References

1. American Psychiatric Association. Personality disorders. In: *Diagnostic and Statistical Manual of Mental Disorders*. 4th ed., text revision. Washington, DC: American Psychiatric Association; 2000:685.

2. Oldham JM, Skodol AE, Bender DS, eds. *Textbook of Personality Disorders*. Washington, DC: American Psychiatric Publishing, Inc.; 2005.

3. Hueston WJ, Werth J, Mainous AG. Personality disorder traits: prevalence and effects on health status in primary care patients. *Int J Psychiatry Med*. 1999;29:63–74.

4. Casey PR, Tyrer P. Personality disorder and psychiatric illness in general practice. *Br J Psychiatry*. 1990; 156:261–265.

5. Hueston WJ, Mainous AG, Schilling R. Patients with personality disorders: functional status, health care utilization, and satisfaction with care. *J Fam Pract*. 1996;42(1):54–60.

6. Shea MT, Pilkonis PA, Beckham E, et al. Personality disorders and treatment outcome in the NIMH treatment of depression collaborative research program. *Am J Psychiatry*. 1990;147(6):711–718.

7. Groves JE. Taking care of the hateful patient. *N Engl J Med*. 1978;298(16):883–887.

8. Devens M. Personality disorders. *Prim Care*. 2007;34(3):623–640.

9. Rost KM, Akin RN, Brown FW, et al. The comorbidity of DSM-III-TR personality disorders in somatization disorder. *Gen Hosp Psychiatry*. 1992;14(5):322–326.

10. Grant BF, Stintson FS, Dawson DA, et al. Co-occurrence of 12-month alcohol and drug use disorders and personality disorders in the United States. *Arch Gen Psychiatry*. 2004;61:361–368.

11. Gross R, Olfson M, Gameroff M, et al. Borderline personality disorder in primary care. *Arch Intern Med*. 2002;162(1):53–60.

12. Grilo CM, Shea MT, Sanislow CA, et al. Two-year stability and change of schizotypal, borderline, avoidant, and obsessive-compulsive personality disorders. *J Consult Clin Psychol*. 2004;72(5):767–775.

13. Gunderson JG, Weinberg I, Daversa MT, et al. Descriptive and longitudinal observations on the relationship of borderline personality disorder and bipolar disorder. *Am J Psychiatry.* 2006;163(7):1126–1128.

14. Linehan MM, Comtois KA, Murray AM, et al. Two year randomized controlled trial and follow-up of dialectical behavior therapy vs therapy by experts for suicidal behaviors and borderline personality disorder. *Arch Gen Psychiatry.* 2006;63(7):757–766.

15. Clarkin JF, Levy KN, Lenzenwger MF, et al. Evaluating three treatments for borderline personality disorder: a multiwave study. *Am J Psychiatry.* 2007;164(6):922–928.

16. Monsen J, Odland T, Faugli A, et al. Personality disorders and psychosocial changes after intensive psychotherapy: a prospective follow-up study of an outpatient psychotherapy project, 5 years after end of treatment. *Scand J Psychol.* 1995;36(3):256–268.

17. American Psychiatric Association Practice Guidelines. Practice guideline for the treatment of patients with borderline personality disorder. American Psychiatric Association. *Am J Psychiatry.* 2001;158(10 Suppl):1–52.

18. Nose, M, Cipriani A, Biancosino B, et al. Efficacy of pharmacotherapy against core traits of borderline personality disorder: meta-analysis or randomized controlled trials. *Int Clin Psychopharmacol.* 2006;21:345–353.

CHAPTER 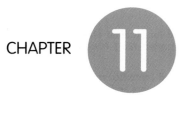 Cultural Considerations in Primary Care Psychiatry

Alan Koike, MD, MSHS • Hendry Ton, MD, MS • David
Gellerman, MD, PhD • Sergio Aguilar-Gaxiola, MD, PhD •
Russell F. Lim, MD

> *A 35-year-old Hmong woman presents to a primary care clinic with complaints of "whole body pain," fatigue, and poor sleep. Further inquiries reveal that she has six children between the ages of 3 and 12, and that she is unable to get out of bed to prepare meals for her family. She speaks Hmong and has had no formal education. She does not speak, read, or write English. She is an animist (believes that animals, plants, rocks, the wind, and water have souls) and complains about a "dab" or unwanted "spirit" that is bothering her and causing her to feel ill.*

CLINICAL HIGHLIGHTS

- Unexplained somatic complaints are commonly endorsed by immigrant and refugee patients, and may be signs of a mental disorder.

- Spiritual beliefs and practices are important to many patients and should be assessed and addressed in order to optimize treatment.

- Language barriers can adversely influence the development of an accurate diagnosis and treatment plan. When possible, translators should be used during

(Continued)

Clinical Significance

Ethnic minority populations are growing at a tremendous rate in the United States. Unfortunately, the growth of health care professionals from some minority groups (e.g., African Americans, Latinos, and Native Americans) is not commensurate with their representation in the general population (2). As the primary care patient population becomes increasingly diverse, it is essential that clinicians better prepare themselves to work with patients from different cultural and linguistic backgrounds. Primary care providers face daunting challenges in providing culturally and linguistically competent care to diverse patient populations. The failure to consider a patient's cultural, spiritual, and linguistic issues can result in a variety of adverse consequences, including miscommunication, poor continuity of care, less preventive screening, difficulties with informed consent, reduced access to care, use of harmful remedies, delayed immunizations, and fewer necessary prescriptions (3).

The Institute of Medicine's (IOM) groundbreaking report, *Unequal Treatment*, found that racial and ethnic minorities—even those with equivalent access to health services—receive lower quality of care than nonminorities for several medical conditions (4). These disparities in health care are associated with worse outcomes and increased mortality. In the area of mental health, the Surgeon General's Supplement to the Report on Mental Health, entitled *Mental Health: Culture, Race and Ethnicity*, identified striking disparities in mental health care for racial and ethnic minorities (5). It reported that minorities have less access, availability, and quality of mental health services. The report further states that a consequence of this disparity is that racial and ethnic minorities bear a disproportionate burden of disability from untreated and examinations to decrease the chance for miscommunication.

- The *Diagnostic and Statistical Manual of Mental Disorders,* 4th edition, text revision (DSM-IV-TR) Outline for Cultural Formulation (OCF) is a useful tool for assessing cultural and linguistic issues (1).

inadequately treated mental health problems. The key message of the report is that culture counts!

Culture influences many aspects of health care, including how patients recognize, acknowledge, and cope with their symptoms; communicate with their providers; accept treatment; and access support systems. A new report by The Joint Commission titled *Hospitals, Language, and Culture: A Snapshot of the Nation* recommends that providers make efforts to address language and cultural issues that create challenges to delivering safe and effective care to diverse populations in the United States (6). Additionally, spirituality is an often overlooked aspect of culture. Spiritual beliefs and practices are important to most patients, yet physicians are often unsure how to address these issues in the context of primary care. This chapter aims to help providers assess spirituality in medical settings, understand the importance of language access in medical care, and provides the OCF as a way to incorporate culture into clinical practice.

Spirituality in Medical Care

The United States is home to a number of diverse religious faiths (7). Surveys have found that 95% of people in the United States believe in God and 84% of Americans claim that religion is important in their lives (8). In the last two decades, the importance of religious faith and spirituality in medicine has been increasingly recognized, such that addressing spirituality in medical education and care is mandated by numerous institutions (9).

Several studies suggest that many patients prefer a clinician who is accepting and attentive to their religious or spiritual beliefs (10). Most patients seem to want their providers to inquire into coping and means of social support and, when indicated, be willing to participate in a spiritually oriented discussion. Patient preferences regarding different spiritual interventions vary depending on the severity of the medical illness as well as the medical setting. For example, studies indicate that most patients do not want a clinician to inquire about their religious beliefs during a routine office visit, but in the context of dying, most would welcome such a discussion (7). In addition, patients' spiritual or religious faith may play a role in their medical decision making, such as consideration of blood transfusions, planning an advance directive, or considering do not resuscitate (DNR) status.

PERFORMING A SPIRITUAL ASSESSMENT

A spiritual history is easily incorporated into the social history. Considering time constraints, a spiritual history should be direct and brief, but elicit sufficient information to determine whether more time is needed for a more in-depth discussion. We also suggest that primary care clinicians incorporate a spiritual history into new patient evaluations and hospital admissions, and to review the spiritual history should there be significant changes in a patient's overall health status or social circumstances. For example, the clinician may ask, "You

Table 11.1 SPIRIT

S: Spiritual belief system
P: Personal spirituality
I: Importance of spirituality in your life
R: Ritualized practices and restrictions
I: Implications for medical care
T: Terminal events planning

From Maugans TA. The SPIRITual history. *Arch Fam Med.* 1996;5:11–16.

mentioned earlier how difficult it has been to deal with diabetes and some of the associated pain symptoms. When you're feeling particularly ill, what keeps you going? Do you consider yourself a religious or spiritual person?"

Several screening tools can be used in the primary care setting to help obtain a spiritual history. We recommend using the SPIRIT questionnaire because it is brief, easy for patients to complete, and will usually provide useful information to the treating clinician (Table 11.1) (11).

The inclusion of the spiritual history in primary care assessments will likely enhance the clinician–patient relationship, expand healthy coping strategies, and improve overall patient care. It is important to recognize recent changes in a patient's perceived religiosity, faith, or church attendance, as these may indicate depression or other mental health disorders. Inquiry into spiritual beliefs and practices should not suggest that clinicians act as spiritual care providers. Physicians are not trained to provide pastoral or spiritual care per se, although encouraging and supporting beliefs and practices already identified by the patient typically would not disrupt or impose upon the clinician–patient relationship (7).

Language: A Hidden Barrier to Quality Care

The Census 2000 revealed that nearly 20% of U.S. residents speak a language other than English when at home. Within this group, nearly 45% speak English "less than very well" (12). This means that persons with limited English proficiency (LEP) are not able to speak, read, write, or understand the English language at a level that allows them to interact effectively with health care providers (13). Limited or lack of communication in health care is associated with disparities in access to services as well as in diagnosis and treatment (4). Research has repeatedly shown that language barriers impede access, compromise quality of care, and increase the risk of adverse health outcomes among patients with LEP. Title VI of the Civil Rights Act of 1964 requires health systems that are recipients of federal financial assistance to provide persons with LEP meaningful access to programs and free language services. Despite this, language barriers continue to be an important obstacle to appropriate care and wide gaps persist due to extra costs and limited availability of interpreters.

> ## Table 11.2 How to Work Effectively with an Interpreter
>
> 1. Greet the patient first, then introduce yourself to the interpreter
> 2. Speak at an even pace and pause after a full thought
> 3. Assume that everything you say will be interpreted
> 4. If you must address the interpreter about an issue, let the patient know what you are going to be discussing
> 5. Avoid the use of slang, technical medical terminology, and complicated sentences
> 6. Ask the interpreter to point out potential cultural misunderstandings that may occur
> 7. Do not hold the interpreter responsible for what the patient says or doesn't say
> 8. Be aware that many concepts have no linguistic or conceptual equivalent in other languages
>
> ---
>
> Adapted from Cynthia E. Roat, MPH, Communicating Effectively through an Interpreter, from the Cross Cultural Health Care Program, December 2007.

USING INTERPRETERS IN THE MEDICAL SETTING

Because one out of six U.S. residents speaks a language other than English, high-quality medical care cannot be provided without proper language access. Qualified interpreters are an integral part of the clinical team and should be respected as part of the health care team. Interpreting involves special skills beyond fluency in another language. Interpreters should be trained and fluent in both the source and target language. Untrained interpreters are at high risk for adding or omitting information, changing the message, or giving inappropriate opinions. Using family members and children as interpreters should be avoided. Other helpful tips for utilizing interpreters in the primary care setting are included in Table 11.2.

When possible, practitioners should use certified translators because a poorly trained interpreter, or the use of a family member as an interpreter often results in poor communication and the development of an ineffective treatment plan (14). Providers should also be trained as early in their training as possible to work with interpreters (15). When possible, health care financing policies should reinforce existing medical research and legal policies. Payers, including Medicaid, Medicare, and private insurers, should develop mechanisms to reimburse for interpretation services for patients who speak limited English (16).

The Outline for Cultural Formulation

Many providers recognize that cultural issues may play an important role in interactions with patients, yet feel ill equipped to address these concerns. The complexity of the interplay between culture and illness can make this process overwhelming. Factual knowledge about cultural groups, while essential, can have limited utility without a framework to organize and to make sense of the information. The OCF, first introduced in 1994, provides clinicians with a systematic approach for assessing the impact of culture on illness and treatment (1). The OCF is made up of five components: (1) cultural identity of the patient,

(2) cultural explanations of the patient's illness, (3) psychosocial environment and levels of functioning, (4) clinician–patient relationship, and (5) overall assessment and treatment plan. This section reviews these different components and offers high-yield questions that can be utilized to elicit important but often overlooked information.

CULTURAL IDENTITY

Cultural identity refers to the multifaceted set of identities that contribute to an individual's understanding of and interactions with his or her environment. While ethnicity is an important part of cultural identity, other factors such as religious and spiritual beliefs, country of origin, sexual orientation, and socioeconomic status may be as or more important to any given person. A devoutly Catholic man born and raised in the Philippines, for example, may have a very different perspective on abortion than an atheist Filipino woman born and raised in the United States. There are several reasons for assessing a patient's cultural identity. Providers gain a better understanding of the patient as a whole person and his or her sociocultural environment. This assessment also helps to identify potential resilience factors and risk factors. Providers may identify conflicting roles that lead to ambivalence or psychosocial distress. Finally, inquiries into areas of identity that are meaningful to the patient help to improve rapport. Table 11.3, Section A, suggests some high-yield questions that may be used to assess the patient's cultural identity.

CULTURAL EXPLANATIONS OF THE PATIENT'S ILLNESS

Primary care providers should be aware that patients may have other explanations for their illnesses that differ from Western medical concepts. Asian models, for example, often include explanations that imbalances of hot and cold energy may cause illnesses, which can be cured by eating foods to make up for the imbalance. Other cultural explanatory models may include supernatural causes, such as spirits, "mal de

Table 11.3 High-Yield Questions

A. **Questions to assess cultural identity**
   1. Do you identify with a particular culture or religion?
   2. Where were you born and raised? How did you come to live in this area?
   3. How comfortable do you feel with being part of "mainstream American" culture?
   4. Please describe the significant activities and groups in your life.

B. **Questions to assess the psychosocial environment**
   1. Who are the important people in your life?
   2. How much do you involve others when making health care decisions?
   3. What would your family expect of you if you were well?
   4. Do you have any contact with the community?

C. **Questions to assist the therapeutic relationship**
   1. In what language do you prefer to communicate?
   2. Some people prefer to see a provider from their own cultural group, and we are happy to honor their preference when we can. What are your preferences with regard to having a provider?
   3. As your doctor, it is important for me to treat you with respect. Are there things that are done in your culture to convey respect? What things would be considered disrespectful for a provider to do?

Table 11.4 Kleinman's Eight Patient-Directed Questions

1. What do you think has caused your problem?
2. Why do you think it started when it did?
3. What do you think your sickness does to you? How does it work?
4. How severe is your sickness? Will it have a short or long course?
5. What kind of treatment should you receive?
6. What are the most important results you hope to receive from this treatment?
7. What are the chief problems your sickness has caused for you?
8. What do you fear most about your sickness?

Kleinman A. *The Illness Narratives: Suffering, Healing and the Human Conditions.* Basic Books; 1988:43–44.

ojo," (evil eye), or "susto" (soul death). Thus, patients may not adhere to their treatment regimens because it does not make sense with their explanation of illness. Arthur Kleinman suggested that clinicians should try to elicit the patient's "explanatory model" of the illness (17). He developed eight questions that can be helpful in discussing unique cultural aspects of illness (Table 11.4). Once the patient's explanatory model is understood, clinicians can develop a collaborative approach that bridges the cultural divide, show an understanding of the patient's point of view, and negotiate an acceptable treatment plan, which will increase both the relevance of and adherence to treatment.

PSYCHOSOCIAL ENVIRONMENT AND LEVEL OF FUNCTIONING

The third component of the OCF can be thought of as stressors and supports for the patient, and can be conceptualized as the role that the patient plays in his or her family and community. Examples of roles that patients could play include the primary breadwinner, parental caregiver, childcare provider, dutiful child, cultural broker, and interpreter. The shame and stigma of mental illness can limit patients' willingness to access community resources because they have to reveal that they have a mental illness. Clinicians need to assess which patients can be referred to programs within their communities and which can or need to be managed by resources outside of the patient's cultural group. It is important to explore with patients their sources of support and what options they have to relieve their stress. Also relevant to the level of functioning and psychosocial environment is who makes decisions about health care. A patient from an individualistic culture may prefer to have more decision-making power, whereas one from a collectivistic culture may be inclined to have family members actively involved in his or her health care decisions. See Table 11.3, Section B, for questions to assess the psychosocial environment.

THE THERAPEUTIC RELATIONSHIP

Stereotypes, cultural misunderstandings, and conflicts in world views that impact social relationships outside of the health care environment play significant roles in the clinical exchange. It is important to be

---

Table 11.5 Using the Outline for Cultural Formulation

- Identify salient features of cultural identity
  - Encourages patient's active participation
  - Is an effective way to build rapport
  - Helps to inform the rest of the cultural formulation

- Develop collaborative explanatory models
  - Improves relevancy of treatment
  - Improves adherence to treatment

- Clarify psychosocial context
  - Identifies key decision makers
  - Clarifies decision-making process

- Examine the impact of the cultural similarities and differences between you and the patient
  - Appreciation of one's own cultural identity and history is the foundation to connect with another's

---

aware of the influence of these cultural factors on the patient–provider relationship. Part of this process requires providers to honestly examine their own cultural identity and beliefs to identify assumptions, biases, and cultural blind spots as well as cultural strengths. See Table 11.3, Section C, for questions to assess the therapeutic relationship.

OVERALL CULTURAL ASSESSMENT FOR DIAGNOSIS AND CARE

The overall assessment should include the key issues identified in the previous four sections of the cultural formulation (Table 11.5). Treatment planning should incorporate strategies that address culturally based problems or build upon cultural strengths.

Practice Pointers

Case 1: Using the Outline for Cultural Formulation
A 35-year-old Hmong woman presents to a primary care clinic with complaints of "whole body pain," fatigue, and poor sleep. Further inquiries reveal that she has six children between the ages of 3 and 12, and that she is unable to get out of bed to prepare meals for her family. She speaks Hmong, and has had no formal education. She does not speak, read, or write English. She is an animist (believes that animals, plants, rocks, the wind, and water have souls) and complains about a "dab" or unwanted "spirit" that is bothering her and causing her to feel ill. She grew up in Laos, lived in a refugee camp in Thailand from 1977 to 2005, and migrated to the United States in 2005.

Discussion: Case 1 can be used to briefly illustrate how the OCF can be used as a guide to assess a patient's culture and its influence on the clinical encounter.

Cultural identity: The primary care provider has determined that her patient strongly identifies with the Hmong culture, and as part of that culture, has animist religious beliefs. The patient feels her most meaningful activity in life is caring for her children and her ability to do so has been significantly compromised by her illness.
Cultural explanations of the patient's illness: During the interview, the doctor finds that the patient had recently been to a shaman who explained that a malevolent spirit, or "dab," is causing her illness. She participated in a shaman ritual to rid her of the evil spirit and has experienced some modest relief since then. The doctor now recognizes that the patient's explanation of her illness is different from his, and that

the patient has had very little contact with or understanding of Western medicine. In addition, the patient is unfamiliar with concepts of mental illness such as depression.

Psychosocial environment and level of functioning: The patient states that her family is the most important thing in her life, and that she feels grateful for the members who have brought her to various healers. She states that her family knows what is best for her in these situations. The clinician understands the need to work closely with the patient's family, as they are her sole source of support, and makes a referral to a local community social service agency that has experience working with Hmong refugees.

The therapeutic relationship: The patient was evaluated with a Hmong-speaking interpreter. Although the doctor is not Hmong, she reassures the patient that she will do her best to try to understand how her cultural beliefs might affect her physical and emotional health. She then asks the patient and the family to teach her about the concept of "dab" and the role of the shaman in Hmong culture.

Overall cultural assessment: Given her cultural identity and recent immigration to the United States, the doctor hypothesized that the patient was not familiar with Western medical concepts. She recognized the importance of having family present to discuss treatment planning and obtained a release of information from the patient to be able to involve the family. The provider also acknowledged significant losses and stresses that the patient experienced at the refugee camps and expressed a commitment to do what she could as a doctor to help alleviate some of the physical and emotional suffering caused by those experiences.

Case 2: Anxiety, chest pain, and the need for an interpreter

A 28-year-old Mexican man presents to an emergency room with chest pain. He has no previous history of heart disease and is otherwise healthy. His electrocardiogram (ECG) indicates a normal sinus rhythm and cardiac enzymes are within normal limits. He is able to speak some English and give brief responses to questions. He is able to communicate his imminent fear of dying, but it is difficult to get a more detailed history due to the patient's LEP.

Discussion: *While it is tempting to obtain the patient's history in English, his LEP makes it essential that the hospital find a qualified Spanish-speaking interpreter. A professional interpreter is provided and the patient reports that he has had brief episodes of chest pain for the past few months. Through the interpreter, you learn that his chest pain starts while he is at rest and is associated with intense anxiety, shortness of breath, tachycardia, and tingling of the extremities, all with a duration of 20 minutes. His symptoms are consistent with panic disorder.*

The key to this case is the access to a qualified professional interpreter, which allows the clinician to make the proper diagnosis of panic disorder. The OCF can then be used to identify other cultural aspects relevant to the patient's care.

Case 3: Cultural considerations and medical decisions

A 25-year-old married, Farsi-speaking, Afghan woman presents to an urgent care clinic with complaints of difficulty breathing, difficulty swallowing, and a choking sensation for the past few months. Upon questioning, she reports other problems including a depressed mood and insomnia as well as decreased energy, concentration, and appetite. She is a mother of two small children and is now 12 weeks pregnant. She feels overwhelmed by the prospect of having another child. The patient is Muslim, but she wants an abortion despite her religious beliefs. Her husband is adamantly opposed to an abortion, stating that "it would be a sin."

Discussion: *If possible, the clinic should obtain a Farsi-speaking interpreter. In this case, the interpreter is a college-educated Iranian American woman, who was born in the United States. A spiritual assessment reveals that the patient is a Sunni-Muslim, but she does not consider herself very religious. While her religion could be a source of support, she feels estranged from her religious leaders because of her wish to have an abortion and does not feel that she can confide in them.*

The patient comes from a male-dominated culture in which the husband is the decision maker of the family, and in which there would be dire consequences if the patient were to act against his wishes. This situation will not be resolved in one visit. At subsequent visits, the provider initially meets with the patient individually, and then brings in the husband to jointly discuss the treatment plan. The physician is aware of the potential cultural differences between the well-educated Farsi-speaking Iranian American interpreter and the Afghan patient and discusses these issues with the interpreter. The physician also reflects on his own feelings regarding abortion and his discomfort with cultures that he perceives as oppressive to women. Recognizing the complex moral and ethical issues of this case, the provider should try to obtain consultation from colleagues and community members familiar with Afghan culture.

Practical Resources

Resources for spiritual issues:
University of Washington School of Medicine: http://depts.washington.edu/bioethx/topics/spirit.html
Jointcommmission.org: http://www.jointcommission.org/PatientSafety/HLC/
Ethnomed: http://ethnomed.org
United States Department of Health and Human Services: http://www.thinkculturalhealth.org/

References

1. American Psychiatric Association. Outline for cultural formulation and glossary of culture-bound syndromes. In: *Diagnostic and Statistical Manual of Mental Disorders.* 4th ed., text revision. Washington, DC: American Psychiatric Association; 2000.

2. Smedley BD, Butler AS, Bristow LR, eds. *In the Nation's Compelling Interest: Ensuring Diversity in the Health Care Workforce. Committee on Institutional and Policy-Level Strategies for Increasing the Diversity of the U.S. Health Care Workforce.* Washington, DC: National Academies; 2004.

3. Flores G, Rabke-Verani J, Pine W, et al. The importance of cultural and linguistic issues in the emergency care of children. *Pediatr Emerg Care.* 2002;18(4):271–284.

4. Smedley BD, Stith AY, Nelson AR, eds. *Unequal Treatment: Confronting Racial and Ethnic Disparities in Health Care.* Washington, DC: National Academies; 2002.

5. U.S. Department of Health and Human Services (USDHHS). *Mental Health: Culture, Race, and Ethnicity: A Supplement to Mental Health: A Report of the Surgeon General.* Rockville, MD: U.S. Department of Health and Human Services, Public Health Service, Office of the Surgeon General; 2001.

6. Wilson-Stronks A, Galvez E. *Hospitals, Language, and Culture: A Snapshot of the Nation.* Oakbrook Terrace, IL: The Joint Commission; 2007.

7. Koenig HG. *Spirituality and Patient Care: Why, How, When, and What.* Philadelphia: Templeton Foundation Press; 2002.

8. Gallup G. *Religion in America—50 years, 1935-1985. The Gallup Report.* Princeton, NJ: Princeton Religion Research Center; 1985.

9. Pulchaski C. Spiritual Assessment in clinical practice. *Psychiatry Ann* 2006;36:150–155.

10. Hebert RS, Jenckes MW, Ford DF, et al. Patient perspectives on spirituality and the patient-physician relationship. *J Gen Intern Med.* 2001;16:685–692.

11. Maugans TA. The SPIRITual history. *Arch Fam Med.* 1996;5:11–16.

12. Shin HB, Bruno R. Language use and English-speaking ability: 2000. *Census 2000 Brief.* Washington, DC: U.S. Census Bureau; 2003.

13. Office of Civil Rights. 2002. Guidance to federal financial assistance recipients regarding Title VI prohibition against national origin discrimination affecting limited English proficient persons. http://www.lep.gov. Accessed December 23, 2007.

14. Brafman AH. Beware of the distorting interpreter. *BMJ.* 1995;311(7004):1439.

15. Phelan M, Parkman S. How to work with an interpreter. *BMJ.* 1995;311(7004):555.

16. Ku L, Flores G. Pay now or pay later: providing interpreter services in health care. *Health Aff (Millwood).* 2005;24(2):435–444.

17. Kleinman A. *The Illness Narratives: Suffering, Healing and the Human Conditions.* New York: Basic Books; 1988:43–44.

CHAPTER 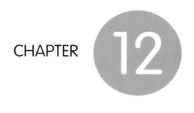 Geriatric Psychiatry—
Dementias

Andreea L. Seritan, MD • Michael K. McCloud, MD, FACP
• Ladson Hinton, MD

A 70-year-old man of Middle Eastern descent with limited English skills presents to the geriatric clinic complaining of memory loss for the past 3 months. He has become easily distracted, forgets important dates and recent events, and was in a minor car accident 2 weeks ago. He is brought in by his daughter who readily gives the history, rushes to answer the interviewer's questions before the patient, and translates the MMSE while at the same time giving clues as to the correct answers.

Clinical Significance

By 2030, one in three U.S. residents will be age 55 or older, and one in five will be at least age 65. Nearly 20% of those aged 55 or older will have psychiatric disorders, including dementias (1). Dementia prevalence increases with age, from 5% of those aged 71 to 79 to 37.4% of those aged 90 and older (2). Given limited access and availability of subspecialty mental health services, elderly patients with dementia and other psychiatric disorders are most often cared for by their primary care clinicians.

Diagnosis

Early diagnosis and treatment of dementias are imperative, as they help to slow cognitive and functional decline. Persons with early-stage dementia are more likely to be able to participate in clinical decision making. Delays in detection of behavior problems result in reactive as opposed to proactive management of dementia and increase reliance on pharmacologic rather than behavioral approaches (3). A simplified algorithm for dementia diagnosis is presented in Figure 12.1.

ESTABLISH PRESENCE OF A DEMENTIA SYNDROME

Dementia implies an acquired, persistent, and progressive impairment in multiple cognitive domains leading to significant functional decline. The *Diagnostic and Statistical Manual of Mental Disorders*, 4th edition, text revision (DSM-IV-TR) diagnostic criteria require involvement of at least two cognitive domains, one of which is memory (5). Other domains noted are mostly cortical functions (also known as "A" functions):

CLINICAL HIGHLIGHTS

- The Mini-Mental State Examination (MMSE) is a useful screening tool for most dementias, but it does not adequately screen for executive dysfunction. Despite a 30/30 score, some patients may still have a dementia syndrome.

- Prior to making a diagnosis of dementia, reversible causes of cognitive dysfunction including medical, medication-induced, and psychiatric conditions should be assessed and treated.

(Continued)

amnesia (memory recall deficit), aphasia (language impairment), apraxia (inability to perform learned motor sequences in the absence of motor impairment), and agnosia (inability to recognize an object in the absence of sensory impairment) (5). A dementing illness is distinguished from congenital mental retardation syndromes by the criterion of acquired impairment.

Although impairments of executive function are common in dementias that involve the frontal cortex or subcortical white matter, they are often overlooked. The MMSE does not adequately screen for executive dysfunction. Some patients with subcortical dementias may still have a 30/30 score. Executive function may be assessed by asking questions about the patient's ability to shop, plan meals, balance the checkbook, keep track of appointments, develop a schedule in advance of an anticipated events, and prioritize things by importance. Collateral information is often crucial. If suspicion exists based on history, several simple tests can be quickly performed in the office to establish whether executive dysfunction is present (Table 12.1) (4).

By contrast, *mild cognitive impairment* (MCI) is defined by deficits in at least one cognitive domain with relatively intact ADLs. In a primary care sample, MCI prevalence was up to 25% in individuals over age 75 (6). MCI is further classified as amnestic (with memory impairment) and nonamnestic, in which other cognitive domains (other than memory) are impaired. Patients with amnestic MCI should be closely followed as they may convert to Alzheimer disease (AD) at a rate of about 15% per year (7). Recent research suggests that neuropsychiatric symptoms, especially depression and apathy, are a predictor of progression to AD (8).

CORTICAL VERSUS SUBCORTICAL DEMENTIAS

After the presence of a dementia syndrome has been established, it is important to further clarify the diagnosis. If either major focal neurologic deficits or a history of cerebrovascular accidents (CVAs) is present together with a sudden onset or a stepwise progressive decline in cognitive function, vascular dementia (VaD) secondary to cortical infarction is most likely present. *Pure* vascular dementias constitute only up to 10% of all dementias, and many persons who have an onset typical of vascular dementia may later present with more gradual deterioration indicative of AD, thus a *mixed* AD-VaD dementia (4).

In other patients, motor slowing (bradykinesia), ataxia, cogwheel rigidity, shuffled gait, tremor, or chorea may be observed. These movement disorders, along with cognitive slowing (bradyphrenia), apathy, retrieval memory deficit but preserved recall initially, and mood disturbances are typical of neurodegenerative or vascular processes involving subcortical structures (4). Neuronal circuits connect the basal ganglia and other subcortical structures with corresponding areas in the frontal lobes. The dementias associated with impairments of these circuits are called *frontal-subcortical dementias*. Examples are Huntington disease (HD), Parkinson disease (PD), progressive supranuclear palsy (PSP),

VASCULAR DEMENTIA

- Neurologic deficits (clinical, neuroimaging)
- Stepwise progression
- Usually presents with a long-standing history of hypertension

FRONTAL-SUBCORTICAL DEMENTIA

- Movement disorders
- Mood disturbance
- Psychomotor and cognitive slowing (apathy)

DEMENTIA WITH LEWY BODIES

- Fluctuating mental status
- Parkinsonism
- Visual hallucinations
- Poor response to antipsychotics

multiple system atrophy, human immunodeficiency virus (HIV) dementia, and subcortical CVAs (Table 12.2) (4).

Dementia with Lewy bodies (DLB), a mixed cortical-subcortical dementia, is the third most frequent cause of dementia, after AD and vascular dementia, and accounts for 15% to 20% of dementias. Onset of the disease varies between 50 and 90 years of age, and dementia usually occurs within 1 year of the onset of parkinsonism. Exquisite sensitivity to antipsychotic side effects and repeated falls are supportive diagnostic features. Delusions, delusional misidentification, mood changes, and rapid eye movement (REM) sleep behavior disorder are other prominent neuropsychiatric manifestations (9).

OVERVIEW ON CORTICAL DEMENTIA AND ALZHEIMER DISEASE

Pure AD constitutes about 35% of all dementias, while mixed AD-VaD accounts for 15% (4). AD is the quintessential amnestic dementia and often presents with anterograde memory loss (difficulty learning new information). Onset is insidious, with early word-finding difficulties progressing slowly to empty but fluent speech, accompanied later by visuospatial impairment. Poor insight into cognitive deficits is typical, while poor judgment and planning may follow as the illness progresses to involve the frontal lobes. Wandering and unsafe driving are other cardinal manifestations.

The MMSE is particularly useful in screening for cortical dementias, especially AD, since it is heavily weighted toward language and memory. Most practitioners use a cut-off score of 24 in screening; however, higher thresholds need to be used in highly educated patients. Difficulty

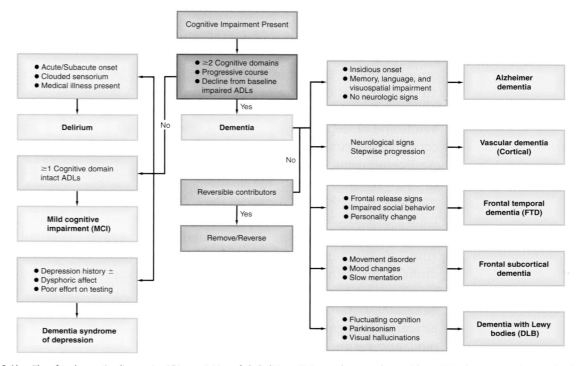

Figure 12.1 Algorithm for dementia diagnosis. ADLs, activities of daily living; CVA, cerebrovascular accident; DLB, dementia with Lewy bodies; FTD, frontotemporal dementia; MCI, mild cognitive impairment.

ALZHEIMER DISEASE

- Memory loss (early word-finding difficulties, anterograde amnesia)
- Language impairment
- Visuospatial skills impairment

FRONTOTEMPORAL DEMENTIA

- Disinhibition (personality change)
- Early loss of social awareness
- Early loss of insight
- Hyperorality
- Stereotyped and perseverative behavior (wandering, mannerisms)

NOT TO BE MISSED

- Dementia with Lewy bodies
- Frontotemporal lobar degeneration
- Dementia syndrome of depression
- Delirium (systemic medical conditions)
- Nutritional deficits (vitamin B_{12}, folate)
- Medication-induced cognitive deficits

with recall (especially if not helped by cues), naming, temporal orientation, and polygon copying are typically found in AD. The clock drawing test examines multiple cognitive domains, including visuospatial skills (Table 12.1) (4).

In addition to VaD with cortical strokes and AD, the other major cortical dementia class is *frontotemporal lobar degeneration (FTLD)*, which accounts for 5% of dementias (4). FTLD is a heterogenous term that includes frontotemporal dementia (FTD or Pick disease), FTD with motor neuron disease (e.g., amyotrophic lateral sclerosis), progressive nonfluent aphasia, semantic dementia, and progressive apraxia. FTLD usually develops between ages 45 and 65, whereas AD usually presents after age 65 (4). The FTD clinical picture is one of profound alteration in social conduct and personality. Memory failures result from executive, organizational, and retrieval deficits rather than from amnesia.

REVERSIBLE CONTRIBUTORS

Completely reversible dementias are rare, although reversible comorbid conditions are common in dementia. Identifying reversible etiologies of cognitive deficits is important, although in some cases (alcohol, vitamin B_{12} or folate deficiency) neuropsychiatric sequelae can only be partially reversed. Replacement of vitamin B_{12} levels below 350 pmol/L is recommended because checking for elevated homocysteine or methylmalonic acid levels may be more expensive and serial blood tests are often necessary. Table 12.3 lists suggested studies for dementia work-up (10). Computerized tomography (CT) will screen for most intracranial mass lesions, hematomas, hydrocephalus, and strokes. Magnetic resonance imaging (MRI) is recommended when white matter disease is suspected, such as with subcortical strokes or multiple sclerosis. Periventricular white matter disease consistent with small vessel ischemia is a commonly reported finding and it does not rule out AD. Functional imaging studies, such as positron emission tomography (PET) or single photon emission computed tomography (SPECT), may indicate impairment before structural changes are visible. Medicare covers PET when used to differentiate AD from FTLD (5). Neuropsychological testing is helpful in distinguishing the dementia syndrome of depression, formerly known as pseudodementia, from other cognitive deficits.

Polypharmacy and drug–drug interactions may lead to adverse events. Anticholinergic medications are generally contraindicated in patients with dementia, since they can worsen cognition. Commonly used medications with anticholinergic properties include antiparkinsonian agents (benztropine, trihexyphenidyl), antipsychotics (chlorpromazine, clozapine), antihistamines (chlorpheniramine, cyproheptadine, diphenhydramine), antispasmodics (dicyclomine, oxybutynin, and tolterodine), and tricyclic antidepressants (TCAs) (11). Benzodiazepines are generally not recommended in patients with dementia, as they can exacerbate cognitive dysfunction and cause paradoxical disinhibition, falls, and respiratory suppression. Although undertreated pain is a common problem, overuse of opioids is not advised either since opioids are associated with delirium.

Table 12.1 Executive Function Testing

TEST	INSTRUCTIONS	DOMAINS TESTED	RESPONSES INDICATIVE OF EXECUTIVE DYSFUNCTION
Clock drawing	"Draw a clock face and put all the numbers in." Then: "Place the hands at 10 minutes after 11"	Planning, attention, language comprehension, visuospatial skills, numerical knowledge, motor skills	Poor number alignment, poor hand placement, stimulus-bound behavior (hands placed at 10 and 11)
MMSE three-step command	"Take this piece of paper in your left hand, fold it in half, and give it back to me"	Sequencing, language comprehension, memory	Poor sequencing, motor perseveration (continue to fold paper multiple times)
Peaks and plateaus Tri-loops (spirals)	"Copy the design and continue to the end of the page"	Motor programming	Motor perseveration (repeat same element, add loops to the spirals)
Luria hand sequence (fist-palm-side)	Examiner demonstrates the fist-palm-side sequence; the patient has to reproduce it within five trials and repeat it five times without error	Sequencing, response inhibition	Motor perseveration, inability to correctly repeat sequence
Verbal fluency	"Name as many animals as you can in 1 minute."	Strategy for word retrieval	Fluency <18 ± 6 animals/minute
Proverb interpretation or finding similarities (e.g., orange-banana, watch-ruler, poem-statue)		Abstraction capacity	Concrete thinking
Trails Part A	"Connect 1-2-3, and so on" (on page with irregular number array)	Set maintenance, response inhibition, vulnerability to interference (timed tests)	Perseveration, connecting only numbers or only letters on Part B
Trails Part B	"Connect 1-A-2-B, and so on" (on page with numbers and letters)		

MMSE, Mini-Mental State Examination.
From Mendez MF, Cummings JL. Diagnosis of dementia; Alzheimer's disease. In: *Dementia: A Clinical Approach*. Philadelphia: Butterworth Heinemann; 2003:8; 41–119.

Biopsychosocial Treatment

SAFETY ISSUES

Treatment planning starts with establishing safety. If local resources are available, home safety assessments are conducted. Environmental hazards, such as gas appliances, firearms, staircases, and steep driveways causing risk of falls, need to be addressed, especially if the patient lives alone. A patient can no longer live independently when the required assistance with ADLs surpasses the level of supervision available, or if incontinence, wandering, and other severe behavioral disturbances occur (12). Department of motor vehicle reporting requirements vary by

Table 12.2 Examples of Frontal-Subcortical Dementias

Basal ganglia calcification (Fahr disease)	Normal-pressure hydrocephalus
Cerebral hypoxia/hypoperfusion	Olivopontocerebellar degeneration
Cerebrovascular accidents (subcortical)	Paraneoplastic syndromes
Creutzfeldt-Jakob disease	Parkinson disease
Dementia pugilistica	Postencephalitic syndromes
Diabetes mellitus (poorly controlled)	Progressive supranuclear palsy
Human immunodeficiency virus dementia	Spinocerebellar ataxias
Huntington disease	Toxic (alcohol, carbon monoxide, lead, manganese, mercury, methanol)
Hypertension	
Hypothyroidism	Traumatic brain injury
Multiple sclerosis	Tumors (primary or metastatic)
Multiple system atrophy	Vasculitis
Neurosyphilis	Vitamin deficiency (B_1, B_{12}, folate)
	Wilson disease

From Mendez MF, Cummings JL. Diagnosis of dementia; Alzheimer's disease. In: *Dementia: A Clinical Approach*. Philadelphia: Butterworth Heinemann; 2003:8; 41–119.

state. Discontinuation of driving should be strongly considered for all patients with AD, even in mild dementia. Family members may need to manage the patient's finances, obtain durable power of attorney for health care and finances, and supervise and administer medications, in order to prevent accidental overdose or questionable adherence. The risk of elder abuse or neglect is considerable for patients with poor

Table 12.3 Suggested Dementia Work-Up

ALWAYS	WHEN SUSPICION EXISTS
BUN/creatinine	CSF studies
CBC	Electroencephalogram
Calcium	Erythrocyte sedimentation rate
CT/MRI	Folate
Electrolytes	Heavy metal screen
Glucose	HIV
Liver function tests	Lyme serology
Thyroid function tests	RPR
Urinalysis	Testosterone
Vitamin B_{12}	Urine toxicology

BUN, blood urea nitrogen; CBC, complete blood count; CSF, cerebrospinal fluid; CT, computerized tomography; HIV, human immunodeficiency virus; MRI, magnetic resonance imaging; RPR, rapid plasma reagin.
From Taylor WD, Doraiswamy PM. Use of the laboratory in the diagnostic workup of older adults. In: *Textbook of Geriatric Psychiatry*. Washington, DC: American Psychiatric Publishing; 2004:179–188.

support networks, the frail, the very old (over age 75 years), and those with a diagnosis of depression or dementia (5).

EDUCATE AND THEN MEDICATE

Although AD is not curable, medication treatment is now the standard of care and it is important to offer hope to caregivers and maintain an optimistic attitude. Family members should be educated about the diagnosis, prognosis, and treatment options, as well as the community resources available. Guidance to local resources, family support groups, educational classes, and "Safe Return" bracelets are some of the benefits the Alzheimer's Association offers.

PHARMACOTHERAPY

Addressing comorbid systemic medical conditions; minimizing cerebrovascular risk factors by adequate control of diabetes mellitus, hypercholesterolemia, and hypertension; and maintaining a healthy diet are basic principles in the pharmacotherapy of dementia. A number of other agents, such as nonsteroidal anti-inflammatory drugs (NSAIDs), hormone replacement, ginkgo biloba, and vitamin E, are not recommended for routine use at this time due to lack of efficacy and potential adverse effects (5).

Cognitive Enhancers

Cognitive enhancers, including cholinesterase inhibitors (ChEIs) and N-methyl-D-aspartate (NMDA) receptor antagonists (memantine), are approved by the Food and Drug Administration (FDA) for AD, but are also used off-label for other dementias, including DLB, VaD, and mixed AD-VaD. DLB involves a greater cholinergic deficit than AD; therefore, patients may be particularly responsive to ChEIs (9). Conversely, patients with FTLD do not respond to ChEIs since the neuropathology of these illnesses may not involve a cholinergic deficit. There is no evidence to date that ChEIs slow down progression of MCI to AD, although patients with apolipoprotein E ε4 allele showed benefit from donepezil at 3 years (7).

Table 12.4 lists properties and dosing of cognitive enhancers (14, 15). Weighing risks and benefits of ChEIs is important, especially given the potential for gastrointestinal side effects (nausea, vomiting, or diarrhea), anorexia and weight loss, dizziness, ataxia, confusion, vivid dreams, agitation, and bradycardia. In patients taking ChEIs, heart rate should be over 60 beats per minute prior to initiation of treatment. The pulse should be regularly monitored, particularly in patients taking beta-blockers, calcium channel inhibitors, or digoxin. Since cholinergics may provoke bronchospasm, patients with severe asthma or chronic obstructive pulmonary disease (COPD) should have a caregiver present when starting ChEIs. Attention should be paid to adverse interactions with prescribed or over-the-counter medications (11).

Treatment of Neuropsychiatric Symptoms

Neuropsychiatric symptoms (NPSs) including psychosis, depression, anxiety, apathy, and behavioral agitation are significant complications

Table 12.4 Cognitive Enhancers: Properties and Uses

AGENT		PROTEIN BINDING	CYP450 ACTIVITY	USUAL DOSE	AVAILABLE FORMULATIONS	OTHER FEATURES	FDA-APPROVED INDICATION
ChEI	Donepezil (Aricept)	96%	CYP 2D6, 3A4 Substrate	5 mg/day for 4–6 weeks, titrate to max. 10 mg/day	5-, 10-mg tab. 5-, 10-mg ODT	Once-daily dosing	Mild to severe AD
	Rivastigmine (Exelon)	40%	None	1.5 mg BID for 2 weeks, titrate by 1.5 mg BID every 2 weeks to max. 6 mg BID (with food)	1.5-, 3-, 4.5-, 6-mg tab. 2-mg/mL sol. 4.6-, 9.5-mg/24 hours patch	Metabolized by cholinesterases Inhibits butyryl cholinesterase	Mild to moderate AD Mild to moderate dementia in PD
	Galantamine (Razadyne)	18%	CYP 2D6, 3A4 substrate	4 mg PO BID for 4 weeks, titrate by 4 mg BID every 4 weeks to max. 12 mg BID	4-, 8-, 12-mg tab. 4-mg/mL sol. 8-, 16-, 24-mg ER tab. (once daily)	Nicotinic cholinergic receptor modulation	Mild to moderate AD
NMDA receptor antagonist	Memantine (Namenda)	45%	None	5 mg/day, titrate by 5 mg/day every week to max. 10 mg BID	5-, 10-mg tab. 2-mg/mL sol.	No hepatic metabolism	Moderate to severe AD

AD, Alzheimer disease; ChEI, cholinesterase inhibitors; ER, extended release; FDA, Food and Drug Administration; NMDA, N-methyl-D-aspartate; ODT, orally disintegrating tablet; PD, Parkinson disease; sol., solution; tab., tablet.

Modified with permission from Kaufer DI, Cummings JL, Ketchel P, et al. Validation of the NPI-Q, a brief clinical form of the Neuropsychiatric Inventory. *J Neuropsychiatry Clin Neurosci.* 2000;12:233–239.

of dementia that afflict about 90% of AD patients (15). Untreated NPSs may lead to excess disability, elevated caregiver burden, risk of harm to the patient or others, elder mistreatment, increased service utilization, and earlier nursing home referral (12). NPSs may be assessed through the Neuropsychiatric Inventory (NPI), a caregiver interview that can also be self-administered in a Brief Questionnaire Form (NPI-Q) (16).

A meta-analysis indicated that treatment with ChEIs decreased behavioral symptoms in AD, although the overall effect was modest (17), while a recent study found no significant impact of donepezil on acute agitation (18). Behavioral symptoms should not be the primary rationale for starting cognitive enhancers. Whenever possible, nonpharmacologic approaches should be utilized first. Symptom-specific pharmacologic approaches are discussed in the following paragraphs.

Psychosis The combined prevalence of delusions and hallucinations in AD patients is 40% to 65%. Delusions accounts for 30% to 50% psychosis and hallucinations for 10% to 20% (9). Delusions of theft, infidelity, and misidentification are most common in the midstages of AD (4). Second-generation antipsychotics are often used for the management of psychotic symptoms and behavioral agitation or aggression. However, a significant risk of increased mortality exists with the use of antipsychotics in elderly patients with dementia, due to cardiovascular, cerebrovascular, and infectious (e.g., pneumonia) events (19). These concerns led to "black box" warnings on the second-generation antipsychotics (5). Therefore, it is important to discuss and document the risks and benefits of antipsychotic use with patients and caregivers of patients who have dementia-related psychosis or agitation. Tapering off the medication after 3 to 4 weeks in nonresponders and periodic attempts (e.g., every several months) to taper and stop antipsychotics in responders may help to minimize adverse effects. In all situations where psychosis suddenly ensues and represents an acute change from baseline, delirium should be high on the differential. Urinary tract infections, dental abscess, and pneumonia are commonly encountered causes of delirium in this patient population.

Depression About 25% of patients with AD may experience major depression, although depressive symptoms may be present in up to 87% of individuals (4). Family or personal history of mood disorders, female gender, preserved insight, and concurrent chronic pain are risk factors for depression in dementia. Diagnosis can be challenging because depression in the context of concurrent dementia has a different natural history and presentation than even geriatric depression without dementia (20).

Depression is also a hallmark of subcortical dementias. In PD, 10% of patients meet criteria for major depressive disorder, while up to 50% have depressive symptoms (21). Most patients with PD and depression also have an anxiety disorder. In Huntington disease, 40% of patients exhibit either depression or mania.

CHAPTER 12 Dementias

Agitation Behavioral agitation is a common distressing symptom that often requires medication management. However, psychosocial interventions should be explored and implemented first. Second-generation antipsychotics is one treatment option, although caution is advised, given the FDA black-box warning discussed above. Mood stabilizers such as divalproex, carbamazepine, and oxcarbazepine may be used as monotherapy or in conjunction with antipsychotics (5). The off-label use of buspirone is sometimes successful in managing anxiety-related agitation (9). For aberrant and purposeless motor behavior in FTLD, SSRIs are the first-line agents used to target serotonergic deficits (13).

Long-term use of benzodiazepines in older demented patients should be avoided, and these potentially harmful medications should be reserved for sedation prior to procedures, such as a tooth extraction or a diagnostic study. Intermediate-duration agents that do not undergo oxidative metabolism and have no active metabolites (e.g., lorazepam or oxazepam) are preferred when absolutely necessary (5).

Apathy Apathy is present in 27% of patients with dementia and may respond to the activating effects of cognitive enhancers or antidepressants with noradrenergic or dopaminergic receptor agonist activity (e.g., sertraline, bupropion, venlafaxine, duloxetine, or desipramine) (12). Profound apathy in patients with medical comorbidity may require the use of psychostimulants, provided there are no cardiovascular contraindications. The use of modafinil, methylphenidate, or dextroamphetamine may be considered (5, 9). Another option is use of anti parkinsonian medications, such as amantadine, L-dopa, pramipexole, or ropinirole.

PSYCHOSOCIAL TREATMENT

Cognitive rehabilitation, memory training, and engagement in pleasurable activities (e.g., crossword or jigsaw puzzles, playing chess or a musical instrument, painting, writing, and conversing in nonnative languages) as long as possible should be strongly encouraged, especially in patients with mild cognitive deficits. Individual or group psychotherapy may be helpful in MCI or early dementia stages. In particular, the use of *problem-solving therapy* in the primary care setting has been proven to help elderly, depressed patients with executive dysfunction (22).

Easy-to-use behavioral plans can be employed with resultant reductions in medication use and maladaptive behavior. Common interventions include sensory stimulation (e.g., sunlight, music), recreational activities, and social interaction (23). The ABC behavioral model assumes that a connection between antecedents (A), maladaptive behaviors (B), and consequences (C) has been learned and will need to be unlearned (23). Modification of reinforcement contingencies may change the behavior. A step-by-step behavioral approach is presented below.

Step 1: **Define the problem** by determining what, where, when, why, and how the behavior manifested. The caregivers are asked to give a detailed description of the behavior, including the context in which it arises, its frequency, and any factors known to trigger, exacerbate, or mitigate it.

WHEN TO REFER

- Diagnostic uncertainty
- Significant comorbid depression
- Safety concerns (inability to care for self, elder abuse, suicidal ideation)
- Behavioral manifestations become difficult to treat
- Significant family caregiver burden

Step 2: **Focus on antecedent control** by identifying unmet needs that the patient attempts to communicate through the behavioral problem. Medical illness, pain, sensory deprivation, and cognitive deterioration, along with psychological comorbidities, may be factors underlying the unwanted behaviors.

Step 3: **Evaluate reinforcers of maladaptive behavior.** Many problem behaviors are reinforced by staff or caregivers, who provide attention when the particular behavior is displayed and withdraw attention when the patient behaves well. Therefore, the patient displays maladaptive behaviors in order to seek attention.

Step 4: **Develop a behavioral plan.** Maximizing the sense of control by giving choices, verbalizing intended physical contact prior to touching the patient, utilizing frequent cues and reminders, giving simple one-step instructions repeatedly and slowly, praising efforts, and selectively redirecting and distracting are strategies that help positively reinforce desired behaviors and extinguish the undesirable ones. Family caregiver and staff education is important so consistent reinforcement can be ensured.

CARING FOR CAREGIVERS

More than 70% of all dementia patients are cared for at home by family members, mostly spouses, of whom approximately two thirds are women (24). Between 40% and 70% of caregivers have clinically significant symptoms of depression, with 25% to 50% meeting criteria for major depressive disorder. Caregiver depression and anxiety may worsen after the placement of the patient in a nursing home. Assessing the physical and mental health of the caregiver is an essential component of providing care for dementia patients. The Zarit Burden Interview (ZBI) is a self-rated 22-item scale that can be used in the office to measure the caregivers' burden (25). Educational programs and family counseling can reduce caregiver burden. Respite care, telephone help lines, and computer chat rooms may be of benefit as well.

Practice Pointers

Case 1: Is it depression or early dementia?

A 70-year-old man of Middle Eastern descent with limited English skills presents to the geriatric clinic complaining of memory loss for the past 3 months. He has become easily distracted, forgets important dates and recent events, and was in a minor car accident 2 weeks ago. He is brought in by his daughter who readily gives the history, rushes to answer the interviewer's questions before the patient, and translates the MMSE while at the same time giving clues as to the correct answers. Medical history includes hypertension and diabetes, both controlled, and no previous history of depression or family history of dementia are noted. The patient appears disinterested in the interview, makes poor eye contact, maintains a blunted affect although is easily irritated, and gives quite a few "I don't know" answers.

Discussion: *The 70-year-old man presenting with forgetfulness scores 18/30 on the MMSE, showing impairments in multiple domains. A more detailed cognitive exam is precluded by the patient's limited cooperation and English skills. Based on the poor effort on interview, irritable and depressed mood, blunted affect, and nonspecific findings on the MMSE, a working diagnosis of depression is made, although cognitive impairment cannot be ruled out. The language barrier makes the MMSE less reliable in this case. Preliminary work-up is negative for any reversible contributors and the patient is started on escitalopram 10 mg/day. At 4-week follow-up, the patient presents with a brighter affect and volunteers more information, including the fact that his oldest son was divorced 3 months prior, and the shame and hurt he is feeling due to this. His repeat MMSE score is 24/30.*

In this case, the therapeutic antidepressant trial was helpful in establishing the presence of a depressive episode in the context of a major family stressor. At this point the clinician still needs to keep in mind the possibility of an early dementia syndrome. Following up in another 4 to 6 weeks to ensure a solid response to antidepressants and repeating the brief cognitive assessment in the office, with referral to a geriatric psychiatrist or neuropsychological testing if still in doubt, are indicated. If the patient is amenable, family or individual therapy will ameliorate the situation, given the recent stressor. Family can be an important ally in the identification and treatment of geriatric depression.

Case 2: Is this typical dementia?

A 75-year-old retired U.S. Navy officer is brought in by his 50-year-old wife, who bitterly complains about his lack of initiative. The patient has an unremarkable medical history and his neurologic exam is normal and his MMSE is 30/30. Additional testing reveals that he can generate 24 animals per minute in a test of verbal fluency but he can only name six words beginning with the letter F in 1 minute (normal range for his age is 18 $\pm$ 6). During the interview, his wife is overbearing, cutting off the patient's responses and answering the questions herself. The patient denies depressed mood and anhedonia but admits that his wife is very "difficult" and that his children no longer visit him since his marriage to her 6 years ago.

Past medical history includes hyperlipidemia and diabetes, with most recent glycohemoglobin of 12.3. He currently takes metformin and lovastatin. A brain MRI reveals white matter hyperintensities, consistent with vascular disease.

Discussion: *The 75-year-old retired executive's presentation poses a diagnostic challenge. Is his apathy part of a dementia or depression picture? Apathy can be a presenting symptom of dementias, especially those involving the frontal lobes. Onset of FTD is usually before age 65, making it less likely in this patient. As discussed, a MMSE score of 30/30 does not preclude a dementia diagnosis. Lower performance on the test of F-word generation can indicate frontal-subcortical impairment, due to retrieval deficits. In the presence of cerebrovascular risk factors, such as diabetes and hyperlipidemia, microvascular changes leading to frontal-subcortical deficits are very likely. Treatment will involve first addressing the medical factors, including adequate control of diabetes. Serial MMSE will help monitor progression of cognitive impairment. If memory changes become prominent, or the MMSE score drops below 24, consider a ChEI.*

Although he is denying depressed mood and diminished interest in pleasurable activities, he should be monitored for depression on a regular basis. The stress related to his family and recent retirement may have a negative impact on the management of his diabetes, dyslipidemia, and cognitive status. In this case, he would likely benefit from a referral for short-term psychotherapy and family therapy.

ICD9

Cognitive Disorder Not Otherwise Specified (NOS)	*294.9*
Delirium Due To [General Medical Condition]	*293.0*
Delirium NOS	*780.09*
Dementia Classified Elsewhere (Axis I) for Axis III conditions below:	*290.10*
Dementia of Alzheimer Type (Axis III)	*331.10*
Dementia with Lewy Bodies (Axis III)	*331.82*
Frontotemporal Dementia (Axis III)	*331.19*
Huntington Disease (Axis III)	*333.40*
Vascular Dementia (Axis III)	*290.40*
Dementia Due to Alcohol	*291.2*
Dementia NOS	*294.80*

Practical Resources

Alzheimer's Association: www.alz.org; 1-800-272-3900
Alzheimer's Disease Education and Referral Center: www.nia.nih.gov/Alzheimers
Family Caregiver Alliance: www.caregiver.org; 1-800-445-8106
National Family Caregivers Association: www.thefamilycaregiver.org

Acknowledgment

The authors thank Jeff Kixmiller, PhD, for his assistance.

References

1. Spar JE, La Rue A. Introduction; mood disorders. In: *Clinical Manual of Geriatric Psychiatry*. Washington, DC: American Psychiatric Publishing; 2006:1–19, 67–172.

2. Plassman BL, Langa KM, Fisher GG, et al. Prevalence of dementia in the United States: The Aging, Demographics, and Memory Study. *Neuroepidemiology*. 2007;29:125–132.

3. Hinton L, Franz CE, Reddy G, et al. Practice constraints, behavioral problems, and dementia care: primary care physicians' perspectives. *J Gen Intern Med*. 2007;22:1487–1492.

4. Mendez MF, Cummings JL. Diagnosis of dementia; Alzheimer's disease. In: *Dementia: A Clinical Approach*. Philadelphia: Butterworth Heinemann; 2003:8; 41–119.

5. American Psychiatric Association. Practice guideline for the treatment of patients with Alzheimer's disease and other dementias, second edition. *Am J Psychiatry*. 2007;164:S25–34.

6. Luck T, Riedel-Heller SG, Kaduszkiewicz H, et al. Mild cognitive impairment in general practice: age-specific prevalence and correlate results from the German study on ageing, cognition and dementia in primary care patients. *Dement Geriatric Cogn Disord*. 2007;24:307–316.

7. Petersen RC, Thomas RG, Grundman M, et al. Vitamin E and donepezil for the treatment of mild cognitive impairment. *N Engl J Med*. 2005;352:2379–2388.

8. Teng E, Lu PH, Cummings JL. Neuropsychiatric symptoms are associated with progression from mild cognitive impairment to Alzheimer's disease. *Dement Geriatric Cogn Disord*. 2007;24:253–259.

9. Cummings JL. Dementia with Lewy bodies; management of neuropsychiatric aspects of dementia. In: *The Neuropsychiatry of Alzheimer's Disease and Related Dementias*. London: Martin Dunitz; 2003:117–132; 281–300.

10. Taylor WD, Doraiswamy PM. Use of the laboratory in the diagnostic workup of older adults. In: *Textbook of Geriatric Psychiatry*. Washington, DC: American Psychiatric Publishing; 2004:179–188.

11. Seritan AL. Prevent drug-drug interactions with cholinesterase inhibitors. *Curr Psychiatry*. 2008;7:57–67.

12. Lyketsos CG, Steinberg M, Tschanz JT, et al. Mental and behavioral disturbances in dementia: findings from the Cache County study on memory in aging. *Am J Psychiatry*. 2000;175:708–714.

13. Woolley JD, Wilson MR, Hung E, et al. Frontotemporal dementia and mania. *Am J Psychiatry*. 2007;164:1811–1816.

14. Marangell LB, Martinez JM, Silver JM, et al. Drug interactions; cholinesterase inhibitors. In: *Concise guide to psychopharmacology*. Washington, DC: American Psychiatric Publishing; 2002:4–9; 171–180.

15. Lyketsos CG, DelCampo L, Steinberg M, et al. Treating depression in Alzheimer's disease. Efficacy and safety of sertraline therapy, and the benefits of depression reduction: the DIADS. *Arch Gen Psychiatry*. 2003;60:737–746.

16. Kaufer DI, Cummings JL, Ketchel P, et al. Validation of the NPI-Q, a brief clinical form of the Neuropsychiatric Inventory. *J Neuropsychiatry Clin Neurosci*. 2000;12:233–239.

17. Trinh NH, Hoblyn J, Mohanty S, et al. Efficacy of cholinesterase inhibitors in the treatment of neuropsychiatric symptoms and functional impairment in Alzheimer's disease: a meta-analysis. *JAMA*. 2003;289:210–216.

18. Howard RJ, Juszczak E, Ballard CG, et al. Donepezil for the treatment of agitation in Alzheimer's disease. *N Engl J Med*. 2007;357:1382–1392.

19. Schneider LS, Dagerman K, Insel PS. Efficacy and adverse effects of atypical antipsychotics for dementia: meta-analysis of randomized, placebo-controlled trials. *Am J Geriatr Psychiatry*. 2006;14:191–210.

20. Lyketsos CG, Lee HB. Diagnosis and treatment of depression in Alzheimer's disease. A practical update for the clinician. *Dement Geriatr Cogn Disord*. 2004;17:55–64.

21. Weintraub D, Stern MB. Psychiatric complications in Parkinson disease. *Am J Geri Psychiatry*. 2005;13:844–851.

22. Alexopoulos GS, Raue P, Arean P. Problem-solving therapy versus supportive therapy in geriatric major depression with executive dysfunction. *Am J Geriatr Psychiatry.* 2003;11:46–52.

23. Cohen-Mansfield J. Nonpharmacologic interventions for inappropriate behaviors in dementia: a review, summary, and critique. *Am J Geriatr Psychiatry.* 2001;9:361–381.

24. Gallicchio L, Siddiqi N, Langenberg P, et al. Gender differences in burden and depression among informal caregivers of demented elders in the community. *Int J Geriatr Psychiatry.* 2002;17:154–163.

25. Zarit SH, Reever KE, Bach-Peterson J. Relatives of the impaired elderly: correlates of feelings of burden. *Gerontologist.* 1980;20:649–655.

13 Sleep Disorders

Julie S. Young, MD, MS • Kimberly A. Hardin, MD, MS, FAASM

> *A 48-year-old man who has been sober for 6 weeks comes to the ambulatory care clinic saying he hasn't "slept a wink" since entering a residential treatment program 4 weeks ago. He stopped drinking alcohol "cold turkey" after his wife of 20 years and two daughters left him due to the patient's refusal to quit drinking. For the past 20 years, he has drank up to one 12 pack of beer nightly and could not fall asleep unless he drank at least two beers before bedtime.*

CLINICAL HIGHLIGHTS

- Insomnia affects more than 30% of the general population.

- Insomnia may present as a symptom of an underlying psychiatric, medical, or substance- or medication-related condition.

- Evaluation of a sleep complaint should include a complete assessment of general medical, psychiatric, and substance misuse–related symptoms. Inquires about sleep hygiene as well as current prescribed and over-the-counter medications should also be initiated.

- The treatment of primary insomnia is multifactorial and should include a stepwise approach that addresses sleep hygiene and environmental

(Continued)

Clinical Significance

Many sleep disorders can adversely affect patient health. Insomnia is widely prevalent and the most commonly encountered sleep disorder in the primary care setting. Although the focus of this chapter is on insomnia, other sleep disorders such as obstructive sleep apnea-hypoapnea (OSAH) and restless leg syndrome (RLS) will be discussed within the context of exploring a differential diagnosis for insomnia.

Insomnia affects greater than 30% of adults in the United States (1, 2). Patient surveys have found that primary care patients with insomnia have 60% higher overall health care costs than those without insomnia. The annual indirect and direct economic burden of insomnia in the U.S. has been estimated to be about $100 billion (3).

Prolonged periods of disrupted sleep can lead to sleep deprivation, or a chronic lack of restorative sleep, which has numerous physical and psychological consequences. Chronic sleep deprivation is associated with hypertension, increased sympathetic cardiovascular activation, blunted hypothalamic-pituitary-adrenal axis function, impaired host defenses, and altered cognitive functioning (4). Inadequate sleep also increases the risk of developing anxiety and mood disorders. Patients with alcohol dependence in remission and comorbid chronic insomnia have a heightened risk of relapse. In sum, insomnia is independently associated with poor health-related quality of life (5).

Diagnosis

Insomnia can lead to cognitive, emotional, and motor dysfunction. The severity of insomnia is determined by the extent to which the sleep problem affects daytime function and is classified as mild, moderate, or

CLINICAL HIGHLIGHTS
(*Continued*)

factors before considering prescription sleep medications.

- Women may have more pronounced sleep disturbance and require additional treatment related to hormonal status.

- Benzodiazepines and anticholinergic agents should be used cautiously in elderly patients.

severe. *Mild insomnia* does not cause daytime dysfunction; *moderate insomnia* usually causes some daytime dysfunction; and *severe insomnia* results in obvious global impairment in daytime functioning. Insomnia is also described by length of symptoms (acute insomnia lasts <3 months, subacute insomnia is present for 3–6 months, and chronic insomnia persists for 6 or more months).

Consequences of impaired cognition include inattentiveness, distractibility, and carelessness. Healthy individuals become prone to mood lability, irritability, decreased frustration tolerance, depressed mood, and anxiety. Motor dysfunction can range from a clinically insignificant decline in fine motor control to an inability to safely operate a motor vehicle.

Despite its impact on overall health and well-being, sleep is often not addressed during routine health visits. Primary care providers do not usually screen for sleep-related problems and patients do not normally bring up the topic unless symptoms are severe. Sleep should be a routine part of the review of systems for all patients who complain of nonspecific symptoms such as fatigue, lethargy, worsening cognitive status, anxiety, or changes in mood. Before pursuing less common paths of diagnostic inquiry, ask about sleep *early* in the interview. Not realizing the significance of sleep to their overall health, patients with even extremely poor sleep may complain about everything *but* sleep, leading you to unnecessary questioning about multiple somatic disorders before you get to the real culprit, disrupted sleep.

A sleep disorder may be diagnosed by using one of four classification systems, each of which includes varying levels of diagnostic precision. The most detailed classifications are the *International Classification of Sleep Disorders* (ICSD-2) and the *Diagnostic Classification of Sleep and Arousal Disorders* (DCSAD), both of which are primarily used by sleep specialists (6, 7). The World Health Organization's *International Classification of Diseases* (ICD-10) (8) includes a more restricted list of specific sleep disorders, but is commonly used in clinical medicine for billing purposes. Although commonly used by psychiatrists, the criteria in the *Diagnostic and Statistical Manual of Mental Disorders,* 4th edition, text revision (DSM-IV-TR) are rarely used by sleep specialists and sleep researchers due to the broad acceptance of existing nosology in the field of sleep medicine, and more importantly, due to its relatively limited scope. ICSD-2 criteria will be used in this chapter (Table 13.1).

Differential Diagnosis

The ICSD-2 lists 10 types of insomnias. These insomnias vary by etiology and require the persistence of difficulty *initiating* or *maintaining* sleep and at least one of nine symptoms of daytime impairment such as fatigue, impaired concentration, or mood irritability. The insomnias can be divided into extrinsic and intrinsic insomnias (Table 13.2). Extrinsic insomnias are due to factors that are external to the patient, while intrinsic insomnias are due to factors that are inherent to the patient.

Table 13.1 General Criteria for the Diagnosis of Insomnia

1. Difficulty initiating or maintaining sleep, awakening too early, nonrestorative or poor quality of sleep
2. Sleep difficulty occurs despite adequate opportunity and circumstances for sleep
3. At least one of the following forms of daytime impairment related to the nighttime sleep difficulty occurs:
   - Fatigue or malaise
   - Attention, concentration, or memory impairment
   - Social or vocational dysfunction or poor school performance
   - Mood disturbance or irritability
   - Daytime somnolence
   - Motivation, energy, or initiative reduction
   - Prone to errors or accidents at work or while operating a car or other machinery
   - Muscle tension, headaches, or gastrointestinal symptoms
   - Preoccupation with sleep or lack of sleep

Adapted from American Sleep Disorders Association, Diagnostic Classification Steering Committee. *International Classification of Sleep Disorders: Diagnostic and Coding Manual.* Westchester, IL: American Academy of Sleep Medicine; 2005.

EXTRINSIC INSOMNIAS

Adjustment Insomnia

In a 1-year period, approximately 15% to 20% of the adult population experience *adjustment insomnia*, or *acute insomnia*, which lasts less than 3 months. The diagnosis of adjustment insomnia requires the presence of an identifiable stressor, which may be psychological (e.g., death of a loved one), interpersonal (e.g., divorce), or environmental (e.g., moving to a new home). Adjustment insomnia usually resolves after the resolution of or adjustment to a stressor. A brief course of a sedative-hypnotic medication coupled with a referral for supportive psychotherapy may be an effective treatment approach.

Inadequate Sleep Hygiene

Sleep hygiene refers to behaviors and activities that promote sleep and discourage wakefulness. The diagnostic criteria for *inadequate sleep hygiene*, a type of insomnia, includes meeting the criteria for insomnia as listed in Table 13.1 for at least 1 month and the presence of at least one of the following: (1) sleep schedule that consists of frequent daytime

Table 13.2 Types of Insomnias

EXTRINSIC INSOMNIAS	INTRINSIC INSOMNIAS
Adjustment sleep disorder[a]	Insomnia due to a mental disorder[a]
Inadequate sleep hygiene	Psychophysiologic insomnia[a]
Insomnia due to a medical condition	Insomnia associated with obstructive sleep apnea
Circadian rhythm sleep disorder ("jet lag")	Insomnia associated with restless leg syndrome
Insomnia due to medications and other substances (alcohol, nicotine, cocaine, methamphetamines)	Insomnia associated with periodic limb movement disorder

[a] The three most common types of insomnias.

From American Sleep Disorders Association, Diagnostic Classification Steering Committee. *International Classification of Sleep Disorders: Diagnostic and Coding Manual.* Westchester, IL: American Academy of Sleep Medicine; 2005.

naps, highly variable bedtimes or rising times, or excess time spent in bed; (2) routine use of alcohol, nicotine, or caffeine, especially preceding bedtime; (3) engaging in mentally stimulating, physically activating, or emotionally upsetting activities close to bedtime; (4) frequent use of bed for activities other than sleep (e.g., watching television); and (5) lack of a comfortable sleeping environment (e.g., too noisy).

Insomnia Due to a Medical Condition

Medical illnesses associated with insomnia are numerous and include common chronic medical disorders (e.g., diabetes or heart failure) to other more reversible systemic conditions (e.g., anemia or a thyroid disorder). Neurologic conditions like dementia, seizures, or stroke make up another major category. Poststroke patients have an increased risk of developing OSAH during the first several months after the stroke. In addition to insomnia, poststroke patients have an increased risk of developing *hypersomnia,* which is associated with prolonged sleep episodes or daytime sleepiness. Parkinson disease and Alzheimer disease are associated with sleep disturbances such as *rapid eye movement (REM) sleep behavior disorder* (RBD), which is characterized by intermittent episodes of elaborate motor activity where dreams may be acted out during REM sleep.

Insomnia Due to Medications and Substances

Multiple drugs can alter sleep quantity and quality. Sedatives and opioids may initially help with sleep onset, but impair sleep architecture and ultimately lead to insomnia. Sedative-hypnotics themselves can disrupt sleep by causing rebound insomnia during withdrawal. Withdrawal from or intoxication with alcohol, marijuana, or other illicit drugs can also cause abnormal sleep patterns. Sleep disturbances may persist for up to 1 to 2 years after ceasing substance use. Table 13.3 lists common medications associated with insomnia.

INTRINSIC INSOMNIAS

Insomnia Due to a Mental Disorder

Insomnia due to a mental disorder is the most common type of insomnia encountered in sleep centers. Several mood, anxiety, psychotic, and neurodevelopmental disorders are associated with sleep problems, and include insomnia as a feature of the disorder. While the many symptoms of psychiatric disorders often vary, sleep disturbance is a common complaint that is more likely to be reported to providers. Table 13.4 lists sleep characteristics among patients with various psychiatric conditions.

Psychophysiologic Insomnia

Psychophysiologic insomnia is characterized by psychological and physiologic hyperarousal at bedtime and occurs in 1% to 2% of the population. Individuals with psychophysiologic insomnia, also known as *learned* or *conditioned insomnia,* are preoccupied with sleep, and often require a combination of behavioral and pharmacologic therapies. The

Table 13.3 Medications Known to Cause Insomnia

CLASS	MEDICATION
Antiepileptics	Lamotrigine
Antidepressants	Bupropion
	Fluoxetine
	Venlafaxine
	Phenelzine
	Protriptyline
Beta-blockers	Propranolol
	Pindolol
	Metoprolol
Bronchodilators	Theophylline
Decongestants	Pseudoephedrine
	Phenylpropanolamine
Steroids	Prednisone
Stimulants	Dextroamphetamine
	Methamphetamine
	Methylphenidate
	Modafinil
	Pemoline

diagnostic criteria for psychophysiologic insomnia include meeting the criteria for insomnia in Table 13.1 for at least 1 month. The patient must also have evidence of conditioned sleep difficulties or hyperarousal at bedtime such as (1) preoccupation and anxiety about sleep; (2) difficulty falling asleep in bed at the desired time, but no difficulty falling asleep during monotonous activities when not intended; (3) sleeping better when away from home; (4) mental arousal characterized by intrusive thoughts; and (5) heightened somatic tension in bed reflected by a perceived inability to relax the body sufficiently to allow the onset of sleep.

Psychophysiologic insomnia differs from adjustment insomnia in its longer duration and lack of a current identifiable stressor. While attempting to fall asleep, those with psychophysiologic insomnia worry excessively about sleep, in contrast to those with generalized anxiety disorder, who tend to ruminate about multiple life stressors. Patients with psychophysiologic insomnia often report improved sleep when varying their bedtime routine or when sleeping in an unfamiliar environment. Those with psychophysiologic insomnia may complain of an inability to "stop thinking" or of "racing thoughts." This is in contrast to thought patterns seen in a manic episode, when thoughts are sped up and difficult to track (flight of ideas), are extremely rapid (racing thoughts), and may include grandiose themes. A patient with mania will not likely complain of daytime fatigue due to sleeplessness.

Table 13.4　Characteristics of Sleep in Various Psychiatric Diagnoses

DSM-IV-TR DIAGNOSIS	COMMON SLEEP COMPLAINTS AND SYMPTOMS
Major depressive disorder	• Difficulty falling asleep (early insomnia) • Frequent awakenings (middle insomnia) • Uncharacteristic early-morning awakening (terminal insomnia) • Hypersomnia ("I sleep all day long so I don't have to face my depression")
Manic episode	• Decreased need for sleep lasting days or weeks • Lack of fatigue despite lack of sleep • Extra work accomplished during usual sleep times ("I stayed up all night and cleaned the whole house")
Posttraumatic stress disorder	• Difficulty falling asleep, which is often associated with anxiety about being abused or traumatized • Physiologic hyperarousal • Very light sleep, with exquisite sensitivity to sounds and other stimuli • Hyperstartled response if awakened by external stimuli • Frequent awakenings • Nightmares
Generalized anxiety disorder	• Prone to *psychophysiologic insomnia* • Difficulty falling asleep due to preoccupation and excessive worry about several stressors
Psychotic disorders	• Hallucinations (e.g., "The voices laugh and scream at me at night, so I can't sleep") • Paranoid thoughts
Attention deficit hyperactivity disorder	• Difficulty falling asleep due to physical hyperactivity • Activating effects of stimulants

DSM-IV-TR, *Diagnostic and Statistical Manual of Mental Disorders,* 4th edition, text revision.

Insomnias Associated with Other Primary Sleep Disorders

OSAH, RLS, and periodic limb movement disorder (PLMD) often initially present as insomnia in the primary care clinic. Table 13.5 includes a summary of the predisposing factors, main clinical features, and treatment options for these conditions.

Subacute and Chronic Insomnia

An estimated 10% of the U.S. population has chronic (>6 months) insomnia. Risk factors for chronic insomnia include the presence of any of the insomnia disorders described above, especially if inadequately treated; female gender; older age (>60 years old); and a familial predisposition to sleep disorders.

PATIENT ASSESSMENT

Evaluation of a sleep complaint includes a focused sleep history, a general physical exam, and pertinent laboratory work. Clarify the sleep complaint by asking about the duration, frequency, and severity of the problem. The following questions might be helpful when considering a sleep disorder:

• When did the problem start?
• How many days a week do you have this problem?

NOT TO BE MISSED

• Recent psychosocial stressors
• Mood disorders (depression and mania)
• Anxiety disorders
• Psychotic disorders
• Medication- and substance-induced insomnias
• Symptoms of inadequately treated general medical conditions (diabetes, thyroid disorders, COPD)
• Primary sleep disorders (OSAH, RLS, and PLMD)

Table 13.5 Predisposing Factors, Clinical Features, and Treatment of Common Primary Sleep Disorders

SLEEP DISORDER	PREDISPOSING FACTORS	CLINICAL FEATURES	TREATMENT
Obstructive sleep apnea-hypoapnea (OSAH)	Nasopharyngeal abnormalities, craniofacial abnormalities, obesity, >40 years old, men > women (2:1), neurologic disorder (e.g., recent stroke)	Repetitive episodes of upper airway obstruction that occur during sleep, usually associated with oxygen desaturation. Episodes include loud snoring or gasps that last 20–30 seconds. Associated with morning headaches and increased daytime sedation	• Nasal continuous positive airway pressure (CPAP) • Behavioral therapies: avoid alcohol, tobacco, and sedative-hypnotics at night; weight loss if overweight; sleep on side, not back • Dental appliances: reposition lower jaw and tongue • Surgical interventions: resection of tonsils, uvula, or part of soft palate
Periodic limb movement disorder (PLMD)	OSAH, restless leg syndrome, narcolepsy, increased age, chronic uremia, TCAs or MAOIs, withdrawal from sedating agents, incidence same in men and women	Periodic episodes of repetitive and stereotyped limb movements during non-REM sleep: extension of the big toe with partial flexion of the ankles, knees, or hips. Muscle contractions last 0.5–5 seconds, with 20- to 40-second interepisode intervals	• Treat underlying problem. • Improve sleep hygiene. • Relaxation therapy • Consider carbidopa, levodopa, pramipexole, FDA-approved sleep agent
Restless leg syndrome (RLS)	Pregnancy (>20 weeks gestation), uremia, iron deficiency anemia, rheumatoid arthritis, renal disease, alcoholism. Peak onset is middle age	Uncomfortable sensations in the legs or arms just prior to sleep onset. Described as "achy," "crawling," "pulling," "prickling," or "tingling." Those who suffer from RLS can have very severe insomnia	• Treat underlying cause • Correct nutritional deficiency (vitamin B_{12}, folic acid, or iron) • Stop or decrease dose of offending medications • Consider: carbidopa or levodopa, pergolide, pramipexole, bromocriptine mesylate, ropinirole

FDA, Food and Drug Administration; MAOIs, monoamine oxidase inhibitors; REM, rapid eye movement; TCAs, tricyclic antidepressants.
From American Sleep Disorders Association, Diagnostic Classification Steering Committee. *International Classification of Sleep Disorders: Diagnostic and Coding Manual*. Westchester, IL: American Academy of Sleep Medicine; 2005.

CHAPTER 13 Sleep Disorders

• What time do you go to bed, and how long does it take to fall asleep?
• Do you wake up during the night?
• What wakes you up?
• How long does it take you to fall back asleep?
• Do you feel rested and refreshed when you awaken?
• Do you take anything to help you to sleep?

After characterizing the sleep complaint, Figure 13.1 can help to systematically rule out and treat common causes of insomnia.

Biopsychosocial Treatment

Treatment of insomnia includes pharmacologic and psychological or behavioral interventions. Since causes of sleep complaints are numerous, treatment starts with an accurate diagnosis and addressing the underlying etiology. First, it is important to identify and address

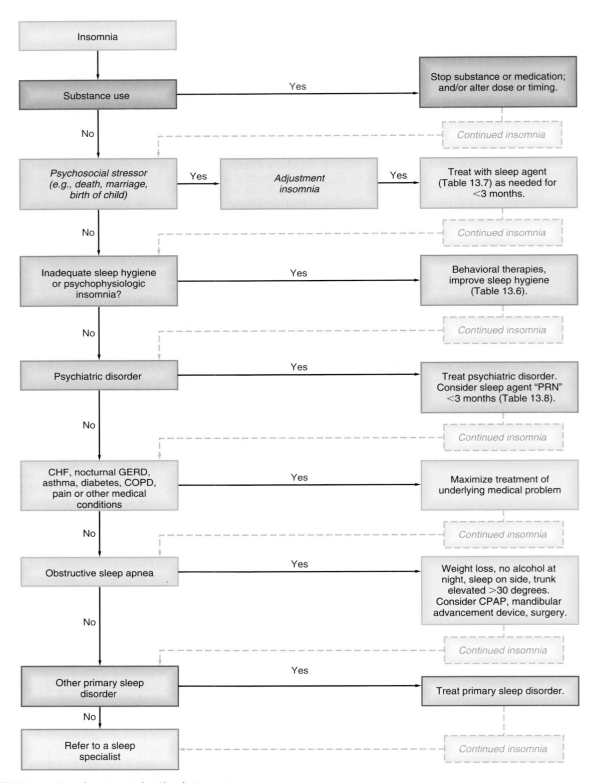

Figure 13.1 Diagnostic and treatment algorithm for insomnia.

modifiable factors such as sleep hygiene, psychosocial stressors, general medical illnesses, and psychiatric disorders prior to starting a sedative-hypnotic agent. Table 13.6 details several biopsychosocial interventions. If the patient has adjustment insomnia or symptoms persist despite addressing acute stressors, the use of a Food and Drug Administration

Table 13.6 Principles and Tips for Good Sleep Hygiene

Sleep diary	• Monitor the amount of sleep during day and night
Regular sleep–wake schedule	• Go to bed at the same time each night • Wake up at same time each morning • Avoid naps during the day
Sleep-promoting nightly ritual	• Plan a relaxing, soothing routine for your last hour of wakefulness (e.g., if the time for "lights out" is 9:45 PM, start winding down by 8:45 PM) • Your last hour could include the following: dimming the lights; screening phone calls for urgent calls; showering, bathing, and doing other usual hygiene routines; changing into your bed clothes; reading relaxing or nonstimulating material; limiting yourself to read only up to your "lights out" time; listening to soothing music or other "white noise"
Avoid stressful or other mentally stimulating activities before bedtime	• Address tomorrow's activities, concerns, or distractions earlier in the day • Unless absolutely necessary, postpone anxiety-provoking conversations that require you to make important decisions, or may cause more conflicts, to a time when you are more alert, rested, and much more likely to make a sound decision
Do not lie in bed "wide awake"	• Trying to will yourself to sleep when you're not sleepy will make you more frustrated, not sleepier • Instead, get out of bed, and engage in mentally and physically nonstimulating activities that will relax, soothe, and, perhaps, even bore you • Do not frequently check the clock
Avoid stimulants, alcohol, and heavy meals at bedtime	• Have your last caffeine- and alcohol-containing food or drink at least 4 hours before you go to bed • Do not smoke within an hour of bedtime, and refrain from smoking if you wake up in the middle of the night • Do not eat a heavy meal within 2 hours of going to bed
Exercise	• Light, aerobic exercise for even 20–30 minutes earlier in the day promotes deep sleep • Avoid exercising within 2 hours of bedtime, since it could actually be activating, and interfere with sleep
Comfortable environment	• Sleep is promoted by darkness, quiet or soothing noises, and a relatively cool temperature (<68°F)

(FDA)-approved sleep aid (or off-label use of sedating medications) may be considered.

PHARMACOTHERAPY

The ideal sleep aid should promote sleep onset and sleep maintenance without next-day side effects such as grogginess, headaches, and fatigue. The FDA has approved three classes of medications for the treatment of insomnia (Table 13.7): benzodiazepine gamma-aminobutyric acid A (GABA$_A$) receptor agonists (BZPs), nonbenzodiazepine GABA$_A$ receptor agonists (non-BZPs), and melatonin receptor agonists. Common BZP side effects include daytime sedation, transient amnesia, cognitive impairment, motor incoordination, dependence, tolerance, and rebound insomnia. In general, BZPs should be limited to healthy patients and used cautiously in the elderly and those with multiple medical problems. Although not FDA approved specifically for insomnia, other medications with sedative properties have been useful in treating some patients with insomnia.

Table 13.7 Food and Drug Administration (FDA)-Approved Drugs for Insomnia

DRUGS	ADULT DOSE (MG)	HALF-LIFE (HOURS)	ONSET (MINUTES)	PEAK EFFECT (HOURS)	MAJOR EFFECTS/CLINICAL COMMENTS
Benzodiazepines (BZPs)					*Caution in elderly patients.* Tolerance to BZPs develops to the sedative, hypnotic, and anticonvulsant effects
Estazolam (ProSom)	1–2	10–24	60	$1/2$–$1\,1/2$	Short-term (7–10 days) treatment for frequent arousals and early-morning awakening. Not as useful for initial insomnia. Avoid in patients with obstructive sleep apnea-hypoapnea. **Caution** in elderly patients and those with liver disease. High doses can cause respiratory depression
Flurazepam (Dalmane)	15–30	47–100	15–20	3–6	Short-term (7–10 days) treatment for middle and terminal insomnia. Increased daytime sedation over time. **Caution** in elderly patients
Temazepam (Restoril)	15–30	6–16		2–3	Short-term (7–10 days) treatment for sleep onset and maintenance. Doses ≥30 mg/day: morning grogginess, nausea, headaches, and vivid dreaming
Nonbenzodiazepines (non-BZPs)					
Eszopiclone (Lunesta)	2–3	6–9	Rapid	1	In elderly start with 1–2 mg. Rapid onset; should be in bed when taking medication. For faster sleep onset, do not ingest with high-fat foods. No tolerance after 6 months
Zaleplon (Sonata)	5–20	1	Rapid	1	Short-term (7–10 days) treatment for initial insomnia
Zolpidem (Ambien, Ambien CR)	5–20	1.4–4.5	30	2–4	Short-term (7–10 days) treatment for initial and middle insomnia (generic form is available). Rapid onset; should be in bed when taking medication. For faster sleep onset, do not ingest with food
Zolpidem CR (Ambien CR)	12.5	1.4–4.5	30	2–4	Short-term (7–10 days) treatment for initial and middle insomnia (generic form is available). Rapid onset; should be in bed when taking medication. For faster sleep onset, do not ingest with food
	6.25–12.5	1.4–4.5	30	2–4	Used for sleep induction and sleep maintenance
Melatonin agonist					
Ramelton (Rozerem)	8	1–2	30	1–$1\,1/2$	Used for initial and middle insomnia. For faster sleep onset, do not ingest with high-fat foods. No tolerance or potential for addiction. **Contraindicated** with fluvoxamine. Should not be used concurrently with melatonin

All sedative-hypnotics should be used with caution and at a lower starting dose when given to the elderly. All sedative-hypnotics should be taken only if the patient plans to go to bed immediately after taking the medication.

Non-BZPs may have a decreased side effect profile when compared to BZPs. Non-BZPs include eszopiclone, zaleplon, zolpidem, and zolpidem extended release. The melatonin receptor agonist ramelteon (Rozerem) also reduces time to fall asleep without next-day psychomotor and memory effects (7). Ramelteon (and melatonin) is associated with less concern for dependence, perhaps due to its less immediate effects on sleep. Limited data exist on the efficacy of non–FDA-approved medications for insomnia such as antidepressants, second-generation antipsychotics, and antihistamines. Table 13.8 summarizes sedating medications that may be useful for patients with insomnia, although selection should be based on the underlying psychiatric conditions. Of the FDA-approved medications, only eszopiclone and zolpidem CR have been approved for use without a specified time limit. The other medications have approved use limited to 35 days or less. Finally, most of the FDA-approved medications for insomnia also carry an FDA black-box warning for complex sleep-related behaviors, which may include sleep driving, making phone calls, and preparing and eating food while asleep. Although dangerous outcomes from these behaviors are rare, primary care practitioners should discuss and document the potential for these behaviors with patients who suffer from insomnia.

PSYCHOSOCIAL TREATMENT

Since pharmacotherapy is not intended for long-term use, nonpharmacologic interventions should be considered before or concurrently with sedative-hypnotic medications. Primary care patients who have insomnia often take sedative-hypnotic agents well beyond the recommended time frame. Discontinuing these medications can lead to increased anxiety and irritability as well as rebound insomnia. The inclusion of a psychosocial treatment approach for insomnia is safe and can be used indefinitely.

Sleep Hygiene Education

Extrinsic factors often cause, worsen, or perpetuate poor sleep. Therefore, it is important to educate patients about the impact of lifestyle and behavioral factors on sleep, and to give specific suggestions to improve sleep hygiene (Table 13.6).

Sleep Restriction

This therapy is based on the premise that those with insomnia can increase their sleep time and sleep efficiency by inducing temporary sleep deprivation through voluntarily reducing their time in bed. For example, people who try to sleep at night and suffer from insomnia should be encouraged to restrict daytime or early evening naps.

Stimulus Control

Stimulus control may be helpful when insomnia is caused by a "bedtime environment" that is conducive to staying *awake* rather than sleeping. A patient's report that he can "never" sleep in his own bed, but sleeps very well in unfamiliar environments, is a clue that he has developed a maladaptive response to his sleep environment. This is a common phenomenon

Table 13.8 Drugs Commonly Used "Off-Label" for Insomnia

DRUG	PERTINENT SIDE EFFECTS	COMMENTS
Antidepressants		
Mirtazapine (Remeron)	Somnolence and increased appetite	May be beneficial if patient has comorbid depression and insomnia. Mirtazapine's sedating effect is inversely dose dependent. As the dose increases, the noradrenergic activity counteracts the sleep-inducing H_1 antihistaminic effect of mirtazapine
Trazodone (Desyrel)	Residual daytime sedation, headache, orthostatic hypotension, priapism, cardiac arrhythmias	One of the most commonly prescribed agents for the treatment of insomnia. May be beneficial if patient has comorbid depression and insomnia. May be an acceptable alternative for patients for whom BzRAs are contraindicated (severe hypercapnea or hypoxemia, or history of substance abuse or dependence). Usually dosed much lower (50–100 mg) than when used for depression
TCAs	Delirium, decreased cognition and seizure threshold, orthostatic hypotension, tachycardia, ECG abnormalities	**Avoid** in hospitalized patients due to their anticholinergic, antihistaminic, and cardiovascular side effects. Not recommended as a treatment for insomnia or other sleep problems unless comorbid depression is present. As with other antidepressants, TCAs are usually used at significantly lower doses than for depression
Antihistamines		
Diphenhydramine (Benadryl)	Residual daytime sedation, weight gain, delirium, orthostatic hypotension, blurred vision, urinary retention	Antihistamines are one of the most commonly used over-the-counter agents for chronic insomnia. If possible, avoid in patients >60 years old
Hydroxyzine (Vistaril)	Residual daytime sedation, weight gain, delirium, orthostatic hypotension, blurred vision, urinary retention	Efficacy as an anxiolytic has been not established. Not FDA approved for insomnia. **Avoid** in patients >60 years old and those with closed-angle glaucoma, prostatic hypertrophy, severe asthma, and COPD
Antipsychotics		
Quetiapine (Seroquel)	Sedation, orthostatic hypotension, metabolic derangements (e.g., weight gain, dyslipidemia, and glucose dysregulation)	The most sedating of the atypical antipsychotics, it is frequently used as a sleep aid. Not recommended for insomnia or other sleep problems unless there is comorbid psychotic or bipolar disorder. Is dosed much lower (25–100 mg) when used for insomnia. Other less expensive sedative-hypnotic agents should be used first

BzRAs, benzodiazepine receptor agonists; COPD, chronic obstructive pulmonary disease; ECG, electrocardiogram; FDA, Food and Drug Administration; TCAs, tricyclic antidepressants (doxepin, amitriptyline, imipramine, nortriptyline, desipramine).

of *psychophysiologic insomnia*. For example, this occurs when wake-promoting activities such as watching TV, studying, and paying bills are done in the bedroom (or on the bed). The treatment focuses on breaking these associations by teaching patients to avoid activities that promote wakefulness in the bedroom (or sleep environment) and to only use the bedroom for sleeping. If sleep is not possible, the patient is encouraged to leave the bedroom until a definitive urge to sleep is present.

CHAPTER 13 Sleep Disorders

WHEN TO REFER

- Refractory insomnia
- Insomnia with a concurrent mood, anxiety, or psychotic disorder
- Suicidal ideation in the context of insomnia
- Need for supportive or cognitive behavioral psychotherapy

Cognitive Behavioral Therapy

Cognitive behavioral therapy (CBT) presumes that cognitive distortions lead to negative emotions and behavior, which may cause or worsen insomnia (8, 9). This therapy includes identifying, challenging, and replacing cognitive distortions and beliefs regarding sleep and loss of sleep with realistic thoughts and beliefs. For example, a college student may catastrophize inability to fall asleep with failing an exam. However, when this belief is examined in detail, the inability to sleep may not necessarily cause her to fail the exam. Previous evidence of such an event may be used to refute this distorted cognition.

Progressive Relaxation Technique

Insomnia is associated with hyperarousal. With this technique, patients are taught how to recognize and control muscular tension through the use of exercises (sometimes using music or audio instructions) to reduce the anxiety and hyperarousal associated with insomnia.

Practice Pointers

Case 1: Insomnia and substance abuse

A 48-year-old man who has been sober for 6 weeks comes to the ambulatory care clinic saying he hasn't "slept a wink" since entering a residential treatment program 4 weeks ago. He stopped drinking alcohol "cold turkey" after his wife of 20 years and two daughters left him due to the patient's refusal to quit drinking. For the past 20 years, he has drank up to one 12 pack of beer nightly and could not fall asleep unless he drank at least two beers before bedtime.

During the first week of sobriety, he had moderate cravings for alcohol and mild tremors that quickly resolved. His sleep was characterized by taking up to an hour to fall asleep and waking up feeling tired and groggy. By the end of his second week of sobriety, he fell asleep soon after going to bed and started to sleep through the night, especially after his wife allowed him to speak to his daughters.

Since the third week of sobriety, he has been living in a house with 23 other people who are in treatment for alcohol or substance dependence. The house has a strict "lights out" time of 10 PM. He shares a room with three other men and sleeps on the lower bunk of a bunk bed. During the first week in the program, his main problems were "falling asleep and staying asleep." Recently, he started getting out of bed to smoke a cigarette on the porch because he felt so restless and anxious about not being able to fall asleep. During the day, he struggles to stay awake during group meetings. He wonders if he's "bipolar" because minor annoyances that never bothered him before, such as a housemate slurping his soup, make him extremely irritable. He also reports a mildly depressed mood that is directly related to his stressors and related insomnia.

Discussion: *Sleep disruption is very common during the first several months after the discontinuation of alcohol and other substances. Since he used alcohol to "self-medicate," the sudden cessation of alcohol may partially explain his prolonged sleep latency during the first week of sobriety. The severe psychosocial stressor of his family's departure from the home also probably contributed to his poor sleep. During the first 2 weeks of sobriety, his differential diagnoses included insomnia due to alcohol withdrawal and adjustment (acute) insomnia. His sleep improved as his minor withdrawal symptoms resolved, and more importantly, after he had the hope of reuniting with his family.*

He started having symptoms of adjustment (acute) insomnia again with increased sleep latency and frequent awakenings (middle insomnia)—immediately after he started facing the new stressors of moving into a residential treatment facility and sleeping in a new, uncomfortable environment. He is also psychologically hyperaroused as he frequently thinks about the separation from his family.

He also has symptoms of psychophysiologic insomnia, *including preoccupation and anxiety about sleep, nodding off unintentionally during the day, and the sense that he needs cigarettes to relax his mind and body. Unfortunately, cigarettes are compounding the problem, since nicotine is a central nervous system stimulant. Although extreme irritability and impulsive behaviors are symptoms of a manic episode, the patient does not report a lack of need for sleep, so bipolar disorder is unlikely. It is also important to rule out other common psychiatric disorders (Table 13.4) such as major depression and/or anxiety disorders.*

For this patient, treatment includes psychoeducation about the effects of psychosocial stressors, alcohol withdrawal, nicotine dependence, environmental factors (new temporary home), and being anxious about not being able to sleep (psychophysiologic insomnia). It would be important to reassure the patient that multiple significant, but modifiable, factors have converged to disrupt his sleep. First, several nonpharmacologic approaches should be tried: sleep hygiene (refraining from cigarette use prior to or during bedtime), environmental triggers (e.g., asking roommates to refrain from discussing the day's events, wearing earplugs, or dimming the alarm clock lights), and behavioral interventions (e.g., refraining from checking the time constantly). The use of CBT may be useful as it would address his depressed mood and related insomnia. In this case, BZP and non-BZP medication should be avoided, as these may trigger alcohol relapse. However, a brief course of one of the non–FDA-approved agents, such as diphenhydramine 25 mg, can be considered.

Case 2: Is there a "medical" cause for this insomnia?

A 53-year-old African-American woman who weighed 232 pounds and was 5'3" tall presented to the ambulatory care clinic complaining of "really bad snoring" and frequent nighttime awakenings, some lasting 30 minutes or more. The patient usually goes to bed feeling "exhausted" and does not have problems falling asleep. However, she awakens 2 to 3 hours later due to a "rumbling" feeling in her stomach, and often feels nauseated. She usually gets up to urinate at this time, but is unsure whether the need to urinate or the gastrointestinal (GI) symptoms wake her up at night. Sometimes her "allergies" act up at that time and she starts coughing. She hasn't had an asthma attack since childhood, but sometimes feels like she's about to have one. However, she calms herself by using deep breathing techniques that she learned at an employee wellness class, and falls asleep again shortly thereafter. She usually awakens feeling fatigued and sleepy several hours later.

She can function relatively well in her job as a bookkeeper in the morning, especially after drinking a cup of regular coffee. By the early afternoon, she can barely keep her eyes open unless she has at least two shots of espresso. The patient often awakens with a pounding headache that is only slightly relieved with ibuprofen. On examination, you note that the patient has a large posterior pharynx and an enlarged neck. Medical history includes moderate hypertension that seems to be well controlled with an angiotensin-converting enzyme inhibitor. At this time, she is opposed to getting a sleep study or using an oral appliance or "any breathing device."

Discussion: *This patient presented with evidence of OSAH: snoring, morbid obesity, daytime somnolence, awakening with a headache, a history of hypertension, and a large posterior oropharynx. Her gastrointestinal symptoms that awaken her from sleep are suggestive of nocturnal gastroesophageal reflux, which is frequently associated with OSAH. Rather than her "allergies" acting up, she's probably coughing because of the reflux, which has gradually worsened after she gained 50 pounds over the past year. The reflux then appears to be triggering symptoms of asthma,* *which she's at risk for due to her childhood history. She's able to stave off an attack as her reflux symptoms resolve by her sitting up in bed and practicing deep breathing techniques. The morning headaches may be due to unrecognized apneic episodes and associated blood pressure spikes throughout the night.*

In addition to OSAH, nocturnal gastroesophageal reflux disease (GERD), GERD-induced asthma, and pulmonary hypertension, the differential diagnosis should include diabetes, hypothyroidism, and Cushing disease. For treatment, review the principles of sleep hygiene with the patient. Help the patient identify a few sleep hygiene problems, and assist her in developing a plan to address them. To prevent nocturnal GERD symptoms, advise the patient not to eat or drink anything within at least 2 hours of bedtime. Consider prescribing a bedtime dose of an antireflux agent. Encourage the patient to continue sitting up in bed and using deep breathing techniques if she continues to wake up with the above GI symptoms. In the meantime, obtain the following screening labs: comprehensive metabolic panel, thyroid-stimulating hormone, complete blood count, and a fasting lipid panel.

In this case, weight loss is paramount. She should be given a referral for nutrition counseling and a weight management program. If symptoms persist after these interventions, consider revisiting the sleep study referral to rule out OSAH and possible treatment with continuous positive airway pressure.

ICD9

Breathing-Related Sleep Disorder	*780.59*
Circadian Rhythm Sleep Disorder	*304.45*
Dyssomnia Not Otherwise Specified	*307.47*
Hypersomnia Due to [General Medical Condition]	*780.54*
Insomnia Due to [General Medical Condition]	*780.52*
Narcolepsy	*347*
Primary Insomnia	*307.42*
Sleep Terror Disorder	*304.46*
Sleepwalking Disorder	*304.46*

Practical Resources

American Academy of Sleep Medicine: www.aasmnet.org
National Heart, Lung, and Blood Institute: www.nhlbi.nih.gov/health/public/sleep/index.htm
National Sleep Foundation: www.sleepfoundation.org
Talk About Sleep: www.talkaboutsleep.com

References

1. Mellinger GD, Balter MB, Uhlenhuth EH. Insomnia and its treatment: prevalence and correlates. *Arch Gen Psychiatry.* 1985;42(3):225–232.

2. Ford DE, Kamerow DB. Epidemiologic study of sleep disturbances and psychiatric disorders: an opportunity for prevention? *JAMA.* 1989;262:1479–1484.

3. National Sleep Foundation. http://www.sleepfoundation.org. Accessed May 15, 2008.

4. National Institute of Health. NIH state-of-the-science conference statement on manifestations and management of chronic insomnia in adults. *NIH Consens Stat Sci Statements* 2005;22:1–30.

5. Katz DA, McHorney CA. The relationship between insomnia and health-related quality of life in patients with chronic illness. *J Fam Pract.* 2002;51(3):229–235.

6. American Sleep Disorders Association, Diagnostic Classification Steering Committee. *International Classification of Sleep Disorders: Diagnostic and Coding Manual.* Westchester, IL: American Academy of Sleep Medicine; 2005.

7. Erman M, Seiden D, Zammit G, et al. An efficacy, safety, and dose-response study of Ramelteon in patients with chronic primary insomnia. *Sleep Med.* 2006;7(1):17–24.

8. Diagnostic Classification Steering Committee. *The International Classification of Sleep Disorders, Revised: Diagnostic and Coding Manual.* Rochester, MN: American Sleep Disorders Association; 1997.

9. World Health Organization. *International Classification of Diseases.* 10th revision. Geneva, Switzerland: World Health Organization; 2007.

14 Suicide and Violence Risk Assessment

Cameron Quanbeck, MD • Pria Joglekar, MD

> *A 76-year-old Caucasian male with chronic obstructive pulmonary disease (COPD), type 2 diabetes, peripheral neuropathy, and osteoarthritis presents with complaints of "horrible insomnia." His wife of 40 years passed away 2 years ago and he is currently living alone. His daughter lives in a nearby town and visits him on a weekly basis. One year prior, his daughter noticed he was having trouble getting around the house to attend to household duties so she hired a home health aide 4 hours a day to assist him. She is concerned because he is depressed and has little energy to participate in pleasurable activities.*

CLINICAL HIGHLIGHTS

- Screening at-risk patients for suicidal thinking in the primary care setting can prevent suicides.

- A number of studies in primary care settings indicate that providers often do not ask depressed patients if they have suicidal thoughts.

- The majority of patients who have committed suicide had contact with a primary care provider within the year before their death and 50% of those who took their own life visited a primary care provider within 1 month.

Assessment and Management of Suicide Risk

CLINICAL SIGNIFICANCE

One in 10 patients seen in primary care settings meets criteria for major depressive disorder. Depression is particularly common in patients presenting for treatment of a chronic medical condition, with a prevalence of about 30% to 40%. Primary care providers see depressed patients routinely and most are managing these patients with antidepressant pharmacotherapy. Suicidal thinking is a feature of depression and suicide is a potential outcome. Clinicians should therefore be familiar with assessing and managing suicide risk.

Primary care clinicians are better positioned than mental health professionals to identify patients at risk and to intervene to prevent suicide. Clinical contact of depressed patients with primary care providers in the time period preceding a suicide is more common than contact with mental health professions. Three of four suicide victims see a primary care provider in the year before suicide, and nearly half of these patients have contact with their primary care physician in the month before their death, particularly older adults (1). In contrast, only 20% of those who die by suicide see a mental health professional in the month prior to their death (2). Although it is not known whether or not these suicides were preventable, this suggests the clinical encounter immediately before suicide can be an opportunity to identify suicide risk and plan appropriate interventions.

Studies suggest that primary care providers could do a better job at identifying patients at risk for suicide. A recent study examined whether or not suicidal thinking was explored in a group of patients who made

(Continued)

CLINICAL HIGHLIGHTS
(*Continued*)

- Patients who commit suicide within a month of seeing a primary care provider are predominately older males with chronic physical illnesses who live alone.

- Suicide risk assessment involves balancing non-modifiable and modifiable risk factors for suicide against factors that protect against suicide. The key modifiable risk factor for suicide is depression, particularly depression coupled with severe anxiety.

- Screening at-risk patients for suicidal thinking is important in assessing suicide risk and will not cause a patient to start thinking about suicide.

- Research has shown that most patients who commit suicide tell family and friends of their wish to die. Therefore, obtaining collateral information from relatives or friends can be an invaluable strategy for detecting patients at high suicide risk.

- If clinicians determine that a patient is at significant acute risk of suicide, they should have a "plan of action" in place that ensures the patient is quickly referred to a mental health professional.

an unannounced visit to a primary care clinic complaining of depressive symptoms and requesting an antidepressant. Fewer than half (42%) of patients were asked about suicidal ideations (3). Another study examined whether or not suicidal thinking was explored by primary care physicians in the last visit prior to suicide in a group of patients who committed suicide within a month of contact. Sixty-two percent of these patients were not asked about suicidal thinking, and in half of these cases, the provider had little knowledge of the patient's life circumstances (4). Suicidal ideation is common in depressed older adults being treated in primary care settings. One in five patients will report suicidal thoughts during a course of treatment for depression, particularly in those with more severe symptoms (5).

SUICIDE RISK ASSESSMENT IN THE PRIMARY CARE SETTING

The striking finding that many of those who commit suicide have seen a primary care provider shortly before their death has led to investigations that attempt to profile the type of patient at risk. One study compared differences between older adults who committed suicide within 30 days of visiting a primary care provider with older primary patients who did not commit suicide. Those who committed suicide had more depressive illness, greater physical illness burden, and functional limitations, and were more likely to be prescribed antidepressants, antianxiety agents, and opiate analgesics (6). A similar study investigated the differences between older men and women who committed suicide shortly after a primary care visit. Male suicides outnumbered female by a ratio of 3:1. Men were more likely to be single or widowed than women. Men were more likely to use hanging as a primary suicide method, whereas women tended to overdose on medications, which suggests care should be exercised in prescribing medications that can be lethal in overdose. In both men and women, the primary complaint involved physical, not psychiatric, symptoms (7). Another study found that older adults were more likely to complain of physical symptoms prior to suicide, whereas younger adults were more likely to seek help for psychiatric symptoms (8).

The assessment of suicide risk is not as simple as asking a patient, "Have you been having suicidal thoughts?" Inquiring about suicidal thinking is important, but is only one piece of performing a suicide risk assessment. The assessment also involves an examination of risk factors for suicide balanced against factors protective against suicide. The more suicide risk factors and fewer protective factors, the greater the risk. There is no specific set of risk factors that have been shown to predict whether or not a patient will commit suicide; because suicide is a very rare event, it is nearly impossible to design and carry out a study with that goal. If primary care providers are aware of key risk and protective factors, however, they can use sound clinical judgment to identify at-risk patients and take steps to reduce the likelihood a suicide will occur.

Nonmodifiable Risk Factors

Certain risk factors are static and cannot be changed with clinical intervention. They include demographic factors (e.g., age, gender, and ethnicity) and certain features of a patient's clinical history. They are important to recognize because they will indicate which type of patient is at highest risk (Table 14.1).

Demographic Risk Factors   Older males are statistically the most likely to die by suicide; elderly men (85 years or older) are at greatest risk with an annual prevalence of 60 suicides per 100,000 (9). Though women attempt suicide three times more often than men, men are four times more likely to die by suicide (10). There are several reasons for the increased risk in men: (1) substance misuse (e.g., alcoholism) is more prevalent among men, (2) men are less willing than women to seek help, (3) men attempt suicide using more lethal methods (e.g., firearms) than women, and (4) females tend to be more socially embedded than men (10). Nevertheless, a significant number of women commit suicide and their risk cannot be discounted. Women with a history of depression and suicide attempts are likely to have poor outcomes postpartum and have increased suicide risk, especially within the first month of delivery (10).

Caucasians and Native Americans are the ethnic groups at highest risk. Their risk of suicide is twice that of African Americans, Hispanics, and Pacific Islanders (10). When examining ethnicity as a risk factor, it is important to also consider age. Suicide rates in all ethnic groups rise sharply from ages 10 to 24, but then plateau into adulthood. Among Caucasian Americans, there is a marked increase in suicide rate in older age, which is not observed in African Americans (9). Thus, African American men commit suicide earlier in life than do Caucasian men (mean ages 34 and 44, respectively) (11). African American females have

---

Table 14.1 Risk Factors for Suicide

Key nonmodifiable risk factors for suicide
- A past suicide attempt, particularly a serious attempt
- Male gender
- Advanced age (>65 years)
- Caucasian or Native American ethnicity
- Divorced, separated, or widowed
- Unemployment (particularly recent loss of job in those <45 years)
- Alcohol dependence (particularly when facing losses)
- Childhood sexual and physical abuse
- Chronic neurologic illness
- A family history of suicide

Key modifiable risk factors for suicide
- Major depressive episode, especially with prominent anxiety symptoms causing insomnia, psychomotor agitation, decreased concentration, and an inability to experience pleasure
- Alcohol abuse
- Hopelessness
- Suicidal ideation and plan (although some patients intent on suicide may deny these thoughts to health care providers)

a remarkably low suicide rate. They are nine times less likely to commit suicide than are Caucasian women. This low suicide rate has been attributed to protective factors of religion and extended kin networks.

Clinical History   The most robust nonmodifiable risk factor for suicide is a previous attempt, particularly a past serious attempt (9). A previous attempt dramatically increases the risk of eventual death by suicide. Previous attempters are 38 times more likely to complete suicide than are nonattempters. Serious attempts can be distinguished from less serious attempts by examining the following factors about the previous attempt: (1) it involved a high degree of intent (e.g., when asked, the patient tells you that, prior to the attempt, he or she fully expected to die and was surprised when he or she did not); 2) it involved a degree of planning, including measures to avoid discovery; and (3) it involved lethal or violent methods that resulted in physical injuries (10).

Patients with a chronic psychiatric disorder are at increased risk for committing suicide. The condition that carries the greatest risk is chronic depression in the form of either major depressive disorder or bipolar disorder. Patients with these disorders are 20 times more likely to commit suicide than those without a mental disorder (10). Substance misuse, particularly alcoholism, also increases suicide risk. Those with alcohol dependence are particularly likely to commit suicide when faced with life stressors caused by their misuse: (1) loss or disruption of a close personal relationship (e.g., divorce), (2) job loss, and (3) legal and financial difficulties (10).

Other important nonmodifiable risk factors include being divorced, separated, or widowed; a family history of suicide; a history of childhood abuse (sexual or physical); unemployment (recent job loss is a common precipitant to suicide in males under the age of 45); and having a chronic physical illness, particularly a neurologic illness (epilepsy, multiple sclerosis, Huntington disease, and brain and spinal cord injuries). Certain nonneurologic illnesses associated with increase suicide risk include human immunodeficiency virus (HIV)/acquired immunodeficiency syndrome (AIDS) and chronic heart, lung, kidney, and prostate diseases (10). In a recent study, older primary care patients ($\geq$65 years) were asked if they were having thoughts they wished they were dead. Those with chronic medical conditions, especially a recent myocardial infarction, were the most likely to report having death wishes (12).

Modifiable Risk Factors

Psychological autopsies (a focused evaluation of the deceased's life and emotional state before death) conducted on suicide victims have found that 90% meet criteria for one or more psychiatric disorders, predominately a major depressive episode (9). A landmark study involving a large sample of patients with recurrent depression found that the presence of certain symptoms was predictive of suicide within the ensuing year. These symptoms were (1) global insomnia (e.g., disruption of all phases of sleep), (2) psychomotor agitation (e.g., restlessness, pacing), (3) severe anxiety, (4) panic attacks, (5) difficulty concentrating, (6) severe anhedonia (e.g., an inability to experience pleasure), and (7) alcohol abuse (13). In examining these data, experts in suicidology reason that depression is difficult to tolerate and there is a wish to escape through death. The added component of severe anxiety creates an intolerable situation that fuels suicidal thoughts and behaviors (9). Depressed patients who are also anxious are more likely to act on suicidal impulses than those with psychomotor slowing (9).

The strong association between anxiety and suicide has been found in other settings. In a retrospective study of psychiatric inpatients who committed suicide, the vast majority (80%) exhibited signs of anxiety and agitation in the week prior to death (9). Primary care patients with anxiety disorders have an increased risk of suicidal ideations and attempts in both the short and long term. Patients with anxiety symptoms coupled with depression have a significantly greater suicide risk than those with depression alone (14). Other key modifiable risk factors for suicide are strong feelings of hopelessness (15); a wish to destroy the lives of survivors (revenge suicide); extreme feelings of worthlessness, shame, or guilt; and polarized thinking (e.g., rigid thinking in which a patient is unable to consider options other than suicide) (10).

Protective Factors

Having strong reasons for living is inversely correlated with hopelessness, suicidal ideations, and depression (10). Those reasons for living include having family and other social support, responsibility for children, and an expectation that current emotional pain is temporary and a hope that things will improve in future (9). Patients with strong religious beliefs are also at a decreased risk of suicide, particularly those who practice Catholicism and Judaism (10). The belief that killing oneself is morally wrong and sinful and results in eternal damnation is a strong deterrent to suicide. A cultural sanction against suicide (the view that suicide is shameful) is another protective factor (9). Other protective factors include rewarding work, a good therapeutic alliance, and healthy and well-developed coping skills (10) (Table 14.2). Older primary care patients (≥65 years) who display a positive affect are less likely than those who do not to report suicidal thinking (16).

Table 14.2 Factors Protective Against Suicide: Reasons to Live

- Strong religious (eternal damnation) or cultural beliefs (shame) against suicide
- A strong social network
- Responsibility for children
- Hope for the future
- Good therapeutic alliance
- A positive affect

ELICITING SUICIDAL IDEATIONS

Any patient presenting with a primary complaint of depression, anxiety, or substance misuse should be screened for suicidal ideation, as they are at elevated risk for self-harm (17). Questions about suicidal ideation should be asked later in a clinical encounter, after rapport with a patient has been established. For example, as part of screening for depression, thoughts of death and suicide should be asked after screening for the other eight depressive symptoms. Figure 14.1 illustrates a line of questioning designed to elicit suicidal ideations in at-risk patients. It is also very important to recognize that asking about suicidal thinking does not "plant" suicidal ideas in a patient's mind (18). It is common for primary care providers to hold this view. One in five primary care providers believed that asking depressed patients about suicidal thinking will cause a patient to begin thinking about it. There is no evidence this is true and, on the contrary, many patients report feeling relieved when they are asked (17).

The intensity and duration of suicidal ideations are predictive of eventual suicide (10). More ominous is the development of a suicide plan. Thirty-four percent of those with suicidal ideations go on to devise a suicide plan. Up to 70% of patients who develop a plan go on to make a suicide attempt, usually within the year after the onset of suicidal thinking (9). A suicide plan dramatically increases risk, especially when the plan (1) is detailed and specific, (2) is formulated to escape detection, and (3) involves a violent and irreversible method (e.g., jumping off a bridge, shooting oneself, or carbon monoxide poisoning). Certain behaviors, such as writing a suicide note and giving away personal possessions, indicate an intensification of suicidal thinking and a strong subjective desire to die (10).

DISPOSITION OF SUICIDAL PATIENTS

As shown in Figure 14.1, screening for suicidal thinking can result in four possible clinical situations: (1) no desire to die or thoughts of death, (2) death wishes but no thoughts of harming self, (3) suicidal ideations without a plan, and (4) suicidal ideations with a plan. In general, patients in categories 1 and 2 can effectively be managed in primary care settings. Patients in the higher-risk categories should be referred to mental health specialists for further assessment, treatment, and monitoring.

Patients who have been having active suicidal ideations without a specific plan should be seen as soon as possible by a mental health professional, ideally the same day. Patients with active suicidal ideation and a specific plan in mind should be sent to the emergency room for immediate evaluation. If an actively suicidal patient is unwilling to go to the emergency room and attempts to leave the clinicians office, a call to the local police department for involuntary detainment may be indicated. Clinicians should familiarize themselves with clinic policies and state laws regarding involuntary commitment and have a low threshold to secure an involuntary hold in those who

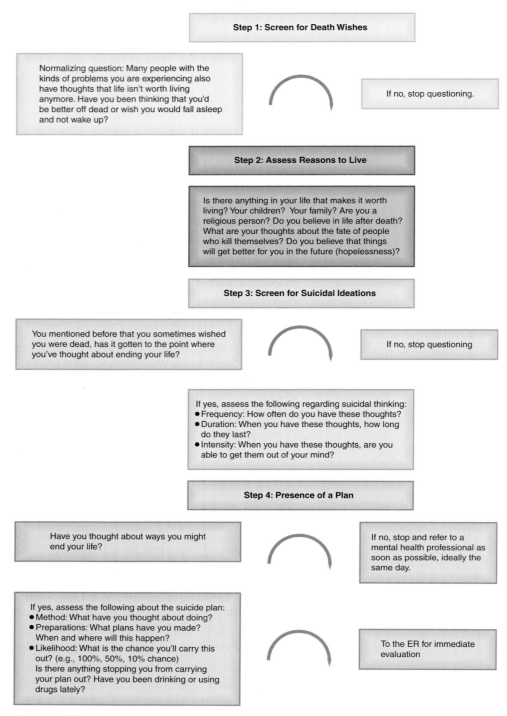

Figure 14.1 Eliciting suicidal thinking in at-risk patients.

are at moderate or high acute risk for suicide and unwilling to get immediate mental health treatment.

MEDICOLEGAL ISSUES

Primary care providers who assume the responsibility for treating a patient with a mental illness will generally be held to the same liability standard as mental health professionals. Consequently, primary care providers who have a patient commit suicide while under their care may be named in malpractice litigation (19). It is critical to ask patients who are having suicidal thoughts about their access to firearms or if they have recently purchased a gun. The risk of suicide in those who have purchased a handgun is nearly 60 times greater than those in the general population (9). If the patient has access to a firearm, steps should be taken to ensure that this access is taken away. Asking the patient or family members to get rid of guns in the home can be an important issue in malpractice litigations (9). Most importantly, if a patient under your care commits suicide and a malpractice suit is brought against you, whether or not you assessed and documented suicide risk will be crucial in determining if the care you provided was negligent.

Another emerging issue in suicide malpractice cases is the use of antidepressant therapy. There is a twofold increase in nonfatal suicide attempts during the first 9 days of treatment with selective serotonin reuptake inhibitors (SSRIs), likely due to the propensity of these agents in some patients to initially increase levels of anxiety and agitation (19). Patients should be closely monitored for the development of suicidal ideations in the first 2 weeks after therapy is initiated. Prescribing practices should be tailored to prevent the possibility of an overdose (e.g., the tricyclic antidepressants are notorious for their lethality). While there may be a short-term risk of emergent suicidality with antidepressant treatment and overdose risk must be considered, it is also important to detect and treat depression effectively. Studies on primary care patients who attempted suicide found that those on antidepressants were not dosed adequately (19).

Practice Pointers

Case 1: Suicide risk assessment

A 76-year-old Caucasian male with COPD, type 2 diabetes, peripheral neuropathy, and osteoarthritis presents with complaints of "horrible insomnia." His wife of 40 years passed away 2 years ago and he is currently living alone. His daughter lives in a nearby town and visits him on a weekly basis. One year prior, his daughter noticed he was having trouble getting around the house to attend to household duties so she hired a home health aide 4 hours a day to assist him. She is concerned because he is depressed and has little energy to participate in pleasurable activities.

He endorses feeling depressed most days, has lost interest in things he used to enjoy, and has had some trouble focusing enough to read the daily paper. On chart review, you note he has lost 10 pounds since he was last seen in the clinic 3 months ago. When you ask him if he has recently thought that life isn't worth living or if he wished he were dead, he breaks eye contact with you and lowers his head. He responds, "No," then pauses and softly says "No" a second time. You provide him with education on depression and he agrees, somewhat reluctantly, to take an antidepressant. He leaves the office with a prescription and a follow-up appointment in 1 week. You continue with your clinic schedule but keep thinking about this patient. Something about his response to your question about death wishes keeps bothering you.

Discussion: *Past research has shown that in the last clinical contact prior to a suicide, most patients will give providers no indication they are about to end their lives and the suicide is unexpected (20). A study of psychiatric inpatients who committed* *suicide in the hospital or immediately after discharge found that the vast majority (77%) denied suicidal thoughts at their last clinical contact (20). This finding extends to primary care settings as well. In only 19% to 54% of primary care encounters did suicidal patients explicitly inform primary care providers of life-ending thoughts and plans (2). Elderly patients, commonly seen in primary care settings, are much less likely than younger patients to endorse having suicidal ideations (9). Although the reasons why many of those who commit suicide did not communicate their intentions to health care professionals can never be known, suicidologists theorize there are several possible reasons. First, patients who are intent on committing suicide may hide their intentions from providers because they don't want to be stopped. Second, clinicians may fail to recognize a patient's distress and make an empathic connection; consequently, a suicidal patient doesn't feel comfortable disclosing these deeply personal thoughts. Third, the clinical encounter may have a temporary calming effect on patients and, in that moment, they are not feeling suicidal, but suicidal impulses return sometime after leaving the office.*

It is very important to be aware that most patients who commit suicide, however, do communicate the desire to end their lives to the people they are closest to. In one study of suicide completers, only 18% told a health care provider of their suicidal ideas, but 60% told a spouse and 50% told a relative of the wish to end their lives (20). It is also critical to recognize that a brief encounter in the office offers a limited view of what is occurring in a patient's life. To get a broader perspective you need to speak with someone who knows the patient well and sees him or her on a regular basis. If you screen an at-risk patient for suicidal thinking and he or she denies suicidal thinking but you are concerned about his or her risk, a call to a family member or friend can be invaluable in preventing a suicide. A patient's recent behaviors and communications outside the office can be important when making an accurate assessment of suicide risk. In practice, it is always ideal to have the patient's permission to contact collateral sources and to protect patient confidentially unless explicitly stated. However, there is an emergency exception to confidentiality. In dangerous situations (e.g., risk of suicide, impending assault, medical emergency), confidentiality can be breached.

After obtaining the permission from the patient, you call his daughter and ask if she's noticed anything different or concerning about him lately. She states, "Oh, doctor, I'm so glad you called; he has been acting different lately. I've noticed that he doesn't watch football anymore, which is something he used to love to do. I have to force him to eat when I visit him and he seems real jittery sometimes. I'm worried about his drinking too. Last week, I found a bunch of empty bottles of vodka in his garage and, when I called him a few days ago, he sounded really out of it. What really scares me is that he's been making changes to his will and just bought my daughter a brand new car. He's spending money that he needs to live on. His health is OK, right? He's not going to die soon, is he?" You reply, "No, but I'm concerned your father may be thinking about ending his life. I'd like you to go to his house immediately and bring him to our emergency room. Call me once you get there and let me know if he is willing to go."

Discussion: *Although an afterthought in the case, this patient has multiple risk factors for suicide (depressed mood, advanced age, loss of his wife, chronic medical illness, possible preparation for suicide, and likely alcohol abuse). Even though the patient reported "no" to wanting to end his life, there is valid justification for concern given the way he answered the question. Referring this patient to the emergency room for a suicide assessment if clinically indicated will very likely prove to be life saving.*

This patient likely has major depressive disorder and should be treated with both psychotherapy and an antidepressant. While on medication for his depression, he should be monitored by both a mental health professional and his primary care provider on a frequent basis for the first 6 months of therapy.

Mr. Green is a 56-year-old patient with type 2 diabetes and hypertension who was recently transferred to your care by a primary care provider who recently retired. He has been scheduled to see you for a routine follow-up. Earlier in the afternoon, you encountered and dealt with an emergent situation with one of your patients and are subsequently running behind schedule. Mr. Green arrived to his appointment on time and has been waiting for over an hour to see you. The clinic receptionist rushes back to see you between patients and expresses concern about his behavior.

Assessment and Management of Violence Risk

CLINICAL SIGNIFICANCE

Violence in primary care settings is common (21). In a survey of general practitioners, two thirds reported experiencing aggressive behavior (verbal abuse, threats to commit violence, or physical assault) from patients in the previous year. Primary care providers who experience work-related violence report that it impairs their job performance because it leads to anxiety and difficulty concentrating in the work environment (22). Primary care providers who are less experienced, work in lower socioeconomic and socially disadvantaged areas, and treat patient populations with a high prevalence of substance misuse and mental health disorders are at increased risk for workplace violence (21).

CLINICAL HIGHLIGHTS

- Most primary care providers report experiencing violent behavior from their patients and these experiences can have a negative impact on work performance.

- Patients with a history of violence and substance abuse are most likely to behave aggressively in the primary care setting; the emergency department is the setting where violence is most common.

- A common precipitant to an assault on a primary care provider is after a patient is told "no."

- Effective strategies to diffuse potential violence include early recognition, avoiding arguments or taking an authoritarian stance, empathizing with the patient's frustration, and providing choices for the patient.

VIOLENCE RISK ASSESSMENT IN THE PRIMARY CARE SETTING

Certain risk factors increase the likelihood a patient will behave aggressively. Past behavior is the best predictor of future behavior. A history of violence is the most powerful long-term predictor of future violence (23). Primary care providers are most often assaulted by patients who misuse substances (24). An important short-term risk factor for violence is recent verbal or physical aggression (25). Symptoms that indicate a patient is at imminent risk for becoming assaultive include (1) psychomotor agitation, (2) a hostile or angry affect, (3) verbal threats to harm others, (4) attacks on objects, (5) intense staring, and (6) a poor therapeutic alliance or resistance to treatment (25, 26).

Past research has identified specific environments, situations, and patient interactions in the health care setting that most frequently trigger a patient assault (27–29). The health care environment with the highest number of assaults is the emergency department (ED). Evening and early morning hours are the highest-risk times, as these are when patients are most likely to be intoxicated. Patients frustrated by long waiting times in the clinic or ED can become angered to the point they resort to violence as a response. Enforcement of hospital rules can precipitate patient violence. Patients who disagree with their physicians or feel dissatisfied with their treatment (including the health care system in general) can become upset and aggressive. Awareness of these common precipitants to patient assault is a key component in efforts to prevent violence (Table 14.3). If a patient becomes aggressive without an identifiable external trigger, the motivation for the violence is often related to psychotic symptoms. A psychiatry consultation should be

> ## Table 14.3 Situations and Interactions within the Health Care System Associated with Violence
>
> - Long waiting times in the emergency department of clinic
> - Disagreement with the physician's treatment plan
> - Dissatisfaction with treatment or the health care system in general
> - Enforcement of hospital and clinic policies and rules
> - Providing care in acute care settings during evening and early morning hours
> - Providing care to patients experiencing psychotic symptoms
>   - Paranoid delusions are most associated with violence
>   - Seen in patients with delirium and major psychotic disorders

obtained for further evaluation and treatment of a possible cognitive (e.g., delirium) or psychotic disorder (e.g., schizophrenia).

Practice Pointers

Case 2: Looking for pre-escalation

Mr. Green is a 56-year-old patient with type 2 diabetes and hypertension who was recently transferred to your care by a primary physician who recently retired. He has been scheduled to see you for a routine follow-up. Earlier in the afternoon, you encountered and dealt with an emergent situation with one of your patients and are subsequently running behind schedule. Mr. Green arrived to his appointment on time and has been waiting for over an hour to see you. The clinic receptionist rushes back to see you between patients and expresses concern about his behavior. She tells you, "At first he seemed all right with having to wait, but he just started yelling at me and demanding to be seen immediately. I keep on telling him that you'll see him soon and ask him to sit down but that just seems to make him angrier. Now he's pacing around the room and staring at me. What should I do?"

Discussion: *Clinicians regarded as experts in de-escalating potentially explosive situations stress the importance of early intervention in the emotional process that can culminate in a physical assault. In this case, the early recognition of pre-escalation, as evidenced by pacing, staring, yelling, demanding, and psychomotor agitation, is paramount. This patient can be offered alternatives to a longer wait time. For example, he can be given the option of making another appointment or provided an accurate time frame for which he will be waiting. An empathic stance also has the potential to diffuse the situation early. For instance, the receptionist might briefly explain the emergent nature of why the doctor is late and say, "I understand your time is important and that this is frustrating for you." Table 14.4 summarizes proactive steps that can be taken in this case to help diffuse the situation and decrease the risk for violent behavior.*

Case 3: Maintenance of safety is paramount

You are working a weekend shift in an urgent care clinic. A nurse approaches you and hands you a patient's chart. She tells you, "This patient, Mr. Johnson, is a big-time drug seeker. He is always coming in here with these bogus pain complaints and demanding OxyContin and other narcotics. You aren't gonna give him any, are you?"

The first thing Mr. Johnson tells you is, "Hey, doctor, I got the worst migraine headache ever. The only thing that will take care of it is a shot of Demerol. Just give me that shot and I'll be out of here." You begin to question Mr. Johnson in detail about the onset, duration, and location of his pain. His answers are vague, nondescriptive, and contradictory. As the interview progresses, he gets increasingly hostile and eventually blurts out, "What's with all

Table 14.4 Clinical Interventions That Can Be Taken to Deescalate a Patient and Prevent a Physical Assault (Based on Practice Pointers Clinical Case)

- *Step 1: Recognize patients who are escalating emotionally*
  - Verbal abuse, psychomotor agitation, hostility, and staring indicate a patient is escalating
  - Appropriate intervention at this stage may avert physical aggression

- *Step 2: Read the situation and the meaning of the behavior*
  - Frustration about coming to the appointment on time and having to wait over an hour
  - Angry about his time being wasted, may feel disrespected

- *Step 3: Connect with the patient*
  - Approach the patient maintaining an adequate distance
    - Agitated patients need increased interpersonal space
  - Speak in a calm voice
  - Instill in patient a sense of control
    - For example: "May I speak with you? You seem very upset right now—can we talk about it?"

- *Step 4: Empathize with the patient and validate emotions*
  - For example: "Sir, I'm really sorry about the long wait. I can imagine it is really frustrating to show up on time and have to wait this long to be seen. I know your time is very important...."

- *Step 5: Depersonalize the situation*
  - Anger can create cognitive distortions that lead to mistaking the intentions of others; for example: "This doctor is putting me off.... He doesn't care about me!"
  - Communicate openly and honestly
    - For example: "You know, the reason I'm so far behind is that I had to deal with an emergency situation earlier this afternoon and send a patient to the hospital. Sometimes these things happen; I hope you understand. I'm doing my best to catch up and get to you."

- *Step 6: Give a patient choices*
  - Asking an escalating patient to make a decision diverts focus from the inciting stimulus and helps in regaining emotional control
  - For example: "Is there anything I can do for you that will make waiting here easier for you? You could take a walk around the building and I could call you when I'm ready to see you, or I could offer you some different magazines and a glass of water...."

the stupid questions? I already told you what I need! Do your goddamn job and give me the shot or I'll sue you!" You exit the room and review Mr. Johnson's medical records. They chronicle numerous urgent care visits for various pain complaints, which are unsubstantiated by objective findings. He demands opiates at each visit and often receives a prescription for a small supply of opiates with instructions to follow up with his primary care physician. He has a past history of heroin dependence and has been arrested in the past for assault. After consulting with a colleague, you determine that he is likely seeking abusable medication and prepare to speak with him about the issue.

Discussion: *Primary care providers should take precautions when preparing to deny a patient's request. Although necessary at times, telling a patient "no" is a common precipitant to assaults on medical staff (25). In this case, giving the patient the narcotics he is demanding may facilitate him leaving the clinic, but will be counterproductive in the long term because the behavior will be reinforced. Table 14.5 details how to approach and manage a patient in this situation in a manner that protects your safety and will not escalate the situation further.*

CHAPTER 14 Suicide & Violent Risk

Table 14.5 Telling a Patient "No": Tips for Protecting Your Safety and Preventing Further Escalation of the Situation

- *Never* enter a room with a potentially violent patient and situate yourself in a position where you can be cornered without a route of escape
- *Always* notify your colleagues about your concerns for possible violence so they are aware and can help if needed
  - Ask another staff member to accompany you if you don't feel safe
  - In some instances, notifying hospital security to stand by is appropriate
- *Avoid* taking an authoritarian stance with a patient; becoming argumentative only serves to fuel the escalating process
  - Agitated and angry patients don't respect your authority; don't think that being a physician protects you from violence
- When denying a request, explain your reasoning to the patient and how you are acting in his or her best interest
  - For example: "Sir, your records indicate that you have a history of heroin use. Giving you narcotic medication for your headache will place you at risk for relapse. I want to do what's best for you. I can offer you some nonnarcotic pain medications instead. What do you think?"

Practical Resources

National Suicide Prevention Lifeline: Sponsored by the U.S. Department of Health and Human Services: The Substance Abuse and Mental Health Administration: www.suicidepreventionlifeline.org; 1-800-SUICIDE or 1-800-273-TALK (8255)
National Institute of Mental Health: www.nimh.nih.gov
American Psychiatric Association Guidelines for Suicide Prevention: http://www.psychiatryonline.com/pracGuide/pracGuideTopic_14.aspx

References

1. Luoma JB, Martin CE, Pearson JL. Contact with mental health and primary care providers before suicide: a review of the evidence. *Am J Psychiatry.* 2002;159:909–916.

2. Blashki G, Pirkis J, Epid A, et al. Managing depression and suicide risk in men presenting to primary care physicians. *Prim Care Clin Office Pract.* 2006;33:211–221.

3. Feldman MD, Franks P, Duberstein PR, et al. Let's not talk about it: suicide inquiry in primary care. *Ann Fam Med.* 2007;5:412–418.

4. Milton J, Ferguson B, Mills T. Risk assessment and suicide prevention in primary care. *Crisis.* 1999;20(4):171–177.

5. Vannoy SD, Duberstein P, Cukrowicz K, et al. The relationship between suicide ideation and late-life depression. *Am J Geriatr Psychiatry.* 2007;15:1024–1033.

6. Conwell Y, Lyness JM, Duberstein P, et al. Completed suicide among older patients in primary care practices: a controlled study. *J Am Geriatr Soc.* 2000;48(1):23–29.

7. Harwood DM, Hawton K, Hope T, et al. Suicide in older people: mode of death, demographic factors, and medical contact before death. *Int J Geriatr Psychiatry.* 2000;15:736–743.

8. Salib E, Tadros G. Elderly suicide in primary care. *Int J Geriatr Psychiatry.* 2007;22:750–756.

9. Simon RI. Suicide risk: assessing the unpredictable. In: *Textbook of Suicide Assessment and Management.* Washington, DC: American Psychiatric Publishing; 2006:1–32.

10. American Psychiatric Association. Practice guidelines for the assessment and treatment of patients with suicidal behaviors. *Am J Psychiatry.* 2003;160(suppl):1–60.

11. Garlow SJ, Purselle D, Heninger M. Ethnic differences in patterns of suicide across the life cycle. *Am J Psychiatry.* 2005;162:319–323.

12. Kim YA, Bogner HR, Brown GK, et al. Chronic medical conditions and wishes to die among older primary care patients. *Int J Psychiatry Med.* 2006;36(2):183–198.

13. Fawcett J, Scheftner WA, Fogg L, et al. Time-related predictors of suicide in major affective disorder. *Am J Psychiatry.* 1990;147(9):1189–1194.

14. Sareen J, Cox BJ, Afifi TO, et al. Anxiety disorders and risk for suicidal ideation and suicide attempts. *Arch Gen Psychiatry.* 2005;62:1249–1257.

15. Beck AT, Brown G, Berchick RJ, et al. Relationship between hopelessness and ultimate suicide: a replication with psychiatric outpatients. *Am J Psychiatry.* 1990;147(2):190–195.

16. Hirsch JK, Duberstein PR, Chapman B, et al. Positive affect and suicide ideations in older adult primary care patients. *Psychol Aging.* 2007;22(2):380–385.

17. Raue PJ, Brown EL, Meyers BS, et al. Does every allusion to possible suicide require the same response? *J Fam Pract.* 2006;55(7):605–612.

18. Schulberg HC, Hyg MS, Bruce ML, et al. Preventing suicide in primary care patients: the primary care physician's role. *Gen Hosp Psychiatry.* 2004;26:337–345.

19. Simon RI, Sadoff RL. Malpractice law: an introduction. In: *Psychiatric Malpractice: Cases and Comments for Clinicians.* Washington, DC: American Psychiatric Press; 1992:23–55.

20. Mays D. Structured assessment methods may improve suicide prevention. *Psychiatric Ann.* 2004;34:367–372.

21. Magin PJ, Adams J, Sibbritt DW, et al. Experiences of occupational violence in Australian urban general practice: a cross-sectional study of GPs. *Med J Aust.* 2005;183:352–356.

22. Coles J, Koritsas S, Boyle M, et al. GPs, violence and work performance—'just part of the job?' *Aust Fam Physician.* 2007;36:189–191.

23. Quanbeck CD. Forensic psychiatric aspects of inpatient violence. *Psychiatry Clin North Am.* 2006;29:743–760.

24. Tolhurst H, Baker L, Murray G, et al. Rural general practitioner experience of work-related violence in Australia. *Aust J Rural Health.* 2003;11:231–236.

25. Quanbeck C, McDermott B. Inpatient settings. In: *Textbook of Violence Assessment and Management.* Washington, DC: American Psychiatric Publishing; 2008:295–318.

26. Lanza ML, Zeiss RA, Rierdan J. Non-physical violence: a risk factor for physical violence in health care settings. *AAOHN J.* 2006;54:397–402.

27. Carmi-Iluz T, Peleg R, Freud T, et al. Verbal and physical violence towards hospital- and community-based providers in the Negev: an observational study. *BMC Health Serv Res.* 2005;5:54.

28. Gates DM, Ross CS, McQueen L. Violence against emergency department workers. *J Emerg Med.* 2006;31:331–337.

29. May DD, Grubbs LM. The extent, nature, and precipitating factors of nurse assault among three groups of registered nurses in a regional medical center. *J Emerg Nurs.* 2002;28:11–17.

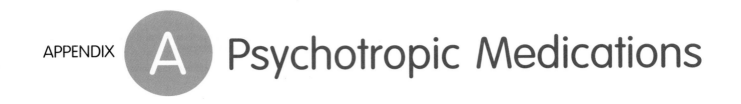

Table 2.3 First-Line Antidepressant Medications

CLASS	INITIAL DOSE (MG/DAY)[a]	THERAPEUTIC DOSE (MG/DAY)	PRACTICAL POINTERS FOR THE PCP[b]
Selective Serotonin Reuptake Inhibitors (SSRIs)			
Sertraline (Zoloft)	50	50–200	Serotonin and dopamine reuptake inhibition Possible early and temporary diarrhea and dyspepsia Relatively low risk for drug interactions
Paroxetine Paroxetine CR (Paxil, Paxil CR)	20 12.5–20	20–60 25–75	High anticholinergic and antihistamine side-effect profile Risk for sedation, weight gain, and dry mouth Short half-life with more risk for discontinuation syndrome High chance for drug interactions Unsafe during pregnancy—class D
Fluoxetine (Prozac)	20	20–60	Long half-life and ideal for intermittently compliant patients Relatively inexpensive High chance for drug interactions
Fluvoxamine (Luvox)	50	50–300	Rarely used due to high side-effect profile
Citalopram (Celexa)	20	20–60	Structurally similar to escitalopram Low risk for drug interactions
Escitalopram (Lexapro)	10	10–20	Structurally similar to citalopram Low risk for drug interactions
Serotonin Norepinephrine Reuptake Inhibitors (SNRIs)			
Venlafaxine XR (Effexor XR)	37.5	75–300	Structurally similar to desvenlafaxine (do not use concurrently) Dual action on serotonin and norepinephrine receptors *Not* consistently "activating" but usually does not cause sedation Sometimes used as an adjunct for chronic pain Not to be used in those with difficult-to-treat hypertension May increase blood pressure and heart rate, especially at higher dosing range (>150 mg/day) Non-XR formulation is rarely used due to side-effect profile and twice-per-day dosing Short half-life with more risk for discontinuation syndrome Reduce dose with renal insufficiency

(Continued)

Table 2.3 First-Line Antidepressant Medications (*Continued*)

CLASS	INITIAL DOSE (MG/DAY)[a]	THERAPEUTIC DOSE (MG/DAY)	PRACTICAL POINTERS FOR THE PCP[b]
Desvenlafaxine (Pristiq)	50	50–100	Structurally similar to venlafaxine (do not use concurrently) Dual action on serotonin and norepinephrine receptors *Not* consistently "activating" but usually does not cause sedation Not to be used in those with difficult-to-treat hypertension Short half-life with more risk for discontinuation syndrome Reduce dose with renal insufficiency
Duloxetine (Cymbalta)	30	30–60	Dual action on serotonin and norepinephrine receptors *Not* consistently "activating" but usually does not cause sedation FDA approved for fibromyalgia and diabetic peripheral neuropathic pain Sometimes used for chronic neuropathic pain Short half-life with more risk for discontinuation syndrome Increased risk for drug interactions
Other			
Bupropion	75–150	300–450	
Bupropion SR (Wellbutrin SR)	100	300–400	Given twice per day Likely dual action on dopamine and norepinephrine receptors Contraindicated with seizure and eating disorders
Bupropion XL (Wellbutrin XL)	150	300–450	Increased risk for seizures in those with alcohol withdrawal Not used for anxiety disorders May worsen anxiety associated with depression No serotonin activity and no related sexual side effects XL formulation is supposed to have slower release and lower side-effect profile (permits higher dosing and lower seizure risk) Less frequently used due to side-effect profile
Mirtazapine (Remeron)	15	15–45	Increases central serotonin and norepinephrine activity (possibly through presynaptic α_2-adrenergic receptor inhibition) Decreased frequency of sexual side effects Increased sedation and sleepiness at mainly *lower* doses Although not indicated for anxiety disorders, it may be helpful Remeron Sol tab is orally dissolving for patients who cannot swallow

FDA, Food and Drug Administration; PCP, primary care physician.

[a] Initial dose should be decreased by half when treating an anxiety disorder or an elderly person.

[b] Drug interactions refer to commonly used medications that are principally metabolized by the P450 2D6 pathway.

Table 3.6 Mood Stabilizers for Bipolar Disorder[a]

	STARTING DOSE[b]	TARGET SERUM LEVEL	TITRATION SCHEDULE	SIDE EFFECTS	MONITORING[b]
Lithium	300 mg BID/TID May be dosed QHS if tolerated	0.6–1.2 mEq/L (acute mania)	Steady-state level reached in 4–5 days Increase by increments of 300–600 mg, as tolerated	Nausea/vomiting, diarrhea, tremor, fatigue, polyuria, acne, worsening psoriasis, diabetes insipidus ECG changes (mainly benign T-wave changes) Hypothyroidism Toxicity (confusion, ataxia, dysarthria, coma) High caution in those with renal insufficiency Potentially lethal due to its narrow therapeutic window Pregnancy category (D)	Check lithium level 5–7 days after each dose change Every 3 months: lithium level, TSH, metabolic panel Lithium toxicity risk increased by: 1. Drugs that decrease glomerular filtration rate, which increase lithium levels (NSAIDs, ACE inhibitors, diuretics) 2. Conditions that cause volume depletion or "dehydration" (e.g., severe vomiting/diarrhea)
Divalproex Sodium (Depakote)	500–1,000 mg BID (25 mg/kg/day for acute mania) Extended release (ER) dosed 500–2,000 mg QHS	85–125 μg/mL (acute mania)	Steady-state level reached in 3–5 days Increase by 500–1,000 mg/day, as tolerated	Sedation Tremor Weight gain Hypersensitivity Thrombocytopenia Transaminitis Hyperammonemia Encephalopathy Pancreatitis Pregnancy category (D)	Baseline, 3-month, 6-month, and annually thereafter: VPA level, CBC, AST, and ALT
Carbamazepine (Tegretol)	ER 200 mg BID	Not established for bipolar disorder	Steady-state level reached in 3–4 days Increase by 200 mg/day (up to 1,600 mg/day), as tolerated	Dizziness Somnolence Stevens-Johnson syndrome Hyponatremia (SIADH) Leukopenia, pancytopenia, thrombocytopenia Hepatitis Drug interactions common Pregnancy category (D)	Baseline, 3-month, 6-month, and annually thereafter: carbamazepine level, CBC, serum chemistry, liver enzymes

| Oxcarbazepine (Trileptal) | 300 mg BID | Not established for bipolar disorder | Increased by 300 mg/day, as tolerated | Fatigue Ataxia Hyponatremia Stevens-Johnson syndrome Pregnancy category (C) | Serum sodium during maintenance treatment (interval not established; consider every 3–4 months) |
| Lamotrigine (Lamictal)[c] | 25 mg/day | Not established for bipolar disorder | 25 mg/day for 2 weeks, then 50 mg/day for 2 weeks, then 100 mg/day for 1 week, then 200 mg/day (dose titration pack available), as tolerated[d] | Rash Stevens-Johnson syndrome Hepatitis Anemia, leukopenia, thrombocytopenia Pregnancy category (C) | Signs of rash |

ACE, angiotensin-converting enzyme; ALT, alanine transaminase; AST, aspartate transaminase; CBC, complete blood count; ECG, electrocardiogram; NSAIDs, nonsteroidal anti-inflammatory drugs; SIADH, syndrome of inappropriate antidiuretic hormone; TSH, thyroid-stimulating hormone; VPA, valproic acid.

[a] Adapted with permission from Scherk H, Pajonk FG, Leucht S. Second-generation antipsychotic agents in the treatment of acute mania: a systematic review and meta-analysis of randomized controlled trials. *Arch Gen Psychiatry.* 2007;64:442–455; and *Physician Desk Reference 2008.*

[b] Starting dose is for average adult patients. Elderly patients and patients with hepatic and renal disease should have lower starting doses. Frequent monitoring is required for those who have severe symptoms.

[c] For bipolar depression and maintenance, not for acute bipolar mania.

[d] Even slower titration when used with divalproex sodium and hepatic enzyme-inducing drugs (alternate dose titration pack is available).

APPENDIX A Psychotropic Medications

Table 4.4 Selective Serotonin Reuptake Inhibitors (SSRIs) and Serotonin Norepinephrine Reuptake Inhibitors (SNRIs) for Anxiety Disorders

SSRIs	STARTING DOSE (MG/DAY)	THERAPEUTIC DOSE (MG/DAY)	HALF-LIFE	DRUG INTERACTIONS
Fluoxetine (Prozac)	10	20–60	Long[a]	2D6 inhibitor
Sertraline (Zoloft)	25	50–200	Medium[a]	(−)
Citalopram (Celexa)	10	20–60	Short	(−)
Escitalopram (Lexapro)	5	10–30	Short	(−)
Paroxetine (Paxil)	10	20–60	Short	2D6 inhibitor
Paroxetine controlled release (Paxil CR)	12.5	12.5–25	Short	2D6 inhibitor
Fluvoxamine (Luvox)	50	150–300	Short	3A4 and 1A2 inhibitor
SNRIs				
Venlafaxine extended release (Effexor XR)	37.5	75–225	Short[a]	(−)
Duloxetine (Cymbalta)	30	60–120	Short	2D6 inhibitor

[a] Including active metabolites.

Table 5.7 First-Line Antipsychotic Medications[a]

	STARTING DOSE	TARGET RANGE[a] (MG/DAY)	PRIMARY CARE TITRATION SCHEDULE	SIDE EFFECTS[b]	MONITORING
Risperidone[c] (Risperdal)	1 mg BID or 2 mg QHS	4–6	Increase up to 2 mg daily, as tolerated	EPS (++) Hyperprolactinemia (+++) Orthostatic hypotension (++) Metabolic abnormalities (++) Sedation (++)	**Initial:** • Baseline weight and body mass index, vital signs, fasting plasma glucose, and lipid profile • Consider doing a pregnancy test and drug toxicology • Brain imaging and a neurologic exam should be done if psychotic symptoms present after the age of 50 • An ECG should be performed on patients who have cardiac disease and start ziprasidone
Olanzapine (Zyprexa)	5–10 mg QHS	10–20	Increase 5 mg every 3–5 days, as tolerated	EPS (+) Orthostatic hypotension (+) Metabolic (+++) Sedation (++)	
Quetiapine[d] (Seroquel)	50–100 mg BID	300–800	Increase 50–100 mg every 2 days, as tolerated (monitor for orthostatic hypotension)	EPS (+/–) Orthostatic hypotension (+++) Metabolic abnormalities (++) Sedation (+++)	**First 4 weeks:** BMI, EPS, vital signs, prolactin (if clinical symptoms of hyperprolactinemia exist) **First 12 weeks:** BMI, EPS, vital signs, fasting glucose, a lipid profile **Quarterly:** BMI **Annually:** BMI, EPS, fasting glucose **Every 3–5 years:** lipid panel
Quetiapine XR (Seroquel XR)	300 mg QHS	400–800	Increase every 1–2 days, as tolerated	EPS (+/–) Orthostatic hypotension (+++) Metabolic abnormalities (++) Sedation (+++)	
Ziprasidone[e] (Geodon)	40 mg BID (with food)[f]	160	Increase every other day to target dose, as tolerated	EPS (+) Orthostatic hypotension (+) Metabolic abnormalities (+) Sedation (++) QTc prolongation (++)	
Aripiprazole (Abilify)	10–15 mg QAM	10–30	Increase dose after 2 days, as tolerated	EPS (+) Orthostatic hypotension (+) Metabolic abnormalities (+) Sedation (+)	
Paliperidone[g] (Invega)	6 mg QAM	6–12	Increase by increments of 3 mg every 5 days, as tolerated	EPS (++) Orthostatic hypotension (+) Metabolic abnormalities (++) Sedation (++)	

BMI, body mass index; ECG, electrocardiogram; EPS, extrapyramidal symptoms.

[a] Dosing information derived from Lehman AF, Lieberman JA, Dixon LB, et al; American Psychiatric Association. Practice guideline for the treatment of patients with schizophrenia, second edition. *Am J Psychiatry.* 2004;161(S2):1–56 and the authors' clinical expert opinion. These doses do not apply to geriatric or pediatric patients.

[b] Metabolic effects include hyperglycemia, weight gain, and hyperlipidemia.

[c] Patient may be able to transition to an intramuscular depot formulation of risperidone.

[d] Because of its low potency, quetiapine is ideal for patients who are sensitive to dopamine blockade, particularly patients sensitive to EPS or patients with psychosis in the context of Parkinson disease.

[e] Contraindications to the use of ziprasidone include persistent QTc >500 msec, recent acute myocardial infarction, and uncompensated heart failure.

[f] Ziprasidone should be taken with food as it increases bioavailability.

[g] Paliperidone is structurally similar to risperidone. Because it is the newest antipsychotic medication, the relative risks for metabolic syndrome and EPS are not fully known.

APPENDIX A   Psychotropic Medications

Table 6.6 Acute and Chronic Pharmacologic Management of Opioid Use Disorders

MEDICATION	ACUTE WITHDRAWAL	CHRONIC MAINTENANCE	CLINICAL INDICATIONS	ADVANTAGES	DISADVANTAGES/ SIDE EFFECTS
Methadone	• Begin: 10–30 mg • Day 2: Same as day 1 • Up-titration: 5–10 mg/day • Peak: 40–60 mg/day • Taper: ↓ 5 mg/ day	60–100+ mg/day	• Inpatient withdrawal • Chronic maintenance	• Proven efficacy • Decreases craving • Does not require with-drawal symp-toms before initiating	• Highly regulated in the U.S. • Potential for abuse and diversion • Constipation • Urinary retention • Increased sweating • Sexual dysfunction
Suboxone	• Begin: 4/1–8/2 mg/day • Day 2: 8/2–16/4 mg/day • Up-titration: ↑ 4 mg/day • Peak: 8/2–32/8 mg/day Taper: • Rapid: ↓ to 0 in 3 days • Moderate: ↓ 2 mg/day • Extended: ↓ 2 mg every third day	16/4–32/8 mg/day	• Inpatient withdrawal • Outpatient withdrawal and maintenance • Rapid withdrawal	• Minimal sedation • Low abuse potential • Every-other-day dosing	• Requires a special DEA license in the U.S. • Patients must have mild withdrawal before initiating • Side effect profile similar to methadone
Clonidine	• Begin: 0.1 mg TID • Peak: 1.2 mg/ day, divided BID or TID	N/A	• Nonopioid treatment of withdrawal • Rapid withdrawal	• Nonaddicting • Does not require with-drawal symp-toms before beginning	• Dose-limiting hypotension and bradycardia • Does not limit craving • Limited efficacy against many symptoms
LAAM	N/A	• 80–140 mg every other day	• Outpatient maintenance	• Every-other-day dosing	• Arrhythmias • Not approved in Europe; not avail-able in the U.S.
Naltrexone	N/A	• 50 mg daily; or • 100, 100, 150 mg every other day	• Outpatient maintenance for highly motivated patients who cannot be maintained on opioids	• No addictive or abuse potential • Every-other-day dosing	• Does not limit craving • Initiation requires prior abstinence • Increased risk of overdose if opioid use resumed • Dysphoria • Anxiety • GI discomfort

DEA, Drug Enforcement Agency; GI, gastrointestinal.

Table 7.6 FDA-Approved Pharmacologic Treatment of Alcohol Dependence

MEDICATION	DOSAGE	SIDE EFFECTS/CAUTION
Naltrexone (ReVia, Vivitrol)	• Start first dose at 25 mg given the possibility of precipitating withdrawal symptoms. If tolerated, subsequent doses may be given at 50 mg • 380 mg IM every 4 weeks	• Must be opioid-free for 7–10 days; otherwise, severe opioid withdrawal may occur • Contraindicated in active opioid users • Caution in patients with depression, suicidal ideation, thrombocytopenia, or liver disease • Pregnancy class C
Acamprosate (Campral)	• 666 mg TID	• May be continued despite alcohol relapse • Requires dose adjustment in renal failure • Caution in patients with depression, anxiety, and suicidal ideation • Pregnancy class C
Disulfiram (Antabuse)	• 250–500 mg/day; start at 125 mg	• Must be abstinent from alcohol for >12 hours prior to use • Toxic reaction of headache, nausea, malaise, and generalized distress when used with alcohol • Severe pharmacokinetic and additive drug–drug interactions are possible with isoniazid and metronidazole • Pregnancy class C

Table 12.4 Cognitive Enhancers: Properties and Uses

AGENT	PROTEIN BINDING	CYP450 ACTIVITY	USUAL DOSE	AVAILABLE FORMULATIONS	OTHER FEATURES	FDA-APPROVED INDICATION
ChEI						
Donepezil (Aricept)	96%	CYP 2D6, 3A4 Substrate	5 mg/day for 4–6 weeks, titrate to max. 10 mg/day	5-, 10-mg tab. 5-, 10-mg ODT	Once-daily dosing	Mild to severe AD
Rivastigmine (Exelon)	40%	None	1.5 mg BID for 2 weeks, titrate by 1.5 mg BID every 2 weeks to max. 6 mg BID (with food)	1.5-, 3-, 4.5-, 6-mg tab. 2-mg/mL sol. 4.6-, 9.5-mg/24 hours patch	Metabolized by cholinesterases Inhibits butyryl cholinesterase	Mild to moderate AD Mild to moderate dementia in PD
Galantamine (Razadyne)	18%	CYP 2D6, 3A4 substrate	4 mg PO BID for 4 weeks, titrate by 4 mg BID every 4 weeks to max. 12 mg BID	4-, 8-, 12-mg tab. 4-mg/mL sol. 8-, 16-, 24-mg ER tab. (once daily)	Nicotinic cholinergic receptor modulation	Mild to moderate AD
NMDA receptor antagonist						
Memantine (Namenda)	45%	None	5 mg/day, titrate by 5 mg/day every week to max. 10 mg BID	5-, 10-mg tab. 2-mg/mL sol.	No hepatic metabolism	Moderate to severe AD

AD, Alzheimer disease; ChEI, cholinesterase inhibitors; ER, extended release; FDA, Food and Drug Administration; NMDA, N-methyl-D-aspartate; ODT, orally disintegrating tablet; PD, Parkinson disease; sol., solution; tab., tablet.

Modified with permission from Kaufer DI, Cummings JL, Ketchel P, et al. Validation of the NPI-Q, a brief clinical form of the Neuropsychiatric Inventory. *J Neuropsychiatry Clin Neurosci.* 2000;12:233–239.

Table 13.7 Food and Drug Administration (FDA)-Approved Drugs for Insomnia

DRUGS	ADULT DOSE (MG)	HALF-LIFE (HOURS)	ONSET (MINUTES)	PEAK EFFECT (HOURS)	MAJOR EFFECTS/CLINICAL COMMENTS
Benzodiazepines (BZPs)					*Caution in elderly patients.* Tolerance to BZPs develops to the sedative, hypnotic, and anticonvulsant effects
Estazolam (ProSom)	1–2	10–24	60	$1/2$–$1^1/2$	Short-term (7–10 days) treatment for frequent arousals and early-morning awakening. Not as useful for initial insomnia. Avoid in patients with obstructive sleep apnea-hypoapnea. **Caution** in elderly patients and those with liver disease. High doses can cause respiratory depression
Flurazepam (Dalmane)	15–30	47–100	15–20	3–6	Short-term (7–10 days) treatment for middle and terminal insomnia. Increased daytime sedation over time. **Caution** in elderly patients
Temazepam (Restoril)	15–30	6–16		2–3	Short-term (7–10 days) treatment for sleep onset and maintenance. Doses ≥30 mg/day: morning grogginess, nausea, headaches, and vivid dreaming
Nonbenzodiazepines (non-BZPs)					
Eszopiclone (Lunesta)	2–3	6–9	Rapid	1	In elderly start with 1–2 mg. Rapid onset; should be in bed when taking medication. For faster sleep onset, do not ingest with high-fat foods. No tolerance after 6 months
Zaleplon (Sonata)	5–20	1	Rapid	1	Short-term (7–10 days) treatment for initial insomnia
Zolpidem (Ambien, Ambien CR)	5–20	1.4–4.5	30	2–4	Short-term (7–10 days) treatment for initial and middle insomnia (generic form is available). Rapid onset; should be in bed when taking medication. For faster sleep onset, do not ingest with food
Zolpidem CR (Ambien CR)	12.5	1.4–4.5	30	2–4	Short-term (7–10 days) treatment for initial and middle insomnia (generic form is available). Rapid onset; should be in bed when taking medication. For faster sleep onset, do not ingest with food
	6.25–12.5	1.4–4.5	30	2–4	Used for sleep induction and sleep maintenance
Melatonin agonist					
Ramelton (Rozerem)	8	1–2	30	1–$1^1/2$	Used for initial and middle insomnia. For faster sleep onset, do not ingest with high-fat foods. No tolerance or potential for addiction. **Contraindicated** with fluvoxamine. Should not be used concurrently with melatonin

All sedative-hypnotics should be used with caution and at a lower starting dose when given to the elderly. All sedative-hypnotics should be taken only if the patient plans to go to bed immediately after taking the medication.

Table 13.8 Drugs Commonly Used "Off-Label" for Insomnia

DRUG	PERTINENT SIDE EFFECTS	COMMENTS
Antidepressants		
Mirtazapine (Remeron)	Somnolence and increased appetite	May be beneficial if patient has comorbid depression and insomnia. Mirtazapine's sedating effect is inversely dose dependent. As the dose increases, the noradrenergic activity counteracts the sleep-inducing H_1 antihistaminic effect of mirtazapine
Trazodone (Desyrel)	Residual daytime sedation, head-ache, orthostatic hypotension, priapism, cardiac arrhythmias	One of the most commonly prescribed agents for the treatment of insomnia. May be beneficial if patient has comorbid depression and insomnia. May be an acceptable alternative for patients for whom BzRAs are contraindicated (severe hypercapnea or hypoxemia, or history of substance abuse or dependence). Usually dosed much lower (50–100 mg) than when used for depression
TCAs	Delirium, decreased cognition and seizure threshold, orthostatic hypotension, tachycardia, ECG abnormalities	**Avoid** in hospitalized patients due to their anticholinergic, antihistaminic, and cardiovascular side effects. Not recommended as a treatment for insomnia or other sleep problems unless comorbid depression is present. As with other antidepressants, TCAs are usually used at significantly lower doses than for depression
Antihistamines		
Diphenhydramine (Benadryl)	Residual daytime sedation, weight gain, delirium, orthostatic hypotension, blurred vision, urinary retention	Antihistamines are one of the most commonly used over-the-counter agents for chronic insomnia. If possible, avoid in patients >60 years old
Hydroxyzine (Vistaril)	Residual daytime sedation, weight gain, delirium, orthostatic hypotension, blurred vision, urinary retention	Efficacy as an anxiolytic has been not established. Not FDA approved for insomnia. **Avoid** in patients >60 years old and those with closed-angle glaucoma, prostatic hypertrophy, severe asthma, and COPD
Antipsychotics		
Quetiapine (Seroquel)	Sedation, orthostatic hypotension, metabolic derangements (e.g., weight gain, dyslipidemia, and glucose dysregulation)	The most sedating of the atypical antipsychotics, it is frequently used as a sleep aid. Not recommended for insomnia or other sleep problems unless there is comorbid psychotic or bipolar disorder. Is dosed much lower (25–100 mg) when used for insomnia. Other less expensive sedative-hypnotic agents should be used first

BzRAs, benzodiazepine receptor agonists; COPD, chronic obstructive pulmonary disease; ECG, electrocardiogram; FDA, Food and Drug Administration; TCAs, tricyclic antidepressants (doxepin, amitriptyline, imipramine, nortriptyline, desipramine).

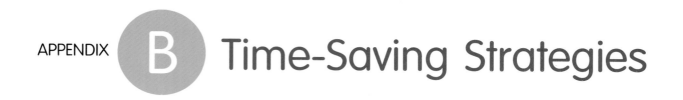

APPENDIX B Time-Saving Strategies

Chapter 1: The Primary Care Psychiatric Interview

Table 1.3 Key Features of the Mental Status Examination (MSE)	
Appearance	• What is the status of the hygiene and grooming and are there any recent changes in appearance?
Attitude	• How does the patient relate to the clinician? • Is the patient cooperative, guarded, irritable, etc., during the interview?
Speech	• What are the rate, rhythm, and volume of speech?
Mood	• How does the patient describe his or her mood? • This should be reported as described by the patient.
Affect	• Does the patient's facial expressions have full range and reactivity? • How quickly does the affect change (lability)? • Is the affect congruent with the stated mood and is it appropriate to topics under discussion?
Thought process	• *How* is the patient thinking? • Does the patient change subjects quickly or is the train of thought difficult to follow?
Thought content	• *What* is the patient thinking? • What is the main theme or subject matter when the patient talks? • Does the patient have any delusions, obsessions, or compulsions?
Perceptions	• Does the patient have auditory, visual, or tactile hallucinations?
Cognition	• Is the patient alert? • Is the patient oriented to person, place, time, and the purpose of the interview?
Insight	• Does the patient recognize that there is an illness or disorder present? • Is there a clear understanding of the treatment plan and prognosis?
Judgment	• How will the patient secure food, clothing, and shelter in a safe environment? • Is the patient able to make decisions that support a safe and reasonable treatment plan?

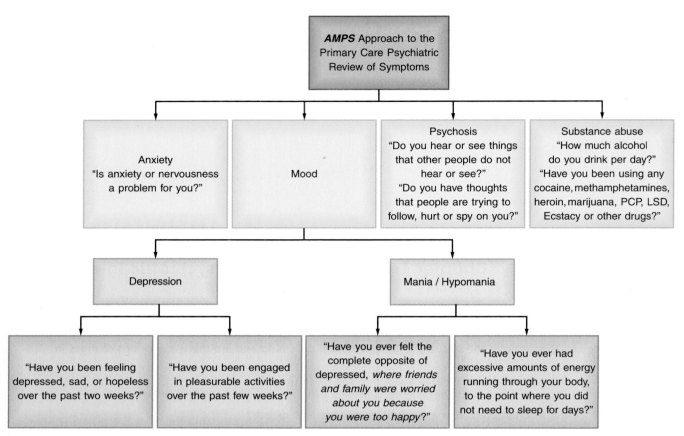

Figure 1.1 Psychiatric review of systems: AMPS screening tool.

Supplemental Psychiatric History Form

Name: _____ **Date:** _____
Reason for Appointment: _____

Past Psychiatric Diagnoses (circle if applicable): anxiety, depression, bipolar disorder, schizophrenia, schizoaffective disorder,alcohol misuse, drug misuse, borderline personality disorder, other mental diagnosis

Have you ever been treated by a psychiatrist or other mental health provider?	Yes / No
Have you ever been a patient in a psychiatric hospital?	Yes / No
Have you ever tried to hurt or kill yourself?	Yes / No
Have you ever taken a medication for psychiatric reasons?	Yes / No

If yes, please list the most recent medication(s) below:
- #1: _____ Did you have any problems with this medication? Yes / No
- #2: _____ Did you have any problems with this medication? Yes / No
- #3: _____ Did you have any problems with this medication? Yes / No
- #4: _____ Did you have any problems with this medication? Yes / No
- #5: _____ Did you have any problems with this medication? Yes / No

Family Psychiatric History: Did your grandparents, parents, or siblings ever have severe problems with depression, bipolar disorder, anxiety, schizophrenia, or any other emotional problems?   Yes / No

Social and Developmental History:
Socioeconomic Status
Are you currently unemployed?   Yes / No
Are you having any problems at home?   Yes / No
Interpersonal Relationships
Are you having any problems with close personal relationships?   Yes / No
Legal History
Have you ever had problems with the law?   Yes / No
Developmental History
Have you ever been physically, verbally, or sexually abused?   Yes / No
What was the highest grade you completed in school?   _____

Anxiety Symptoms, Mood Symptoms, Psychotic Symptoms, Substance Use
Is anxiety or nervousness a problem for you?   Yes / No
Mood Symptoms
- Have you been feeling depressed, sad, or hopeless over the past two weeks?   Yes / No
- Have you had a decreased interest level in pleasurable activities over the past few weeks?   Yes / No
- Have you ever felt the complete opposite of depressed, *when friends and family were worried about you because you were too happy?*   Yes / No
- Have you ever had excessive amounts of energy running through your body, to the point where you did not need to sleep for days?   Yes / No
- Do you have any thoughts of wanting to hurt or kill yourself or someone else?   Yes / No
Psychotic Symptoms
Do you hear or see things that other people do not hear or see?   Yes / No
Do you have thoughts that people are trying to follow, hurt or spy on you?   Yes / No
Substance Use
How many packs of cigarettes do you smoke per day?   _____
How much alcohol do you drink per day?   _____
Have you ever used cocaine, methamphetamines, heroin, marijuana, PCP, LSD, Ecstacy or other drugs?   Yes / No

Figure 1.2 Supplemental Psychiatric History Form.

Chapter 2: Mood Disorders—Depression

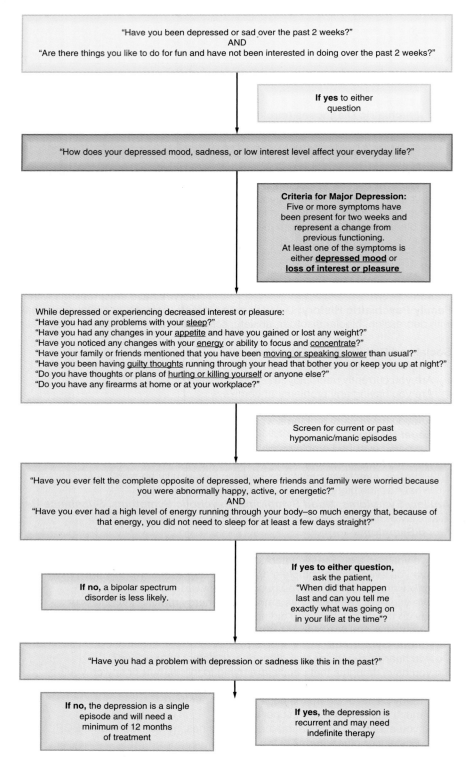

Figure 2.1 Diagnosing depression in the primary care setting.

Patient Health Questionnaire (PHQ-9)
Nine Symptom Depression Checklist

Name: _____   Date: _____

Over the *last 2 weeks*, how often have you been
bothered by any of the following problems?
(Please circle your answer.)

	Not at All	Several Days	More than Half the Days	Nearly Every Day
1. Little interest or pleasure in doing things	0	1	2	3
2. Feeling down, depressed, or hopeless	0	1	2	3
3. Trouble falling or staying asleep, or sleeping too much	0	1	2	3
4. Feeling tired or having little energy	0	1	2	3
5. Poor appetite or overeating	0	1	2	3
6. Feeling bad about yourself—or that you are a failure or have let yourself or your family down	0	1	2	3
7. Trouble concentrating on things, such as reading the newspaper or watching television	0	1	2	3
8. Moving or speaking so slowly that other people could have noticed. Or the opposite— being so fidgety or restless that you have been moving around a lot more than usual	0	1	2	3
9. Thoughts that you would be better off dead or of hurting yourself in some way	0	1	2	3

Add Columns, [_____] + [_____] + [_____]

Total Score*, [_____]   *Score is for healthcare provider incorporation

10. If you circled *any* problems, how *difficult* have these problems made it for you to do your work, take care of things at home, or get along with other people? (Please circle your answer.)	Not Difficult at All	Somewhat Difficult	Very Difficult	Extremely Difficult

A score of: 0–4 is considered non-depressed; 5–9 mild depression; 10–14 moderate depression;
15–19 moderately severe depression; and 20–27 severe depression.

Figure 2.2 Patient Health Questionnaire (PHQ-9) nine-symptom depression checklist. (PHQ is adapted from PRIME MD TODAY. PHQ Copyright ©1999 Pfizer Inc. All rights reserved. Reproduced with permission. PRIME MD TODAY is a trademark of Pfizer Inc.)

APPENDIX B   Time-Saving Strategies

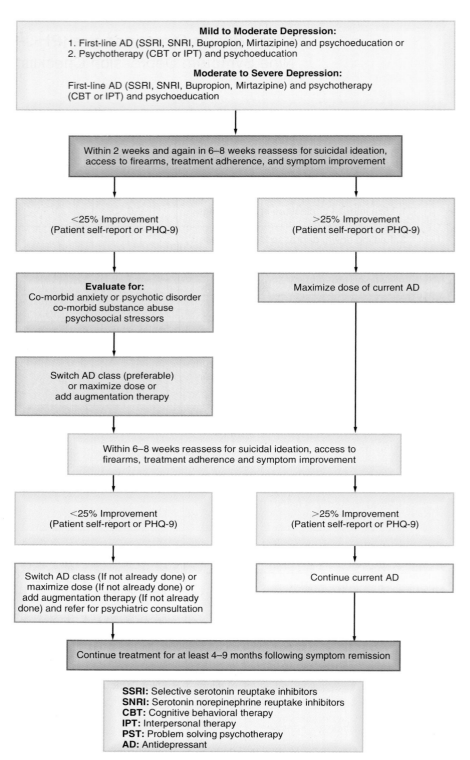

Figure 2.3 Primary care treatment algorithm for depression.

THE MOOD DISORDER QUESTIONNAIRE

Instructions: Please answer each question to the best of your ability.

	YES	NO
1. Has there ever been a period of time when you were not your usual self and...		
...you felt so good or so hyper that other people thought you were not your normal self or you were so hyper that you got into trouble?	○	○
...you were so irritable that you shouted at people or started fights or arguments?	○	○
...you felt much more self-confident than usual?	○	○
...you got much less sleep than usual and found you didn't really miss it?	○	○
...you were much more talkative or spoke much faster than usual?	○	○
...thoughts raced through your head or you couldn't slow your mind down?	○	○
...you were so easily distracted by things around you that you had trouble concentrating or staying on track?	○	○
...you had much more energy than usual?	○	○
...you were much more active or did many more things than usual?	○	○
...you were much more social or outgoing than usual, for example, you telephoned friends in the middle of the night?	○	○
...you were much more interested in sex than usual?	○	○
...you did things that were unusual for you or that other people might have thought were excessive, foolish, or risky?	○	○
...spending money got you or your family into trouble?	○	○
2. If you checked YES to more than one of the above, have several of these ever happened during the same period of time?	○	○
3. How much of a problem did any of these cause you—like being unable to work; having family, money, or legal troubles; getting into arguments or fights? *Please circle one response only.* No Problem Minor Problem Moderate Problem Serious Problem		
4. Have any of your blood relatives (i.e., children, siblings, parents, grandparents, aunts, uncles) had manic-depressive illness or bipolar disorder?	○	○
5. Has a health professional ever told you that you have manic-depressive illness or bipolar disorder?	○	○

If the patient answers:

1. **"Yes"** to 7 or more of the 13 items in question number 1;

AND

2. **"Yes"** to question number 2;

AND

3. **"Moderate"** or **"Serious"** to question number 3;

you have a positive screen. All three of the criteria above should be met. A positive screen should be followed by a comprehensive medical evaluation for bipolar spectrum disorder.

Figure 3.1. The mood disorder questionnaire (6). (© 2000 by American Psychiatric Publishing, Inc. Reprinted with permission. This instrument is designed for screening purposes only and is not to be used as a diagnostic tool.)

Table 3.3 Medications and Medical Conditions Associated with Mood Disturbances

Medications
- Antidepressants
- Corticosteroids
- Dopamine agonists
- Isoniazid
- Interferon
- Opioids
- Sedatives-hypnotics
- Stimulants
- Sympathomimetics

General Medical Conditions
- Adrenal disorders
- CNS infections (e.g., HIV, herpes, syphilis)
- Brain tumor
- Huntington disease
- Multiple sclerosis
- Parkinson disease
- Porphyria
- Seizure disorder
- Stroke
- Systemic lupus erythematosus
- Thyroid disorder
- Traumatic brain injury
- Vasculitis
- Vitamin B_{12} deficiency
- Wilson disease

Substance Conditions
Intoxication
- Alcohol
- Amphetamines
- Cocaine
- Caffeine
- Phencyclidine
- Hallucinogens

Withdrawal
- Alcohol
- Barbiturates
- Benzodiazepines

Other Psychiatric Conditions
- Schizoaffective disorder
- Schizophrenia
- Major depressive disorder
- Attention deficit hyperactivity disorder
- Borderline personality disorder
- Narcissistic personality disorder

CNS, central nervous system; HIV, human immunodeficiency virus.

Chapter 4: Anxiety Disorders

Table 4.1 GAD-7

How often during the past 2 weeks have you felt bothered by:

1. Feeling nervous, anxious, or on edge?	0	1	2	3
2. Not being able to stop or control worrying?	0	1	2	3
3. Worrying too much about different things?	0	1	2	3
4. Trouble relaxing?	0	1	2	3
5. Being so restless that it is hard to sit still?	0	1	2	3
6. Becoming easily annoyed or irritable?	0	1	2	3
7. Feeling afraid as if something awful might happen?	0	1	2	3

Each question is answered on a scale of:
0 = not at all
1 = several days
2 = more than half the days
3 = nearly every day

A score of 8 or more should prompt further diagnostic evaluation for an anxiety disorder.

From Spitzer RL, Kroenke K, Williams JB, et al. A brief measure for assessing generalized anxiety disorder: the GAD-7. *Arch Intern Med.* 2006;166:1092–1097.

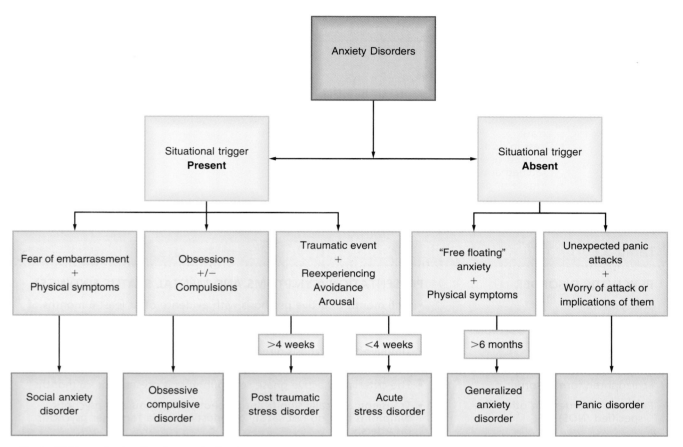

Figure 4.1 Diagnostic algorithm for anxiety disorders.

Chapter 5: Psychotic Disorders

Table 5.3 Definition of Psychotic Symptoms

POSITIVE SYMPTOMS	WHAT ARE THEY?	OFTEN CONFUSED WITH...
Hallucinations	• Sensory perception in the absence of sensory stimuli. May occur with any of the senses (visual, auditory, olfactory, skin sensations, etc.)	• Perceptual distortions or illusions: sensory misperception in the presence of stimuli (e.g., mistakenly identifying a chair as a person) • ''Mystical experiences,'' often part of a spiritual belief system • May be due to medical disorders (temporal seizures, migraine auras, uremia, hepatic encephalopathy, etc.)
Delusions	• Fixed belief that is at odds with reality (delusions of persecution, grandeur, parasites, etc.)	• Beliefs due to environmental, social, cultural, or spiritual/religious background (e.g., belief in God's influence over health or destiny, transfer of the soul with blood transfusions, breaking a mirror brings bad luck, etc.)
Bizarre delusions	• Not physically possible (e.g., people walking through walls or traveling back in time)	• Nonbizarre delusions are possible, but untrue—for instance, a patient feeling that ''a celebrity is in love with me''
Thought disorder	• Disorders of thought process or *how* one thinks. Patients may have difficulty with logical construction of thoughts (tangential, word salad, flight of ideas, loosening of associations, neologisms, etc.) or expression of their thoughts in unintelligible ways	• Delirium, dementia, aphasia, mania

(Continued)

Table 5.3 Definition of Psychotic Symptoms (*Continued*)

POSITIVE SYMPTOMS	WHAT ARE THEY?	OFTEN CONFUSED WITH...
Bizarre behaviors	• Inability to dress, act, or interact in socially appropriate ways. Behaviors may be crude (cursing, solicitous), offensive, violent, or erratic • Dress in poorly fitting clothing, wear makeup smeared over the face or buttons mismatched and zippers undone • Urinate or defecate in unusual places, even if a bathroom is nearby	• Social trends (intergenerational conflicts), unusual fashions, fads, or social groups with nonconformist behaviors

Table 5.6 Differentiating Psychiatric Causes of Psychosis

PSYCHOTIC DISORDER	PRESENTATION (SYMPTOMS AND MENTAL STATUS FINDINGS)
Schizophrenia	• One month of active psychosis with evidence of at least 6 months of intermittent or attenuated psychotic symptoms and diminished social or occupational function
Brief psychotic disorder	• Time-limited psychosis directly related to a distressing event in a person's life
Schizophreniform disorder	• The criteria for active phase schizophrenia is present for <6 months
Psychotic disorder not otherwise specified (NOS)	• Transient, clinically significant psychotic symptoms and psychotic symptoms that do not satisfy diagnostic criteria for other psychotic disorders.
Schizoaffective disorder	• Co-occurring psychotic symptoms and mood disturbance that may be difficult to distinguish from mood, psychotic, dissociative, somatic, or personality disorders • Psychotic symptoms are present during periods of normal mood • Categorized as depressed or bipolar type
Delusional disorder	• "Nonbizarre" delusion(s) that may actually occur in the real world
Bipolar disorder	• *Episodic* mood disorder usually characterized by depressive or manic symptoms • Psychotic symptoms may occur during either depressive or manic episodes and usually remit upon treatment of the mood abnormality
Major depressive disorder	• *Episodic* periods of depression and temporally associated psychotic symptoms • Psychotic symptoms may occur during a depressive episode and usually remit upon treatment of the mood abnormality
Posttraumatic stress disorder (PTSD)	• PTSD is often associated with hypervigilance, which can be confused with paranoia, and re-experiencing symptoms in severe form may include outright perceptual disturbances (e.g., auditory or visual hallucinations)
Borderline personality disorder	• Personality disorder characterized by dysregulation of affect and tendency toward brief periods of psychotic symptoms during distress
Dissociative disorders	• Disorders characterized by disruption of a continuous sense of self, including amnestic episodes or transition to altered behaviors and expressions
Substance intoxication or withdrawal	• Illicit drugs like cocaine, methamphetamine, heroin, and even alcohol can cause psychotic symptoms in the context of both intoxication and withdrawal
Malingering	• Intentionally produced symptoms for external gain (e.g., disability insurance or to avoid legal prosecution)

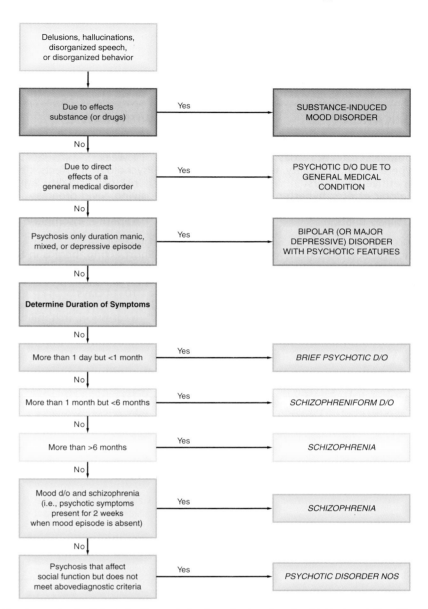

Figure 5.1 Diagnostic algorithm for psychosis. (Adapted with permission from the American Psychiatric Association. *Diagnostic and Statistical Manual of Mental Disorders*. 4th ed., text revision. Washington, DC: American Psychiatric Publishing, Inc.; 2004.)

APPENDIX B Time-Saving Strategies

Chapter 6: Substance Use Disorders—Stimulants and Opioids

Table 6.3 Intoxication and Withdrawal

	INTOXICATION	WITHDRAWAL
Stimulants	Time course: 24–48 hours Psychological effects: restlessness, agitation, hyperactivity, irritability, impulsiveness, repetitive behaviors Physiologic effects: hypertension, tachycardia, tachypnea, hyperthermia, pupillary dilation	Time course: peak in 2–4 days, resolution in 1 week Psychological effects: depression, increased risk of suicidality, agitation, paranoia, craving, vivid dreams Physiologic effects: fatigue, increased appetite, insomnia or hypersomnia
Opioids	Time course: 6–24 hours Psychological effects: drowsy/sedated, impaired memory, impaired attention Physiologic effects: pupillary constriction, decreased respiratory rate, decreased bowel sounds, slurred speech	Time course: Short-acting: begins in 6–8 hours, resolves in 7–10 days Long-acting: begins in 1–3 days, resolves in 10–14 days Psychological effects: restlessness, depression, irritability Physiologic effects: myalgias and arthralgias, diarrhea, abdominal cramping, lacrimation, rhinorrhea, piloerection, yawning, insomnia, temperature dysregulation

Table 6.8 FRAMES Guideline to Motivational Interviewing

- *Feedback* is given regarding the negative consequences of substance use behaviors, including future risk
- *Responsibility* for change emphasizes personal choice
- *Advice* is given about behavioral change, from reduction to abstinence
- *Menu* of treatment options reinforces personal responsibility and choice
- *Empathic* and nonjudgmental counseling style
- *Self-efficacy* encourages a sense of optimistic empowerment and positive change

Adapted from Miller WR, Sanchez VC. Motivating young adults for treatment and lifestyle change. In Howard G, ed. *Issues in Alcohol Use and Misuse by Young Adults.* Notre Dame, IN: University of Notre Dame Press; 1994:55–82.

Chapter 7: Substance Use Disorders—Alcohol

Table 7.3 Brief Screening Instruments for Alcohol Use Disorders

CAGE Questionnaire[a,b]

1. Have you ever felt that you should **C**ut down on your alcohol use?
2. Have people **A**nnoyed you by asking about or criticizing your alcohol use?
3. Have you ever felt **G**uilty about your alcohol use?
4. Have you ever used alcohol as an **E**ye-opener first thing in the morning to avoid unpleasant feelings?

Alcohol Use Disorder Identification Test-Consumption (AUDIT-C)[c,d]

1. How often do you have a drink containing alcohol?

Never	0
Monthly or less	1
2–4 times a month	2
2–3 times a week	3
4 or more times a week	4

2. How many drinks containing alcohol do you have on a typical day when you are drinking?

1 or 2	0
3 or 4	1
5 or 6	2
7 to 9	3
10 or more	4

3. How often do you have six or more drinks on one occasion?

Never	0
Less than monthly	1
Monthly	2
Weekly	3
Daily or almost daily	4

[a] One affirmative answer should prompt further questioning about alcohol use and two or more affirmative answers increase the chance of alcohol use disorders.
[b] From U.S. Preventive Services Task Force. Screening and behavioral counseling interventions in primary care to reduce alcohol misuse: recommendation statement. *Ann Intern Med.* 2004;140(7):554–556.
[c] A score of 4 or more most likely indicates alcohol abuse or dependence and warrants further investigation.
[d] From Fiellin DA, Reid MC, O'Connor PG. Screening for alcohol problems in primary care: a systematic review. *Arch Intern Med.* 2000;160:1977–1989.

Table 7.7 Brief Intervention for Alcohol Use Disorders

STEPS	COMMENTS	SAMPLE STATEMENTS
1. Assessment and direct feedback	Ask about alcohol use (CAGE, AUDIT-C) Provide education and feedback about the connection between alcohol use and legal, occupational, or relationship problems	"Your liver disease is likely to be related to alcohol use. Would you like me to give you some information about your hepatitis and alcohol use?" "I am very concerned about your drinking and how it is affecting your health."
2. Goal setting	Individually tailored goals based on collaboration between the patient and the provider Goals may change depending on readiness for change Goals should be realistic and include psychotherapy, social support, and use of medications when indicated	"What are your thoughts about alcohol use?" "Although I would advise complete alcohol cessation, how realistic is that for you?" "Although the use of medications is important in your recovery, it is critical to attend AA and monitor for triggers that may lead to relapse."

(Continued)

APPENDIX B   Time-Saving Strategies

Table 7.7 Brief Intervention for Alcohol Use Disorders (*Continued*)

STEPS	COMMENTS	SAMPLE STATEMENTS
3. Behavioral modification	Identify situational triggers, finding other enjoyable activities and adaptive coping skills Includes relapse prevention	"What causes you to start drinking?" "What else can you do when you feel alone, stressed, or frustrated?" "Who can you talk to when you feel that you have failed to cut down on drinking?"
4. Self-help	Encourage self-discipline and increased self-awareness about alcohol use disorder	"Would you like an information booklet about alcohol addiction?" "Do you know where you can get help for your drinking problem?"
5. Follow-up and reinforcement	Often considered the most important aspect of the treatment plan Provide praise, reassurance, and encouragement during periods of sobriety Returning to appointment is a sign of patient motivation and efforts, even if relapse occurs	"I'm very glad to see you come back to talk more about your alcohol use." "How did your plan to stop or reduce your drinking work?"

Modified from Bertholet N, Daeppen JB, Wietlisbach V, et al. Reduction of alcohol consumption by brief alcohol intervention in primary care: systematic review and meta-analysis. *Arch Intern Med.* 2005;165:986–995.

Chapter 8: Unexplained Physical Symptoms— Somatoform Disorders

Table 8.1 Somatoform Disorders: Diagnostic Criteria

DSM-IV-TR	DEFINITION
Somatization disorder	• Many unexplained physical complaints before age 30 • Four pain, two gastrointestinal, one sexual, and one pseudoneurologic symptom
Undifferentiated somatoform disorder	• One or more unexplained physical complaints • Duration of at least 6 months
Conversion disorder	• One or more unexplainable, voluntary motor or sensory neurologic deficits • Directly preceded by psychological stress
Pain disorder	• Pain in one or more sites that is largely due to psychological factors
Hypochondriasis	• Preoccupation with a nonexistent disease despite a thorough medical work-up • Does not meet criteria for a delusion
Body dysmorphic disorder	• Preoccupation with an imagined defect in physical appearance
Somatoform disorder not otherwise specified (NOS)	• Somatoform symptoms that do not meet criteria for any specific somatoform disorder

All the above disorders (1) cause significant social/occupational dysfunction, (2) are not due to other general medical or psychiatric conditions; and (3) are not intentionally produced or related to secondary gain.
From American Psychiatric Publishing, Inc. *Diagnostic and Statistical Manual of Mental Disorders,* 4th ed., text revision. Washington, DC: American Psychiatric Association; 2000.

Table 8.2 CARE MD – Treatment Guidelines for Somatoform Disorders

CBT/Consultation	• Follow the CBT treatment plan developed by the therapist and patient
Assess	• Rule out potential general medical causes for the somatic complaints • Treat co-morbid psychiatric disorders
Regular visits	• Short frequent visits with focused exams • Discuss recent stressors and healthy coping strategies • Overtime, the patient should agree to stop over utilization of medical care (e.g. frequent emergency room visits, or excessive calls and pages to the primary care provider)
Empathy	• "Become the patient" for a brief time • During visits, spend more time listening to the patient rather than jumping to a diagnostic test • Acknowledge patient's reported discomfort
Med-psych interface	• Help the patient self-discover the connection between physical complaints and emotional stressors ("the mind-body" connection) • Avoid comments like, "your symptoms are all psychological" or "there is nothing wrong with you medically"
Do no harm	• Avoid unnecessary diagnostic procedures • When possible, minimize unnecessary requests for consultation to medical specialists • Once a reasonable diagnostic work up is negative, feel comfortable with a somatoform disorder diagnosis and initiate treatment

From McCarron R. Somatization in the primary care setting. *Psychiatric Times.* 2006;23(6):32–34.

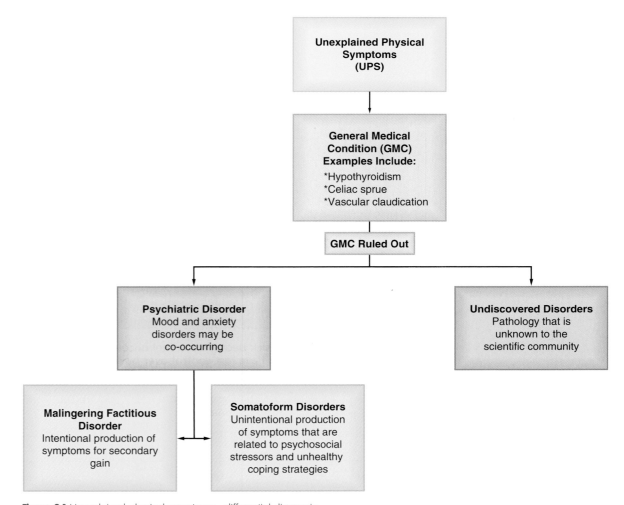

Figure 8.1 Unexplained physical symptoms—differential diagnosis.

Chapter 9: Eating Disorders

Table 9.1 DSM-IV-TR Criteria

EATING DISORDER (SUBTYPES)	CRITERIA
Anorexia nervosa • Restricting • Binge eating/ purging	All four criteria need to be met for diagnosis • Refusal to maintain body weight at or above normal weight for age and height (<85% expected body weight) • Intense fear of gaining weight even though underweight • Disturbed thoughts about body weight or shape and denial of symptom severity • Amenorrhea

Bulimia nervosa
• Purging
• Nonpurging type
	• Binge eating characterized by
	  ○ Eating an amount of food larger than most people would consume in a similar period of time and circumstance
	  ○ Loss of control during the binge
	• Recurrent inappropriate compensatory behaviors (i.e., exercise, diuretics, laxatives, purging) to prevent weight gain
	• Binge eating and behaviors occur at least twice a week for 3 months
	• Self-evaluation unduly influenced by body shape and weight

Binge eating disorder	• Recurrent episodes of binge eating characterized by
	  ○ Eating larger amount of food than normal during short period of time
	  ○ Lack of control over eating during binge period
	• Binge eating episodes are associated with
	  ○ Eating until uncomfortably full
	  ○ Eating large amounts of food when not physically hungry
	  ○ Eating more rapidly than normal
	  ○ Eating alone because of embarrassment by how much food is consumed
	  ○ Feeling disgusted, depressed, or guilty after overeating
	• Binge eating occurs at least 2 days a week for 6 months
	• Binge eating not associated with regular inappropriate compensatory behavior

Eating disorder NOS	• Disordered eating that does not meet full criteria for anorexia nervosa or bulimia nervosa

Modified from American Psychiatric Association. *Diagnostic and Statistical Manual of Mental Disorders.* 4th ed., text revision. Washington, DC: American Psychiatric Publishing, Inc.; 2000.

Table 9.3 SCOFF: Validated Screening Questions for Eating Disorders in Primary Care Settings

• Do you make yourself **s**ick because you feel uncomfortably full?
• Do you worry that you have lost **c**ontrol over how much you eat?
• Have you recently lost more than **o**ne stone (14 pounds or 6.3 kg) in a 3-month period?
• Do you belief yourself to be **f**at when others say you are too thin?
• Would you say that **f**ood dominates your life?

Two positive answers are highly predictive of either anorexia nervosa or bulimia nervosa.

From Morgan JF, Reid F, Lacey H. The SCOFF questionnaire: assessment of a new screening tool for eating disorders. *BMJ.* 1999;319:1467–1468.

Chapter 10: Personality Disorders

Table 10.3 Feelings of Countertransference and Reactions to Avoid

PROVIDER'S FEELING	PERSONALITY DISORDER	POTENTIAL PROVIDER PITFALLS	SUGGESTED ACTION
Anger (patient is viewed as manipulative)	• Borderline • Antisocial • Narcissistic	Overreaction to provocation, retaliation (e.g., verbal/physical abuse of patient, substandard care, inappropriate comments in charting)	• Be aware of feelings • Process in Balint groups • Strictly adhere to evidence-based standard of care
Fear of patient (physical or legal threat)	• Antisocial • Paranoid	Immediate emotional or physical overresponse (out of proportion to threat)	• Maintain personal safety • Document thoroughly
Sympathy	• Borderline (sympathy by some providers associated with negative views by other providers may represent *splitting* by the patient) • Dependent	Overindulgence or tendency to rescue the patient	• Provide regular, structured, and scheduled visits with the same provider that do not run over scheduled time • Manage splitting in interdisciplinary meetings to make sure all members of team are acting in accordance with treatment plan and not providing "special" treatment
Self-doubt	• Narcissistic	Putting down the patient instead; questioning your own abilities in a nonrealistic way	• Be aware of your behavior • Examine your abilities in a realistic way • Process in Balint groups
Frustration	• Borderline • Avoidant • Dependent	Patients may not follow through with treatment recommendations or rely overly on provider	• Set clear expectations • Ally yourself with patient's family/friends to assist (as permitted by privacy restrictions)
Attraction	• Histrionic • Borderline	Inappropriate relationship with patient	• Consider using a chaperone for exams requiring examination of genitalia • Do not see patient after hours or in social settings

Table 10.5 Using E MC² as Part of the Treatment for Borderline Personality Disorder

Empathy – Try to fully understand the details of one's turbulent and chaotic life.

"Manage," not "cure" – Personalities are formed early and can be difficult to modify. Improvement may be gradual and temporary with frequent "relapses" of behavior.

Countertransference – Consider why you are feeling a certain way before you respond to a patient.

Comorbidity – Screen for other psychopathology (e.g., mood, anxiety, and substance use disorders).

Chapter 11: Cultural Considerations in Primary Care Psychiatry

Table 11.3 High-Yield Questions

A. **Questions to assess cultural identity**

1. Do you identify with a particular culture or religion?
2. Where were you born and raised? How did you come to live in this area?
3. How comfortable do you feel with being part of "mainstream American" culture?
4. Please describe the significant activities and groups in your life.

B. **Questions to assess the psychosocial environment**

1. Who are the important people in your life?
2. How much do you involve others when making health care decisions?
3. What would your family expect of you if you were well?
4. Do you have any contact with the community?

C. **Questions to assist the therapeutic relationship**

1. In what language do you prefer to communicate?
2. Some people prefer to see a provider from their own cultural group, and we are happy to honor their preference when we can. What are your preferences with regard to having a provider?
3. As your doctor, it is important for me to treat you with respect. Are there things that are done in your culture to convey respect? What things would be considered disrespectful for a provider to do?

Table 11.5 Using the Outline for Cultural Formulation

- Identify salient features of cultural identity
  - Encourages patient's active participation
  - Is an effective way to build rapport
  - Helps to inform the rest of the cultural formulation

- Develop collaborative explanatory models
  - Improves relevancy of treatment
  - Improves adherence to treatment

- Clarify psychosocial context
  - Identifies key decision makers
  - Clarifies decision-making process

- Examine the impact of the cultural similarities and differences between you and the patient
  - Appreciation of one's own cultural identity and history is the foundation to connect with another's

Chapter 12: Geriatric Psychiatry—Dementias

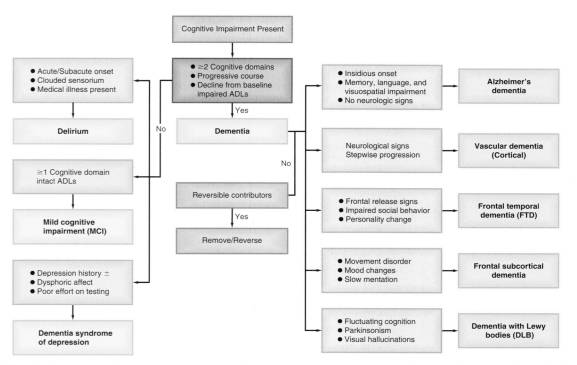

Figure 12.1 Algorithm for dementia diagnosis. ADLs, activities of daily living; CVA, cerebrovascular accident; DLB, dementia with Lewy bodies; FTD, frontotemporal dementia; MCI, mild cognitive impairment.

Table 12.3 Suggested Dementia Work-Up

ALWAYS	WHEN SUSPICION EXISTS
BUN/creatinine	CSF studies
CBC	Electroencephalogram
Calcium	Erythrocyte sedimentation rate
CT/MRI	Folate
Electrolytes	Heavy metal screen
Glucose	HIV
Liver function tests	Lyme serology
Thyroid function tests	RPR
Urinalysis	Testosterone
Vitamin B_{12}	Urine toxicology

BUN, blood urea nitrogen; CBC, complete blood count; CSF, cerebrospinal fluid; CT, computerized tomography; HIV, human immunodeficiency virus; MRI, magnetic resonance imaging; RPR, rapid plasma reagin.

From Taylor WD, Doraiswamy PM. Use of the laboratory in the diagnostic workup of older adults. In: *Textbook of Geriatric Psychiatry*. Washington, DC: American Psychiatric Publishing; 2004:179–188.

Chapter 13: Sleep Disorders

Table 13.4 Characteristics of Sleep in Various Psychiatric Diagnoses

DSM-IV-TR DIAGNOSIS	COMMON SLEEP COMPLAINTS AND SYMPTOMS
Major depressive disorder	• Difficulty falling asleep (early insomnia) • Frequent awakenings (middle insomnia) • Uncharacteristic early-morning awakening (terminal insomnia) • Hypersomnia ("I sleep all day long so I don't have to face my depression")
Manic episode	• Decreased need for sleep lasting days or weeks • Lack of fatigue despite lack of sleep • Extra work accomplished during usual sleep times ("I stayed up all night and cleaned the whole house")
Posttraumatic stress disorder	• Difficulty falling asleep, which is often associated with anxiety about being abused or traumatized • Physiologic hyperarousal • Very light sleep, with exquisite sensitivity to sounds and other stimuli • Hyperstartled response if awakened by external stimuli • Frequent awakenings • Nightmares
Generalized anxiety disorder	• Prone to *psychophysiologic insomnia* • Difficulty falling asleep due to preoccupation and excessive worry about several stressors
Psychotic disorders	• Hallucinations (e.g., "The voices laugh and scream at me at night, so I can't sleep") • Paranoid thoughts
Attention deficit hyperactivity disorder	• Difficulty falling asleep due to physical hyperactivity • Activating effects of stimulants

DSM-IV-TR, *Diagnostic and Statistical Manual of Mental Disorders,* 4th edition, text revision.

Table 13.6 Principles and Tips for Good Sleep Hygiene

Sleep diary	• Monitor the amount of sleep during day and night
Regular sleep–wake schedule	• Go to bed at the same time each night • Wake up at same time each morning • Avoid naps during the day
Sleep-promoting nightly ritual	• Plan a relaxing, soothing routine for your last hour of wakefulness (e.g., if the time for "lights out" is 9:45 PM, start winding down by 8:45 PM) • Your last hour could include the following: dimming the lights; screening phone calls for urgent calls; showering, bathing, and doing other usual hygiene routines; changing into your bed clothes; reading relaxing or nonstimulating material; limiting yourself to read only up to your "lights out" time; listening to soothing music or other "white noise"
Avoid stressful or other mentally stimulating activities before bedtime	• Address tomorrow's activities, concerns, or distractions earlier in the day • Unless absolutely necessary, postpone anxiety-provoking conversations that require you to make important decisions, or may cause more conflicts, to a time when you are more alert, rested, and much more likely to make a sound decision
Do not lie in bed "wide awake"	• Trying to will yourself to sleep when you're not sleepy will make you more frustrated, not sleepier • Instead, get out of bed, and engage in mentally and physically nonstimulating activities that will relax, soothe, and, perhaps, even bore you • Do not frequently check the clock

(Continued)

Table 13.6   Principles and Tips for Good Sleep Hygiene (*Continued*)

Avoid stimulants, alcohol, and heavy meals at bedtime	• Have your last caffeine- and alcohol-containing food or drink at least 4 hours before you go to bed • Do not smoke within an hour of bedtime, and refrain from smoking if you wake up in the middle of the night • Do not eat a heavy meal within 2 hours of going to bed
Exercise	• Light, aerobic exercise for even 20–30 minutes earlier in the day promotes deep sleep • Avoid exercising within 2 hours of bedtime, since it could actually be activating, and interfere with sleep
Comfortable environment	• Sleep is promoted by darkness, quiet or soothing noises, and a relatively cool temperature (<68°F)

Chapter 14: Suicide and Violence Risk Assessment

Table 14.4   Clinical Interventions That Can Be Taken to Deescalate a Patient and Prevent a Physical Assault (Based on Practice Pointers Clinical Case)

- *Step 1:* Recognize patients who are escalating emotionally
  - Verbal abuse, psychomotor agitation, hostility, and staring indicate a patient is escalating
  - Appropriate intervention at this stage may avert physical aggression

- *Step 2:* Read the situation and the meaning of the behavior
  - Frustration about coming to the appointment on time and having to wait over an hour
  - Angry about his time being wasted, may feel disrespected

- *Step 3:* Connect with the patient
  - Approach the patient maintaining an adequate distance
    - Agitated patients need increased interpersonal space
  - Speak in a calm voice
  - Instill in patient a sense of control
    - For example: "May I speak with you? You seem very upset right now—can we talk about it?"

- *Step 4:* Empathize with the patient and validate emotions
  - For example: "Sir, I'm really sorry about the long wait. I can imagine it is really frustrating to show up on time and have to wait this long to be seen. I know your time is very important...."

- *Step 5:* Depersonalize the situation
  - Anger can create cognitive distortions that lead to mistaking the intentions of others; for example: "This doctor is putting me off.... He doesn't care about me!"
  - Communicate openly and honestly
    - For example: "You know, the reason I'm so far behind is that I had to deal with an emergency situation earlier this afternoon and send a patient to the hospital. Sometimes these things happen; I hope you understand. I'm doing my best to catch up and get to you."

- *Step 6:* Give a patient choices
  - Asking an escalating patient to make a decision diverts focus from the inciting stimulus and helps in regaining emotional control
  - For example: "Is there anything I can do for you that will make waiting here easier for you? You could take a walk around the building and I could call you when I'm ready to see you, or I could offer you some different magazines and a glass of water...."

Step 1: Screen for Death Wishes

Normalizing question: Many people with the kinds of problems you are experiencing also have thoughts that life isn't worth living anymore. Have you been thinking that you'd be better off dead or wish you would fall asleep and not wake up?

If no, stop questioning.

Step 2: Assess Reasons to Live

Is there anything in your life that makes it worth living? Your children? Your family? Are you a religious person? Do you, believe in life after death? What are your thoughts about the fate of people who kill themselves? Do you that things will get better for you in the future (hopelessness)?

Step 3: Screen for Suicidal Ideations

You mentioned before that you sometimes wished you were dead, has it gotten to the point where you've thought about ending your life?

If no, stop questioning

If yes, assess the following regarding suicidal thinking:
- Frequency: How often do you have these thoughts?
- Duration: When you have these thoughts, how long do they last?
- Intensity: When you have these thoughts, are you able to get them out of your mind?

Step 4: Presence of a Plan

Have you thought about ways you might end your life?

If no, stop and refer to a mental health professional as soon as possible, ideally the same day.

If yes, assess the following about the suicide plan:
- Method: What have you thought about doing?
- Preparations: What plans have you made? When and where will this happen?
- Likelihood: What is the chance you'll carry this out? (e.g., 100%, 50%, 10% chance)
Is there anything stopping you from carrying your plan out? Have you been drinking or using drugs lately?

To the ER for immediate evaluation

Figure 14.1 Eliciting suicidal thinking in at-risk patients.

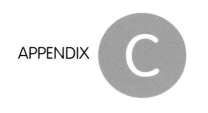

Anxiety Disorders

Acute Stress Disorder	308.3
Acute Stress Reaction	308
Adjustment Disorder (Mixed Anxiety and Depressed Mood)	309.28
Agoraphobia without Panic Disorder	300.22
Anxiety State, Unspecified	300
Generalized Anxiety Disorder	300.02
Panic Disorder with Agoraphobia	300.21
Panic Disorder without Agoraphobia	300.01
Phobia, Specific (Acrophobia, Animal, Claustrophobia, Fear of Crowds)	300.29
Phobia, Unspecified	300.2
Posttraumatic Stress Disorder	309.81
Social Phobia (Social Anxiety Disorder)	300.23

Dementia and Delirium

Cognitive Disorder Not Otherwise Specified (NOS)	294.9
Delirium Due to [General Medication Condition]	293.0
Delirium NOS	780.09
Dementia Classified Elsewhere (Axis I) for Axis III Conditions Below:	290.10
Dementia of Alzheimer Type (Axis III)	331.10
Dementia with Lewy Bodies (Axis III)	331.82
Frontotemporal Dementia (Axis III)	331.19
Huntington Disease (Axis III)	333.40
Vascular Dementia (Axis III)	290.40
Dementia Due to Alcohol	291.2
Dementia NOS	294.80

Eating Disorders

Anorexia Nervosa	307.1
Bulimia Nervosa	307.51
Eating Disorder NOS	307.50

(Continued)

Mood Disorders

x =
- 0 Unspecified
- 1 Mild
- 2 Moderate
- 3 Severe, without Psychosis
- 4 Severe, with Psychosis
- 5 In Partial or Unspecified Remission
- 6 In Full Remission

Major Depression	
Single Episode	296.2x
Recurrent Episode	296.3x
Depressive Disorder NOS	311
Dysthymic Disorder	300.4
Adjustment Disorder with Depressed Mood	309.0
Mood Disorder Due to [General Medical Condition]	293.83
Bipolar I Disorder	
Single Manic Episode	296
Most Recent Episode Hypomanic	296.4
Most Recent Episode Manic	296.4x
Most Recent Episode Mixed	296.6x
Most Recent Episode Depressed	296.5x
Most Recent Episode Unspecified	296.7x
Bipolar II Disorder	296.89
Bipolar Disorder NOS	296.8
Mood Disorder Due to [General Medical Condition]	293.83

Personality Disorders

Paranoid Personality Disorder	301.0
Schizoid Personality Disorder	301.20
Schizotypal Personality Disorder	301.22
Antisocial Personality Disorder	301.7
Borderline Personality Disorder	301.83
Histrionic Personality Disorder	301.50
Avoidant Personality Disorder	301.82
Dependent Personality Disorder	301.6
Obsessive Compulsive Personality Disorder	301.4
Personality Disorder NOS	301.9
Narcissistic Personality Disorder	301.81

Psychotic Disorders

Schizophrenia	295.xx
Paranoid Type	0.30
Disorganized Type	0.10
Catatonic Type	0.20
Undifferentiated Type	0.90
Residual	0.60
Delusional Disorder	297.10
Psychotic Disorder NOS	298.9
Psychotic Disorder with Delusions Due to [General Medical Condition]	293.81
Psychotic Disorder with Hallucinations Due to [General Medical Condition]	293.82
Schizoaffective Disorder	295.70
Schizophreniform Disorder	296.40
Shared Psychotic Disorder	297.3

(Continued)

Somatoform Disorders (Unexplained Physical Symptoms)

Body Dysmorphic Disorder	300.7
Conversion Disorder	300.11
Hypochondriasis	300.7
Pain Disorder	
Associated with Medical and Psychological Factors	307.89
Associated with Psychological Factors	307.8
Somatization Disorder	300.81
Somatoform Disorder Not Otherwise Specified (NOS)	300.82
Undifferentiated Somatoform Disorder	300.82
Factitious Disorder	
With Combined Psychological and Physical Signs and Symptoms	300.19
With Predominantly Physical Signs and Symptoms	300.19
With Predominantly Psychological Signs and Symptoms	300.16
Factitious Disorder NOS	300.19
Malingering	V65.2

Sleep Disorders

Breathing-Related Sleep Disorder	780.59
Circadian Rhythm Sleep Disorder	304.45
Dyssomnia NOS	307.47
Hypersomnia Due to [General Medical Condition]	780.54
Insomnia Due to [General Medical Condition]	780.52
Narcolepsy	347
Primary Insomnia	307.42
Sleep Terror Disorder	304.46
Sleepwalking Disorder	304.46

Substance Use Disorders

Alcohol Abuse	305.00
Alcohol Dependence	303.90
Alcohol-Induced Anxiety Disorder	291.8
Alcohol-Induced Mood Disorder	291.8
Amphetamine Abuse	305.70
Amphetamine Dependence	304.40
Cocaine Abuse	305.60
Cocaine Dependence	304.20
Hallucinogen Dependence	304.50
Hallucinogen Abuse	305.30
Opioid Abuse	305.60
Opioid Dependence	304.00
Other Substance Abuse	305.90
Other Substance Dependence	304.90
Other Substance-Induced Delirium	292.81
Phencyclidine (PCP) Abuse	305.90
Phencyclidine (PCP) Dependence	304.90
Polysubstance Dependence	304.90
Sedative, Hypnotic, or Anxiolytic Abuse	305.40
Sedative, Hypnotic, or Anxiolytic Dependence	304.10
Substance-Induced Anxiety Disorder	292.89
Substance-Induced Mood Disorder	292.84

Index

Page numbers in *italics* denote figures (*f*) and tables (*t*).